Terrorism, Violent Radicalization, and Mental Health

Terrorism, Violent Radicalization, and Mental Health

Edited by

Kamaldeep Bhui
Professor of Psychiatry, University Department of Psychiatry
& Nuffield Department of Primary Care Health Sciences,
University of Oxford, Oxford, UK

Dinesh Bhugra
Emeritus Professor of Mental Health and Cultural Diversity,
Institute of Psychiatry, Psychology and Neuroscience (IoPPN),
King's College London, UK

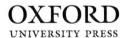

OXFORD
UNIVERSITY PRESS

OXFORD

UNIVERSITY PRESS

Great Clarendon Street, Oxford, OX2 6DP,
United Kingdom

Oxford University Press is a department of the University of Oxford.
It furthers the University's objective of excellence in research, scholarship,
and education by publishing worldwide. Oxford is a registered trade mark of
Oxford University Press in the UK and in certain other countries

© Oxford University Press 2021

The moral rights of the authors have been asserted

First Edition Published in 2021

Impression: 1

Published in the United States of America by Oxford University Press
198 Madison Avenue, New York, NY 10016, United States of America

British Library Cataloguing in Publication Data
Data available

Library of Congress Control Number: 2020944415

ISBN 978–0–19–884570–6

DOI: 10.1093/med/9780198845706.001.0001

Printed and bound by
CPI Group (UK) Ltd, Croydon, CR0 4YY

Contents

Contributors

Neil Krishan Aggarwal
New York City Psychiatrist and An
Advisor to the DSM-5 Cultural Issues
Subgroup, New York, USA

Shamila Ahmed
Senior Lecturer in Criminology,
Academic Enterprise Coordinator,
School of Social Sciences, University
of Westminster, London, UK

Lord John Alderdice
Senior Research Fellow and Director
of the Centre for the Resolution
of Intractable Conflict, Harris
Manchester College, University of
Oxford, Oxford, UK

Reem Alksiri
World Psychiatric Association,
Scientific Section on Psychological
Aspects of Torture and Persecution,
Switzerland

Dinesh Bhugra
Emeritus Professor of Mental
Health and Cultural Diversity,
Institute of Psychiatry, Psychology
and Neuroscience (IoPPN), King's
College London, London, UK

Kamaldeep Bhui
Professor of Psychiatry, University
Department of Psychiatry & Nuffield
Department of Primary Care Health
Sciences, University of Oxford,
Oxford, UK

Anna Bonnel
Psychologist, Polarization Clinical
Team, Centre intégré universitaire
de santé et de services sociaux
du, Centre-Ouest-de-l'île de
Montréal, Canada

Eke Bont
PhD Candidate, Law and
Criminology, Royal Holloway
University, London, UK

Michael Chartrand
Service de police de la Ville de
Montréal (SPVM), Montréal, Canada

Anthony F. Chen
World Psychiatric Association,
Scientific Section on Psychological
Aspects of Torture and Persecution,
Switzerland

Caitlin Clemmow
Honorary Senior Lecturer in Security
and Crime Science at the Jill Dando
Institute of Security and Crime
Science, University College London,
London, UK

Frank Farnham
Consultant Forensic Psychiatrist at
Barnet Enfield and Haringey NHS
Trust, London, UK

Donato Favale
Erasmus Student, Department of
Clinical and Experimental Medicine,
Foggia, Italy

Muhammad Fraser-Rahim
Executive Director, Quilliam International and Assistant Professor, The Citadel (The Military College of South Carolina), Charleston, SC, USA

Paul Gill
Associate Professor, Jill Dando Institute of Security and Crime Science, University College London, London, UK

Ghayda Hassan
Université du Québec à Montréal, Montréal, Canada

Richard Horne
Social Worker, Polarization Clinical Team, Centre intégré universitaire de santé et de services sociaux du, Centre-Ouest-de-l'île de Montréal, Canada

Yasmin Ibrahim
Professor of Digital Economy and Culture, Queen Mary University, London, UK

Edgar Jones
Professor Edgar Jones, Institute of Psychiatry, Psychology and Neuroscience, King's College London, London, UK

Mohammed Hassan Khalid
McNair Scholar, University of Maryland, Baltimore County, USA

Myrna Lashley
Lady Davis Institute and McGill University, Quebec, Canada

Anousheh Machouf
Psychologist, Polarization Clinical Team, Centre intégré universitaire de santé et de services sociaux du, Centre-Ouest-de-l'île de Montréal, Canada

Marie-Hélène Rivest
Social Worker, Polarization Clinical Team, Centre intégré universitaire de santé et de services sociaux du, Centre-Ouest-de-l'île de Montréal, Canada

Cécile Rousseau
Professor, Division de psychiatrie sociale et culturelle, Division of Social and Cultural Psychiatry, McGill University, Montréal, Canada

Christian Savard
Psychologist, Polarization Clinical Team, Centre intégré universitaire de santé et de services sociaux du, Centre-Ouest-de-l'île de Montréal, Canada

Alice Sibley
MSc Student King's College London, London, UK

Carl H.D. Steinmetz
Managing Director at Expats & Immigrants B.V., Amsterdam, Netherlands

Sara Thompson
Department of Criminology, Ryerson University, Toronto, Canada

Serge Touzin
Lady Davis Institute,
Montréal, Canada

Antonio Ventriglio
Honorary researcher at the
Department of Clinical and
Experimental Medicine,
Foggia, Italy

Thomas Wenzel
World Psychiatric Association,
Scientific Section on Psychological
Aspects of Torture and Persecution,
Switzerland

Tarek Younis
Lecturer in Psychology, Middlesex
University, London, UK

Abbreviations

ADHD	attention-deficit–hyperactivity disorder		ISIS	Islamic Republic of Iraq and Syria
AI	artificial intelligence		JCC	juvenile correctional counsellors
AIVD	*Algemene Inlichtingen en Veiligheidsdienst*		LGBT	lesbian, gay, bisexual, and transsexual
ANC	African National Congress		MRTA	Revolutionary Movement Tupac Amaru
ASD	autism spectrum disorder			
BNP	British National Party		NCTV	National Coordinator for Security and Counter-terrorism
BOP	Bureau of Prisons			
CVE	Countering Violent Extremism		NHS	National Health Service
			PIRA	Provisional IRA
DSM	Diagnostic and Statistical Manual of Mental Disorders		PTSD	post-traumatic stress disorder
			PVE	preventing violent extremism
EDL	English Defence League		RAN	Radicalisation Awareness Network
ERG 22+	Extremism Risk Guidance			
ETA	Euskadi Ta Askatasuna		RCMP	Royal Canadian Mounted Police
EU	European Union			
FBI	Federal Bureau of Investigation		SPJ	Structural Professional Judgement
ICE	Immigration and Customs Enforcement		START	National Consortium for the Study of Terrorism and Responses to Terrorism
IMC	Independent Monitoring Commission			
IPA	interpretative phenomenological analysis		SVPT	sympathy for violent protest and terrorism
IRA	Irish Republican Army		UAE	United Arab Emirates
IS	Islamic State		UGC	user-generated content
			UN	United Nations

Section 1

Introduction and background

Chapter 1

Violent radicalization and terrorism: A societal challenge for all citizens

Kamaldeep Bhui and Dinesh Bhugra

1.1 **Background**

Terrorism is mentioned in the press on an almost daily basis. More recently, there was establishment and then demise of ISIS (Islamic State of Iraq and Syria); before that, Al-Qaeda; and, historically, a myriad of distinct non-state-actor campaigns against governments. These show that each terrorist group or campaign emerges in the context of very specific social, cultural, and political contexts, as evidenced by the rich offerings in this book for world experts studying different groups and types of extremism and terrorism. Identities, be they along regional, national, religious, or tribal lines, are often the fracture points. Terrorism is, by its intent and methods, a political activity that resorts to violence and risks the death of innocents. It also strikes fear and powerlessness into the hearts of governments, democratic or not, in order to bring to light a perceived injustice or abuse of liberties, and recognition. The situation is even more complex in that some groups identified as terrorists, with hindsight and the lens of history, appear to be better recognized as freedom fighters (African National Congress [ANC] in South Africa for example, or the Irish Republican Army [IRA] in Northern Ireland), and especially when these groups do engage with political rather than violent protest. Clearly, these movements justify their use of violence on the basis of what is at stake for certain sectors of society, often their sectors and in-groups. Yet, not everyone takes that path. More research is needed on the make-up of those engaging in violence generally, those engaging in terrorist violence, and those who perhaps organize terrorist threats, and then those more remote actors who support such activities from afar. What is it that moves people from citizenship through escalating levels of commitment? Is even this question founded on a falsifiable premise? This volume seeks to bring together distinct disciplinary and ideological narratives of what causes terrorism, the role of propensity to violence and a process called radicalization, and the influence of cognitive, emotional, social, cultural, and historical factors.

1.2 **Ethical dilemmas**

With such a controversial topic, there is much scope for misunderstanding, indignation, unintended offence, and for efforts to research and understand causation and prevention as in some way mitigating the human and social cost of criminal activities falling under the aegis of terrorism actions. That is not the intention of this book. Given the complexity of the topic, better knowledge and understanding is the only way to truly develop effective solutions to many public health and social and political dilemmas facing nation states, societies, and humanity in general. Even studying such phenomenon means interacting with people at various stages or phases of the proposed pathway to commit terrorist acts. Criminology research is thus bedevilled with ethical dilemmas of who can be followed-up and for how long, and whether the usual conditions of confidentiality in research can be upheld, given the risk of incrimination through discovering information in the research process, and perhaps also becoming victim to misinformation, recrimination, and violence. The safety of researchers is at stake, but the willingness of people involved in terrorism to reveal such sentiments is highly suspect.

1.3 **The prevalence–impact paradox**

Terrorism is very rare. Homicide is rare. Understanding causation in rare events and testing prevention is bedevilled by small numbers of events and if each is contextualized and driven by different factors, generalizable findings are unlikely. The growth in terrorism studies has been well evidenced since 9/11. Yet, as illustrated in this volume repeatedly, terror threats have persisted for hundreds of years in various forms. The use of violence for political gain through warfare between nations, and asymmetric violence emerging from less powerful or marginalized groups to harm the interests of larger groups has escalated. Historians argue that terrorism involving self-destructive acts dates back to the early tenth and eleventh centuries, with various permutations in different countries and eras depending on the cultural idioms and practices that are co-opted and modified to promote violence in protest. Most events are actually in low- and middle-income countries, and perpetrators are more commonly in Muslim-majority nations, as are victims, i.e. more Muslim people die from terrorism than other groups. Although often related to an issue of religious doctrine or ideology—the position of US and UK governments—many, and indeed the majority of, people of Muslim faith and heritage decry such an interpretation, proposing that terrorists use religious rhetoric to recruit and justify political actions to remedy social and cultural adversities and perceived and real persecution. In contrast, despite terrorism being rare, the profile it is given in higher-income countries, i.e. the Global North, often distorts the numbers of people and the locations of most victims, and counterterrorism actions and investment seems disproportionate.

1.4 **Moral injury**

Counterterrorism responses arise to protect the national states' sovereignty when challenged, and to reassure fearful citizens of the intentions of the government to protect them and create safe environments for them and their children to flourish, have secure employment and wealth, and generally a good life. Nonetheless, the fear invoked and the restrictions imposed on citizens are tangible, and the deaths of victims, even if few, touches a nation and the families and communities of those killed. The sense of powerlessness, injustice, and fractured moral frameworks following such incidents are much harder to heal and build than restoring infrastructures, creating memorials and monuments, and redeveloping sites, or even physical healing from fractures. The impact that is often not discussed is moral injury, something we struggle to heal from if there is no easy remedy or fair resolution. This angers and leads to counterterrorism measures that can be draconian and destructive, further fuelling the justifications of those claiming political or religious or identity-related persecution for violence.

One of the responses of the Global North is to seek explanations for why terrorism happens, what might drive terrorists to commit acts of violence on innocents, whether there are effective preventive opportunities and interventions, what actions minimize the risk of attacks from known terrorist groups or individual actors, and how to respond to such attacks, including the handling of perpetrators.

1.5 **Radicalization**

One explanation is to invoke the notion of radicalization as a process to explain how people born and raised in high-income countries, afforded the benefits of good education, employment, and security in those countries, then come under the influence of nefarious groups and individuals to come to develop extremist views and then under further influence use violence to attack and kill people in these countries. The process is hypothetical and lacking empirical evidence of how people in populations enter consecutive stages of the hypothesized process to occupy a high-risk category. Even then, how a person goes on to commit acts of violence is difficult to predict. Decades of research in forensic settings demonstrates how hard it is to identify who will and will not be violent. Studies of people with mental illness and populations struggle to identify people who go on to take their lives. Accounts from convicted terrorists do show the influences to which they were exposed that may have led them down a particular path, within their reflections when no longer under the influence of such groups. This information is important at that individual level, and, if generalities can be understood, the information will help inform prevention and de-radicalization. The difficulty is that such personal biographies and narratives over decades are highly idiosyncratic and unlikely to be easily comparable. Yet lessons can be learnt.

1.6 **The mind**

All actions are behavioural and mediated by cognition and emotion, so one could argue that psychological processes and social influences on those processes are relevant to understand what drives people to such actions. The forensic research literature is full of examples of epidemiological, social, environmental, genetic, imaging, and neuropathological studies of violent offenders, with less on terrorist offenders specifically. There are clearly processes that lend themselves to violence, including lack of empathy, personality disorders as they are known, impaired judgement, impulsivity, anger and paranoia, and perhaps certain mood states that encourage pessimism and negative evaluations of future options; furthermore, failed problem solving or the skills and ability to influence through social and political means will also be important. Yet not one of these factors can in isolation explain a complex and rare behaviour such as terrorism. Paradoxically, organizing terrorism actions and enacting them requires careful preparation and orchestration when these are group driven and on a mass scale. Impairments in reason or function are not likely to be so evident, not least if the activities are surreptitious and criminal, and need to be concealed for fear of discovery and conviction. Thus, studies of the criminal mind, or the psychological and psychiatric correlates of violent offending are relevant but lack specificity when applied to terrorist offending. At the same time, any suggestion that mental illnesses or psychological states are relevant or might be manipulated to both radicalize and deradicalize is met with scepticism, not least as the search for such evidence again is misunderstood to justify or explain away terrorism. Yet, more recent work suggests that impaired judgement and psychological functioning and mood states may well be associated or clustered in some types of terrorist offender with other characteristics that also confer risk, although invoking causality requires much more research and better evidence than we currently have.

1.7 **Calls for interdisciplinary critique**

As there are so many types of terrorist offender, and terrorism contexts, it is unlikely a single explanation or paradigm for action or understanding can apply in all situations. Nonetheless, research into the variations, as well as commonalities, can help illuminate what types of prevention, counterterrorism, and deradicalization processes may be helpful, as well as what social and international policies might be conducive for effective actions, and actions that minimize harms such as racism, Islamophobia, and harsh social and immigration policies for some sectors of society. Our thesis is that solutions and responses will need to be tailored to particular groups, at particular times, in particular contexts, and tailoring of responses requires a constant adjustment and refinement as terrorist groups and campaigns change their narratives of persuasion and justification and their means to commit terrorist acts.

Cultural psychiatry has evolved as a discipline, originally grounded in ethnography and anthropology and qualitative research and increasingly adopting methods of epidemiology, systematic reviews, and clinical trials, too. The particular contribution of cultural psychiatry is to embrace a number of important variables of interest, characteristics of people and diverse populations such as their religious beliefs and practices, their cultural and ethnic and national identity, and explanatory models of illness and misfortune, as well as implicit rules of living in society and forming and protecting the in-group. Alongside this, studies of migration and globalization have led to better ways to evaluate the impact of acculturation and shifts in societal values where people or places are in transition.

Yet many disciplines have major contributions to make, and the authors of this book represent a rich and powerful body of researchers, commentators, policy shapers, and politicians who have committed themselves to address this challenging problem. Thus, in Chapter 2, Neil Krishnan Aggarwal demonstrates persuasive use of technologies and how psychiatrists and other professionals have to make judgements about militant and non-militant groups and cultural justifications for violence. The sophistication with which cultural heritage and latent identities are deployed to engage, motivate, and convert the interested to activists are outlined using first-language access to digital and other media. In Chapter 3, Shamila Ahmad's perspective is refreshingly grounded in criminology and emotional resilience as a response to terror, seeking to ensure criminal justice responses are just. Denials of injustice, suffering, and erosion of human rights in the 'war on terror' are otherwise exploited by terrorists as a counter-narrative to the 'war on terror'. In Chapter 5, Alice Sibley shows how another extremist group, The English Defence League, recruits people into its ranks. Recruitment seems to rely on reducing the differentiation between Muslims and terrorists as categories of people, with narratives of threat, conspiracy, cultural change, and loss of belonging rather than reference to political parties, economic hardship, or age and gender. In Chapter 10, Gill et al. show the need for complexity in understanding violent radicalization, deploying notions of equifinality, i.e. violent radicalization has many paths to it, and multiple trajectories to multiple outcomes originating from poor mental health. Poor mental health may be related but is neither necessary nor sufficient, and is not a predictable determinant of violent radicalization. In Chapter 4, Edgar Jones argues for more community connections and social capital to counter-extremists, but he exposes the tension in counterterrorism actions that can alienate communities. Tarek Younis takes this argument further in Chapter 14, illustrating how the health service in the UK is being co-opted into counterterrorism measures, inappropriately and risking role confusion for doctors and health professionals more generally. Yet, Rousseau et al., from Montreal, highlight in Chapter 12 innovative pilot work for how a public health service for young people can, working closely with security agencies and using models of cultural consultation developed in cultural psychiatry, provide useful mental health interventions and safe practice and protection for children and adolescents and their families. In Chapter 11, Lashley et al. illustrate work in Canada on the training needed by police to engage the public, secure their support, and at the same time pose a useful counterterrorism response. From surveys of people in three Canadian cities, Lashley et al. argue for police cultural competence as a powerful necessity in counterterrorism roles. In Chapter 15, Carl Steinmetz, uses the response from the Danish government and contrasts this with the response from the British and other governments, and illustrates how a policy and community response are not necessarily at odds with counterterrorism and security measures. In Chapter 16, he proposes how collectivism and individualism lead to different drivers and different solutions to counterterrorism, and that a culturally grounded approach can optimize community participation in averting future threats and responding to potential threats. It is important to recognize that not all countries or cultures will use the same methods and the same methods will not work across borders, but it is critical to learn from each other and use relativist approaches. In Chapter 8, Eke Bont examines the biographies of former IRA operatives and shows a shift in their belief in violence as a solution; specifically, she investigates moral injury among former IRA operatives and humanizes their struggles for freedom, liberty, and political engagement after leaving violence behind. Politicians and mental health professionals often differ in their approaches and alliances in responding to terrorist threats, and rarely are they able to get an insider's view of terrorism as experienced by people from the same in-group as the terrorist campaigners. Lord John Alderdice, a politician, and also a psychiatrist and psychoanalyst, was involved in the peace campaign in Northern Ireland, and played a pivotal role in securing sustained peace. His analysis of group relations, described in Chapter 17, is at the heart of the terrorism process and makes compelling reading, not least as it is grounded in the harsh realities faced by him and his colleagues in Northern Ireland.

In Chapter 7, Wenzel et al. also use a psychoanalytic lens to explore the internal and interpersonal and group processes that underlie terrorism, echoing themes in the chapters by Alderdice (Chapters 15 and 16), Ahmad (Chapter 3) and Jones (Chapter 4). They invoke 'chosen trauma' as the driving force behind extremist actions and propose transitional justice as a mechanism to reduce the risk of further conflict and violence. The digital power of some terrorist groups enables them to be even more influential in the propagation of terrorism, a theme picked up in Chapter 6 by Yasmin Ibrahim, who illustrates how the sharing economic and social media are aligned, creating an architecture for the online production of terror. Ibrahim explores the moral and ethical considerations of the sharing economy and digitalization of human communications and existence. Finally, we are very privileged to have a rare insight into the depth workings of Quilliam. Chapter 13 by Fraser-Rahim and Khalid offers an in-depth biography, a first-hand account, written with a person who has been a terrorist. They illustrate how Quilliam works with terrorist offenders using powerful biographical narrative methods to reveal and mitigate misjudgements and erroneous motivations. In Chapter 9, Donato and Ventriglio set out a range of theories of terrorism and radicalization, especially drawing on sociological and cultural theories, grounding the evidence from the literature in brief biographies, further reinforcing the complexity with which we are now grappling.

The work of this volume is rich, synthesizing distinct and contrasting perspectives that are interlinked. Yet any such work must always be incomplete, as is any study of a new phenomenon that warrants further research, understanding, and commensurate timely policy and practical advice. The disjuncture between contrasting perspectives is a reflection of the many facets and perspectives through which terrorism studies have developed, and then specifically the motivations and responses of health agencies as having a legitimate if not critical contribution. There is an urgent need to explore various facets of radicalization and terrorist acts both from an aetiological perspective and also by preventing and managing these so that processes of cultures in conflict, acculturation, and alienation can be explored and suitable support given when and where indicated to mitigate and prevent extremism and violent extremism.

Political, social, and health perspectives on causation and complexity in terrorism research

Chapter 2

In defence of Islam: How the Islamic State justifies violence

Neil Krishan Aggarwal

2.1 Introduction

What draws people to the media of the Islamic State (IS)? Any textbook on terrorism, violent radicalization, and mental health must contend with IS's growth and development. If terrorism can be defined as the real or perceived use of violence against civilians for political or ideological reasons [1], then IS qualifies as an Islamist militant group. By an *Islamist militant group*, I refer to non-state actors struggling to overthrow a political system through violence and govern all aspects of life for Muslims and non-Muslims, based on literal interpretations of texts from the corpus of Islamic law [2].

IS has distinguished itself from other terrorist groups since its origins in 2003. It is the first terrorist group to integrate physical and digital warfare in real time by releasing violent videos for download from Internet sites in conjunction with attacks [3]. No other terrorist group has held as much territory as during its peak strength in 2014, when it ruled an area comparable in size to the country of Jordan [4]. It controlled over four million people and a third of the territory in Iraq and Syria, amassing millions of dollars from smuggling oil on the world market, taxing inhabitants, and kidnapping hostages for ransom to become the richest terrorist group in history [5], with an estimated annual budget of more than $1 billion and over $2 trillion in combined assets [6]. It has enslaved thousands of Muslim and non-Muslim women and children [7], destroyed priceless antiquities [8], and contributed to some of the largest population transfers after World War II: over 220,000 Iraqis and five million Syrians have received refugee status after fleeing IS violence, and over three million Iraqis and six million Syrians remain internally displaced [9, 10]. Between 30,000 and 42,000 fighters from over 85 countries joined IS, mostly from countries with high levels of economic development, low income inequality, and highly developed political institutions, leading to speculations that foreigners are attracted by the group's use of social media [11, 12].

Indeed, IS has run a social media empire. In 2015, IS produced 123 media products in Arabic and 8 in English in just 7 days, with videos comprising 24 of these releases [13]. Crisp audiovisual production, images captured from flying drones, and media products in nearly a dozen languages have inspired militants to immigrate and expand IS's self-styled caliphate [14]. Supporters in IS territories used to share media rapidly across social media [15]; after Facebook, YouTube, and Twitter cracked down on IS content under pressure from governments worldwide, the group switched to encrypted messaging applications like WhatsApp, Kik, Surespot, and Telegram [16, 17]. The high ratio of audiovisual to literary products targets millennial youth who prefer to watch videos rather than read texts [18]. Despite this volume of data, we have little understanding of the psychological processes through which IS media persuades people. Some suggest that IS media uses canonical Islamic texts to justify violence against disbelievers [19]. Others suggest that sensationalist images of violence and excitement seeking explain its appeal [20, 21].

While these works advance our knowledge about IS's techniques of persuasion, key questions remain: firstly, how has the group tried to persuade others through media now that it has lost all territory? Most research articles [19–21] use videos from the time of the group's maximal strength from 2014 until 2017, but its number of militants is diminished to ~14,000–18,000, including about 3000 foreigners, as of this writing in May 2019 [22]. Secondly, are references to religious texts and images of violence its only techniques of persuasion or are there others? Research articles [19–21] use inductive analyses, but how can we understand IS's media techniques through the established scholarship on the psychology of persuasion more generally?

This chapter introduces and applies a methodology from the psychology of persuasion to analyse IS videos. By persuasion, I use Robert Cialdini's definition of 'social influence' through which media influences people by seven mechanisms: (1) drawing contrasts between 'us' and 'them'; (2) imposing obligations of action upon the audience; (3) establishing initial propositions for the audience to accept; (4) presenting evidence of what other people know to be true as social proof to influence actions; (5) liking the characters delivering the messaging; (6) invoking authority; and (7) claiming that future scarcity should motivate present actions [23]. By using deductive analysis, we can identify which mechanisms of persuasion are present in IS media [24]. Indeed, a review of hundreds of media products throughout IS's evolution from 2003 to 2017 shows that IS's most prevalent mechanisms of persuasion are to invoke authority through scriptural references or historical prototypes, draw contrasts between Muslim believers and non-disbelievers from other religions, and impose an obligation to act upon the audience, with videos after 2005 casting militants as likeable characters that audiences can relate to [24].

A sceptic could ask: how does analysing the psychology of media persuasion relate to culture or psychiatry? Well, culture can be defined as one's conception of one's place in the world based on sharing meanings, practices, and symbols with a group [25]. Society entrusts psychiatrists with determining whether an individual's violent thoughts, emotions, and behaviours toward oneself or others can be attributed to psychopathology, but militant groups justify violence as politically necessary without any link to mental illness [26]. Militant groups use the Internet to transform how individuals and groups conceive of their place in the world in online communities that transcend geographies [27, 28]. In assuming that political violence stems from individual-level psychopathology rather than cultural justifications, mental health professionals risk ignoring how militants normalize violence through shared meanings, practices, and symbols. Without this clarification, it is unclear if known or suspected militants should receive social, health, or criminal justice interventions.

This study examines IS's mechanisms of persuasion in an Arabic-language video titled 'Meanings of Constancy—Wilāyat Al-Shām, Al-Barakah' [29]. Militant videos are informative data sources for cultural analysis because they depict meanings, practices, and symbols that groups use to justify violence [30]. This video serves as a case study on IS's depiction of losses and attempts to persuade viewers to act violently. The Syrian village of Baghuz marked the last territory under IS rule, where hundreds of militants took thousands of civilians as human shields against the American- and European-backed Syrian Democratic Forces at the beginning of 2019 [31, 32]. IS announced the release of this video in issue 173 of the Arabic weekly periodical *Al-Naba* ('*The News*'), published in March 2019 [33]. *Al-Naba* is IS's oldest continuing periodical, containing reports about militant operations and commentaries on current events [34]. The video was streamed from Jihadology.net, a password-protected research archive of jihadist primary source materials on the Internet [35]. Consistent with methods to analyse militant videos deductively, I classify the video's assumptions, arguments, and conclusions according to Cialdini's seven mechanisms of persuasion [24]. Except for verses of the Quran, for which I reference A. J. Arberry's classic translation, all translations from Arabic into English are mine and follow principles of dynamic formal equivalence that convey the spirit of the original text colloquially in the target language [36]. All transliterations follow the standard format of the *International Journal of Middle Eastern Studies*.

2.2 'Meanings of Constancy—Wilāyat Al-Shām, Al-Barakah'

The video lasts 14 minutes and 18 seconds. Three text slides appear in succession: (1) the standard Islamic benediction to God—'In the Name of God, the Merciful, the Compassionate'; (2) a slide with the phrase 'Islamic State'; and (3) the location as 'Barakah Province'. Here is the first mechanism of persuasion: IS invokes political authority by claiming that its territory is a province (*wilāyah*), even though no country in the world recognizes it.

The video has three sequences. Sequence 1 from 00:16 to 00:60 consists of five video clips: (1) a young man sitting on the ground with others who asks, 'What is our offense? What is our crime? That we have wanted to implement the law of God!'; (2) two men driving in a white van and enforcing public morality; (3) a line of men praying behind their weapons; (4) an elderly man sitting on the ground who reads the Quran; and (5) an aerial shot of people milling around tents.

The first four video clips persuade viewers by offering evidence of what people know to be IS's strict rules on expressing devotion. The fifth video clip persuades viewers by offering evidence of poverty. At 00:43, text in Arabic appears with the phrase 'Meanings of Constancy—Wilāyat Al-Shām, Al-Barakah'. The message is clear: IS's inhabitants will practise religion, even if they must suffer.

Sequence 2, from 00:60 to 12:58, consists of four men who speak directly to viewers. Because the second, third, and fourth men persuade viewers through the same mechanisms of persuasion as the first, I only analyse the text of the first speaker as a representative example. The first speaker is identified as 'Brother Abu 'Abdul 'Azīm'. This is his *nom de guerre* (*kunya*), indicating that he has a son named "Abdul 'Azīm." He also appears in the first video clip.

He begins by invoking religious authority: 'In the name of God, praise be to God, prayers and peace upon the prophet of God' (until 1:02). Next, he draws a contrast between 'us' Muslims and 'those' disbelievers: 'My brothers! There is the measure of this world (*muqayas dunyawī*) and the measure of the Afterlife (*muqayas ukhrawī*). The measure of this world is that one plus one equals two. So if we are a thousand, and a hundred get killed, then we say that we lost a hundred. This is the measure of this world' (until 1:19). In contrast, the measure of the Afterlife is based on religion. He says,

> As for the measure of the Afterlife, this is God's measure—mighty and majestic is He—and it differs. So what does God—praise be to Him, and may He be exalted—say about the Men of the Pit (*ahl ul-ukhdūd*)? What does he call their killing? He says—praise be to Him, and may He be exalted—in [the chapter titled] The Constellations (*al-burūj*):

By heaven of the constellations, by the promised day, by the witness and the witnessed, slain were the Men of the Pit, the fire abounding in fuel, when they were seated
over it and were themselves witnesses of what they did with the believers. They took
revenge on them only because they believed in the All-mighty, the All-laudable, God.
(chapter 85, verses 1–8) (until 2:24) [37, p. 331]

With the phrase 'My brothers!' Abu 'Abdul 'Azīm treats viewers as fellow members of a Muslim ingroup. He contrasts Muslims from a disbelieving outgroup by
invoking the religious authority of Chapter 58 of the Quran. The verse describes
an incident whereby disbelievers slew the Muslims who believed in God. By
using traditional honorifics in Arabic after the word 'God', such as 'mighty and
majestic is He', 'praise be to Him', and 'may He be exalted', IS reinforces his piety.

Abu 'Abdul 'Azīm then imposes certain initial propositions on his audience:

What is our offense? What is our crime? Why are we bombed from airplanes? Why
have all the disbelieving nations of the world gathered to kill us? What is our offense?
What is our crime? Why do they surround us? Why do they bomb us day and night
while the world is silent despite their gathering to battle and kill us? What is our offense? What is our crime? That we have wanted to implement the law of God! There is
no place in the world where the reality of the Quran and Hadith is found except for this
people. (until 2:52)

IS embraces its lack of international recognition by any government and alleges
that its enemies do not believe in the Word of God as enshrined in the Quran
or the example of His prophet Muhammad as enshrined in the collection of
biographical texts known as Hadith. IS positions itself as the only people in the
world committed to implementing God's law on earth.

As further proof to persuade people to his way of thinking, Abu 'Abdul 'Azīm
invokes religious authority by quoting the Quran. He says,

Listen to me, to the rest of the verses in the chapter The Constellations so that you know
the measure of the Afterlife and God's measure, mighty and majestic is He.

God to whom belongs the Kingdom of the heavens and the earth, and God is Witness
over everything. Those who persecute the believers, men and women, and then have
not repented, there awaits them the chastisement of Gehenna [Hell], and there awaits
them the chastisement of the burning. Those who believe, and do righteous deeds, for
them await gardens underneath which rivers flow; that is the great triumph. (chapter
85, verses 9–11) (until 4:21) [37, pp. 331–2]

God is the greatest. God tells us in this fragment that the Men of the Pit were killed.
They were burned. They were enslaved. According to the considerations of this world,
they were destroyed. But what did God—praise be to Him, and may He be exalted—call
this killing and this burning? God—may He be exalted—said, 'Those who believe, and do
righteous deeds, for them await gardens underneath which rivers flow; that is the great
triumph. Surely thy Lord's assault is terrible. Surely it is He who originates, and brings
again, and He is the All-forgiving, the All-loving, Lord of the Throne, the All-glorious,
Performer of what He desires'. (chapter 85, verses 11–16) (until 5:11) [37, p. 332]

Here, Abu 'Abdul 'Azīm invokes the Quran to make two arguments: (1) disbelievers who kill believers in this world will face Hell in the Afterlife, and (2) believers who do righteous deeds in this life will enjoy God's mercy in the Afterlife. Unlike traditional Muslim scholars, who spend years learning the social, historical, and linguistic contexts of religious scriptures, contemporary Islamists interpret current affairs through the Quran without considering the contexts of their revelation [38]. As a result, Abu 'Abdul 'Azīm equates persecuted believers in the Quran from the seventh century with IS's besieged militants today. This passage also reveals IS's distinct conception of psychology whereby a sense of self transcends the positivist, materialist world and endures into the Afterlife after the demise of the physical body [26].

IS also casts Abu 'Abdul 'Azīm as a likeable character with whom viewers can relate. 'This encirclement is suffocating', he says, smiling resignedly into the camera. 'He gives us our reward, and praise is for God. One day at a time. We see and we live according to the circumstances of the prophet—peace and prayers upon him. If you entrust God the right to His trust, then he rewards you all like he rewards the birds. You eat when you are hungry and you set out in groups. So praise be to God, the Lord of the worlds. And spread the good news. Victory is near' (until 6:34). The camera briefly pans away from him to show a bearded militant feeding destitute children.

This text exhibits several mechanisms of persuasion. Firstly, Abu 'Abdul 'Azīm offers evidence of what we all know, that multiple forces have encircled IS's last village. Nonetheless, he reiterates his commitment to live strictly according to IS's interpretation of scripture, presenting himself as a steadfast, likeable character. He acknowledges genuine hardships, and the footage of a bearded man feeding children conveys that IS will not abandon its most vulnerable adherents. Nonetheless, Abu 'Abdul 'Azīm calls viewers to trust in God and forge bonds with others on the same path who he likens to birds flying together as they await victory. Herein lie the meanings of constancy.

Sequence 2 features three other speakers: Brother Abu 'Abdul 'Azīz from 7:41 to 10:52, Brother Abu 'Abdul Rahman from 10:54 to 12:12, and Brother Abu Abdullah from 12:14 to 12:57. Each man invokes religious authority by referencing the Quran, contrasts 'us' Muslims with 'those' disbelievers, and establishes propositions that IS's enemies oppose it for trying to implement God's law on earth. Sequence 3 begins from 12:59 and ends the video, showing two men from IS's religious police (al-hisba) driving a white van throughout the village to enforce public morality.

Lettering on the driver's door identifies the men as belonging to IS's Office of Religious Police. IS bureaucratized public virtue by employing officers who ensured that its inhabitants in Iraq, Libya, and Syria adhered to authoritarian religious mores for men and women, by punishing men for incorrect beard lengths, failing to pray, and possessing drugs and alcohol, and assaulting women who did not veil themselves from head to toe [39]. By offering audiovisual proof of IS enforcing its exacting codes of conduct, the video persuades viewers that the group has opted to live by the measure of the Afterlife rather than the measure of this world.

2.3 **Discussion**

This chapter has analysed the psychological mechanisms of persuasion in an IS video on the fall of its last territory. Consistent with the group's other media since 2003, 'Meanings of Constancy—Wilāyat Al-Shām, Al-Barakah' has invoked authority by citing the Quran, drawn contrasts between Muslim believers and non-Muslims disbelievers, and casted militants like Abu 'Abdul 'Azīm as likeable characters. Audiovisual footage presents evidence of what people already know as proof of IS's strict enforcement of public morality, the military blockage around IS's last village, and the suffering of vulnerable populations such as children. With the start of the global War on Terror in 2001, scholars have struggled to do empirically driven research on terrorism: terrorists typically distrust outsiders as potential government informants, precluding participant observation [40], and governments have prosecuted researchers after interviewing terrorists for violating national security laws [41]. With such challenges, studying textual sources offers an insider perspective to avoid imposing our worldview onto others [42], consistent with a central concern in cultural psychiatry and psychiatric anthropology of differentiating normal from abnormal behaviours in societies that differ from ours [43].

This video illustrates IS's meanings, practices, and symbols that justify and normalize violence. IS propagates meanings such as the dichotomy between the 'measure' of this world and the Afterlife, that the world has arrayed its forces against the group for attempting to implement God's law, and that its believers are persecuted today just as God's believers were persecuted in the Quran fourteen centuries ago but will find true reward after death. Contemporary psychiatry and psychology assume that the healthy individual prioritizes oneself over others, achieves full autonomy, defines goals independently, and chooses to maximize material benefits [44]. If autonomy—the act of complying literally with one's 'self (*auto*) law (*nomy*)'—marks this secular individualistic self, then IS encourages shared meanings, practices, and symbols centred on *allonomy*, the act of complying with the law of the other (*allo*) [24]. This law of the other is IS's interpretations of the Quran and the Hadith. IS's video reinforces this cultural ideal by depicting militants praying behind militants, elderly men reading the Quran, and the religious police continuing to enforce public morality during war and poverty. Abu ʿAbdul ʿAzīmʾs reference to the symbol of birds who eat when they are hungry and flock together further reinforces a cultural ideal of collectivism over individualism within IS's norms. The social sciences—anthropology, economics, political science, psychology, and sociology—emerged as discourses of knowledge after the Enlightenment when Western European societies encouraged the secularization of political systems and the relegation of religion to private life [45]. IS's video critiques not just secular society, but also secular individuals, presenting an alternate vision that justifies violence to implement God's law on earth.

This study has two key limitations. Firstly, analysing the psychological mechanisms of persuasion tells us how IS justifies violence but cannot explain why people ultimately take up arms. Case in point: I have no inclination to fight on IS's behalf despite watching 'Meanings of Constancy—Wilāyat Al-Shām, Al-Barakah' a half dozen times to write this chapter. Therefore, we need more work that clarifies how militant videos fit within individual trajectories of militancy. This is no easy task, as researchers who have tried to study how individuals consume militant videos have faced censure from Institutional Review Boards for exposing human subjects to violent content [46]. Secondly, it is likely that the mechanisms of persuasion in this video are representative, but not exhaustive, of all such mechanisms in IS media. IS has released subsequent videos, including 'Meanings of Constancy From al-Bāghuz #2—Wilāyat Al-Shām, Al-Barakah' [47], which depicts battle scenes. IS likely produces multiple media products with different mechanisms of persuasion to broaden its appeal among different types of people.

Despite these limitations, the analysis of IS media according to mechanisms of persuasion offers a systematic method to explore how terrorist groups justify violence. This has important implications as societies grapple with IS and other types of extremism. Firstly, even though IS's former head and self-styled caliphate was killed during an American military intervention in October 2019 [48], the group has continued to produce media. Examining how this media continues to attract recruits can help researchers and policymakers to understand a group's shifts in mechanisms of persuasion over time [24]. Comparing the mechanisms of persuasion in militant media with responses from known or suspected militants either through interviews or focus groups can help researchers hone counter-messaging strategies.

Secondly, comparing the psychology of persuasion across different terrorist groups allows researchers and policymakers to keep making the point that justifications for violence are not specific to any single religious, racial, or ethnic group. Anti-Semitic attitudes in Europe led to a disturbing increase in the number of attacks against Jews in 2018: France reported a 74% increase since 2017 to over 500 incidents, and Germany had a 10% increase to 1646 incidents [49]. Indeed, a comparison of media produced by Islamist, White Nationalist, and Zionist militant groups shows that all use common deception-based mechanisms of persuasion such as drawing contrasts between 'us' and 'them', imposing obligations of action upon the audience, invoking authority, and claiming that future danger should motivate present actions [50]. It would be worth exploring whether counter-messaging techniques that are useful against one group could be extended to other groups.

As governments and non-governmental organizations struggle to devise counter-narratives, exploring communication techniques to counter mechanisms of violent persuasion offers a tangible way for psychiatry to contribute to the science, policy, and practice of counterterrorism. The analysis of militant media reveals our own assumptions about the self and other, individuals and groups, peace and violence, secularism and religiosity, and desirable goals toward a successful life in a world that increasingly connects us to others with vastly different worldviews.

References

1. **Horgan J.** The psychology of terrorism. London: Routledge; 2014.
2. **Mishal S, Rosenthal M.** Al Qaeda as a dune organization: toward a typology of Islamic terrorist organizations. Studies in Conflict & Terrorism 2005;**28**:275–93.
3. **Glasser SB, Coll S.** The web as weapon. The Washington Post. 9 August 2005.
4. **Chulov M, Borger J.** Syria: ISIS advance on Aleppo aided by Assad regime air strikes, US says. The Guardian. 2 June 2015.
5. **Sprusansky D.** Understanding ISIS: frequently asked questions. Washington Report on Middle East Affairs 2014;**33**:19–20.
6. **Gerges FA.** A history of ISIS. Princeton, NJ: Princeton University Press; 2016.
7. **Callimachi R.** ISIS enshrines a theology of rape. The New York Times. 13 August 2015.
8. **Stack L.** Islamic State blows up temple at Palmyra ruins in Syria. The New York Times. 24 August 2015.
9. **Office of the United Nations High Commissioner for Refugees.** Iraq emergency. Available from: http://www.unhcr.org/en-us/iraq-emergency.html [accessed 21 July 2017].
10. **Office of the United Nations High Commissioner for Refugees.** 2017 Syria emergency. Available from: http://www.unhcr.org/en-us/syria-emergency.html [accessed 21 July 2017].
11. **Benmelech E, Klor EF.** What explains the flow of foreign fighters to ISIS? Cambridge: National Bureau of Economic Research; 2016.
12. **Cook J, Vale G.** From Daesh to 'diaspora': tracing the women and minors of Islamic State. London: International Center for the Study of Radicalisation; 2018.

13. **Zelin A.** Picture or it didn't happen: a snapshot of the Islamic State's official media output. Perspectives on Terrorism 2015;**9**:85–97.
14. **Shane S, Hubbard B.** ISIS displaying a deft command of varied media. The New York Times. 30 August 2014.
15. **Berger JM.** The metronome of apocalyptic time: social media as carrier wave for millenarian contagion. Perspectives on Terrorism 2015;**9**:61–71.
16. **Berger JM.** Tailored online interventions: the Islamic State's recruitment strategy. CTC Sentinel 2015;**8**:19–23.
17. **Callimachi R.** A news agency with scoops directly from ISIS, and a veneer of objectivity. The New York Times. 14 January 2016.
18. **Gates S, Podder S.** Social media, recruitment, allegiance and the Islamic State. Perspectives on Terrorism 2015;**9**:107–16.
19. **Boutz J, Benninger H, Lancaster A.** Exploiting the Prophet's authority: how Islamic State propaganda uses Hadith quotation to assert legitimacy. Studies in Conflict & Terrorism 2019;**42**:972–96.
20. **Andersen JC, Sandberg S.** Islamic State propaganda: between social movement framing and subcultural provocation. Terrorism and Political Violence 2018, DOI: 10.1080/09546553.2018.1484356.
21. **Venkatesh V, Podoshen JS, Wallin J, Rabah J, Glass D.** Promoting extreme violence: visual and narrative analysis of select ultraviolent terror propaganda videos produced by the Islamic State of Iraq and Syria (ISIS) in 2015 and 2016. Terrorism and Political Violence 2018, DOI: 10.1080/09546553.2018.1516209.
22. How many IS foreign fighters are left in Iraq and Syria? BBC News. 20 February 2019.
23. **Cialdini R.** Influence: science and practice, third edition. New York: HarperCollins; 1993.
24. **Aggarwal NK.** Media persuasion in the Islamic State. New York: Columbia University Press; 2019.
25. **Mezzich JE, Caracci G, Fabrega Jr H, Kirmayer LJ.** Cultural formulation guidelines. Transcultural Psychiatry 2009;**54**:383–405.
26. **Aggarwal NK.** Mental health in the war on terror: culture, science, and statecraft. New York: Columbia University Press; 2015.
27. **Kirmayer LJ, Raikhel E, Rahimi S.** Cultures of the internet: identity, community, and mental health. Transcultural Psychiatry 2013;**50**:165–91.
28. **Bhui K, Ibrahim Y.** Marketing the 'radical': symbolic communication and persuasive technologies in jihadist websites. Transcultural Psychiatry 2013;**50**:216–34.
29. **The Islamic State.** Meanings of constancy—Wilāyat Al-Shām, Al-Barakah. Available from: https://jihadology.net/2019/03/11/new-video-message-from-the-islamic-state-meanings-of-constancy-wilayat-al-sham-al-barakah/ [accessed 10 May 2019].
30. **Chen H.** Exploring and data mining the dark side of the Web. Heidelberg: Springer-Verlag GmBH; 2012.
31. Islamic State: 'Thousands of civilians' still trapped in Baghuz. BBC News. 16 February 2019.
32. SDF attack Islamic State group's Syria enclave Baghuz. BBC News. 10 March 2019.
33. *Maānī Al-Thabāt Min Al-Bāghūz.* Al-Naba 2019;**10**:7.

34. **Khalaf R, Jones S.** Selling terror: how ISIS details its brutality. Financial Times. 17 June 2014.

35. **Wood G.** Don't shut down the internet's biggest jihadist archive. The Atlantic. 12 December 2018.

36. **Nida E.** Principles of translation. In: **Venuti L,** ed. The translation studies reader. New York: Routledge; 2000, pp. 126–40.

37. **Arberry AJ.** The Koran interpreted: a translation. New York: Touchstone; 1996 (first published 1955 by George Allen & Unwin).

38. **Duderija A.** Neo-traditional Salafi Qu'ran-Sunna hermeneutics and its interpretational implications. Religious Compass 2011;**5**:314–25.

39. **Callimachi R.** For women under ISIS, a tyranny of dress code and punishment. The New York Times. 12 December 2016.

40. **Altie MB, Horgan J, Thoroughgood C.** In their own words? Methodological considerations in the analysis of terrorist autobiographies. Journal of Strategic Studies 2012;**5**:85–98.

41. **Bhui KS, Hicks MH, Lashley M, Jones E.** A public health approach to understanding and preventing violent radicalization. BMC Medicine 2012;**10**:16.

42. **Aggarwal NK.** The Taliban's virtual emirate: the culture and psychology of an online militant community. New York: Columbia University Press; 2016.

43. **Devereux G.** Normal and abnormal. In: **Littlewood R, Dein S,** eds. Cultural psychiatry and medical anthropology: an introduction and reader. London: The Athlone Press; 2000, pp. 213–89.

44. **Kirmayer LJ.** Psychotherapy and the cultural concept of the person. Transcultural Psychiatry 2007;**44**:232–57.

45. **Foucault M.** The archaeology of knowledge and the discourse on language. Sheridan A, tr. New York: Vintage Books; 2012 (first published 1969 by Editions Gallimard).

46. **Cottee S, Cunliffe J.** Watching ISIS: how young adults engage with official English-language ISIS videos. Studies in Conflict & Terrorism 2020;**43**:183–207.

47. The Islamic State. Meanings of constancy from al-Bāghuz #2—Wilāyat Al-Shām, Al-Barakah. Available from: https://jihadology.net/2019/03/21/new-video-message-from-the-islamic-state-meanings-of-constancy-from-al-baghuz-2-wilayat-al-sham-al-barakah/ [accessed 4 May 2019].

48. **Callimachi R, Hassan F.** Abu Bakr al-Baghdadi, ISIS leader known for his brutality, is dead at 48. The New York Times. 27 October 2019.

49. **Kingsley P.** Anti-Semitism is back, from the Left, Right and Islamist extremes. Why? The New York Times. 4 April 2019.

50. **Karandikar S.** Persuasive propaganda: an investigation of online deceptive tactics of Islamist, White, and Zionist Extremists. In **Chiluwa IE, Samoilenko SA,** eds. Handbook of research on deception, fake news, and misinformation online. Hershey: IGI Global; 2019, pp. 538–55.

Chapter 3

The undeniable reality of the 'War on Terror', radicalization, and sanity

Shamila Ahmed

3.1 Introduction

Psychology has long explored the relationship between beliefs, ideology, politics, identity, and violence [1, 2]. More recently, this has been extended to investigate the relationship between mental illness and radicalization. Research confirms that, among imprisoned terrorists, the prevalence of mental illness is as low as, or lower than in, the general population [3]. There is no associated generalizable link between terrorist activities and specific mental illnesses, such as bipolar disorder or schizophrenia [4, 5]. However, these approaches examined the impact of pre-existing mental illnesses on radicalization and failed to explore how societal and institutional structures intersect with experiences of mental functioning and health to facilitate radicalization. This problematic approach has been highlighted by the Radicalisation Awareness Network (RAN). According to RAN [6], 'when trauma exists in the background (personal, familial and/or communal) of an individual turning towards radicalization, it is easy to focus on the trauma rather than the structural issues associated with the trauma.'

This chapter contends that an exploration of the intersectionality of structural issues and trauma, where one examines the relationship between 'structure, mental health (agency–emotions–trauma) and radicalization', can offer a greater understanding of the radicalization process. Such an approach acknowledges the capacity for injustice, inequality, victimisation, and suffering, and so on, to impact on mental health. And through doing so, it offers the possibility of understanding how the structures that are prevalent and constructed as part of the 'War on Terror' can produce secondary victimization and impact in a way that undermines belief in a 'just world', thereby fracturing existing emotional health and positive beliefs to provide a cognitive and emotional opening to radicalization.

3.2 **States of denial**

Stanley Cohen's *States of Denial* offers insight into the complexity of the relationship between structure, agency, emotions and trauma [7]. According to Cohen, denial is an unconscious defence mechanism against the horrors of acknowledging the suffering, injustice, and other unpleasant phenomenon that exist in the world. However, what happens when denial is no longer able to operate as a form of defence? This chapter explores how Islamist narratives, such as those of Al-Qaida [8], which highlight the existence of structures that cause suffering, inequality, and injustice in the 'War on Terror', make denial impossible. It is argued that the lack of services to support the negative emotions such acknowledgment evokes leads to these emotions forming a crucial part of the radicalization process.

Within this Freudian meta-narrative perspective, the psyche blocks off information that is literally unthinkable or unbearable, therefore preventing these thoughts from reaching conscious knowledge [7]. In doing so, denial makes it possible to cope with the guilt, fear, anxiety, and other disturbing emotions aroused by reality. Denial is also adaptive, and it is this adaptive capacity that allows individuals to maintain a sense of clarity, sanity, and normality across multiple events and their particular realities [7]. However, there are moments when images of pain and suffering cut right through us and, in these moments, it is possible to see and feel pain and suffering [7]. In such instances where denial is not possible, conscious acknowledgement has the capacity to invoke emotions and motivate behaviours. Cohen [7] contends that some individuals experience suffering at all times and not just at certain image-induced moments, and these individuals become investigative journalists and medical, legal, or human rights professionals. However, Cohen [7] argues that where individuals become emotionally overwhelmed and there is a "romantic identification" with the victim and those experiencing suffering, this can lead to a lapse of judgement about the actions required to achieve a sense of justice. It is also possible to contend that the suffering of others can be manipulated into motivating individuals to commit acts of violence through portraying violence as the only remedy to alleviate suffering. As will be detailed further on, Islamist groups use these very processes to radicalize individuals, and it is their acute understanding of how the structures in the 'War on Terror' impact emotions, agency, and trauma that allows them to provide a narrative perceived as compassionate, understanding, and empathetic of the reality of those that are progressively radicalized.

3.3 **Forms of denial and the 'War on Terror'**

According to Cohen [7], states frequently use literal, interpretive, and implicatory denial. Literal denial is used to deny a fact or knowledge of a fact; interpretive denial is where states confer a different meaning to something, most often utilizing an 'ideological construction'; and implicatory denial is used to denote when 'there is no attempt to deny either the facts or its conventional interpretation. What are denied or minimised are the psychological, political or moral implications that conventionally follow' [7].

The 'War on Terror' was produced foreign and domestic policies that deny the impact of social control and state agency on human rights, state crimes, and mass victimization [9–11]. The 'War on Terror' has been built into the ideological façade of the state and academics have attempted to demonstrate the psychological, political, and moral impact of the war [12, 13]. For example, the 'War on Terror' impacts on emotions and human suffering, locally and globally [14]. The various mechanisms of control and prevention introduced and sustained by states have altered our collective understandings of identity, suffering, injustice, and so on.

Cohen's [7] work demonstrates how states frame, justify, and legitimize actions through sophisticated techniques of denial. One can also elude to how just as victims of state crime are not 'seen as victims', those labelled as potential 'terrorists' are depicted as threats that deserve no human rights and the use of absolute state force [15–17]. These forms of denial prevalent in the 'War on Terror' have enormous consequences for not only leading to actions that cause harm and suffering, but also for facilitating radicalization by increasing recruits who see the suffering inflicted by counterterrorist strategies.

3.4 **Islamist narratives as counter-discourses to denial**

The following research offers some insight into the relationship between 'structure, mental health (agency–emotions–trauma), and radicalization' through exploring how denial, and therefore a lack of recognition can impact on radicalization. Research by Čehajić and Brown [18] revealed that where Serbian participants acknowledged their group's actions, including genocidal acts committed in Bosnia and Herzegovina between 1992 and 1995, this acknowledgement was found to positively impact on intergroup contact after the conflict. The relationship between acknowledgement and forgiveness and reconciliation has overwhelming empirical support [19–21], and is a central component of the success of truth and reconciliation policies and restorative justice policies [18, 22, 23].

Unlike these policies, which exist to provide a platform for all voices—indeed recognizing how the existence of such platforms is fundamental to allowing an individual the humanity to be heard—the 'War on Terror' discourse operates to marginalize other discourses and voices, and through doing so, it impedes the possibility of alternative solutions to the conflict. Orli Fridman [24] defines these voices to be those of 'individuals and groups who choose to address issues of morality and responsibility against war and violence in their society and to speak about them out loud as they force alternative attitudes into the public sphere'. According to Cohen [7, p. 95], such groups work to highlight how language works to produce a numbing effect, making denial possible. Through seeking to disperse a counter-discourse, refuting the ideological construction of the 'War on Terror', questioning the legitimacy and, more importantly, highlighting its oppressive nature and mass implications for justice, equality, and human rights, it could be argued that Islamist groups constitute one of these groups.

3.4.1 Cognitive denial

According to Cohen [7], denial can be cognitive, which involves not acknowledging the facts; emotional, whereby one does not feel and is not disturbed; moral, which involves not recognizing wrongness; or active, where no attempt is made to respond to knowledge. The 'War on Terror' and radicalization incorporate cognitive, emotional, moral, and active modes of denial. Although denial is adaptive, thereby allowing individuals to deny suffering, inequality, and injustice in order to maintain their sanity [7], the 'War on Terror' has made suffering, inequality, and injustice part of Muslims daily lives, and Islamist groups highlight the existence of these very entities [25–27]. Islamist groups counter-discourse to the 'War on Terror' is based on demonstrating the injustice, inhumanity, and suffering caused by states, and therefore dispersing narratives aimed at exposing facts that shatter the cognitive mode of denial. This then leads to the fundamental question of, 'If denial operates as a self-defence mechanism and within the "War on Terror" the capacity for denial has been diminished because states have created a reality where individuals are emotionally overwhelmed and Islamist groups disperse narratives to counter-denial and invoke overwhelming emotions, then how do individuals cope with such a diminished self-defence capacity and what is the impact of this on their sanity?'

3.4.2 Emotional denial

Islamist narratives highlight the lack of recognition towards Muslim suffering and the marginalization of Muslims in the 'War on Terror'. Being denied recognition at an individual level and group level can affect beliefs and push individuals towards more extremist views [28]. Gavrielides and Santiago [29] argue that social marginalization leads individuals to radicalization because radicalization gives them the opportunity to get their point across.

Key to understanding the relationship between denial, recognition, and acknowledgment is noticing emotions and responses. Research demonstrates how a lack of recognition and acknowledgment elicits negative affective responses, including resentment, hatred, and rage [30]. Islamist narratives are based on shattering the emotional mode of denial and eliciting these negative effective responses. The narratives incorporate vast amounts of information that break cognitive denial, and exposure to information about suffering, injustices, and atrocities leads to individuals being emotionally overwhelmed, which, as previously stated, Cohen suggests can lead to an obscured sense of judgement on how to achieve justice and reduce suffering [7].

Emotions and responses are also shaped by group membership and group identification. Research demonstrates that having the capacity for secondary emotions such as pride, love, guilt, and remorse makes us human, and these emotions are typically selected more often for the ingroup than for the outgroup [31]. The 'War on Terror' has facilitated belonging and unity to the ummah, with the Muslim diaspora now uniting through their shared experiences of injustice, suffering, and oppression [14, 32]. Victimization has therefore become a point of unity for the ummah, with research highlighting how reactions to ingroup victimization also occur among group members who did not experience the events personally [33, 34]. The transitional nature of marginalization, criminalization, and otherization has affected British Muslims belonging to the ummah, with research finding that prior to joining extremist groups, recruits 'had a very strong connection to other Muslims across the globe' [35, p. 110].

Although the 'War on Terror' has facilitated an alternative understanding of the Muslim diaspora, with perceptions and experiences of suffering exacerbating negative emotions, Islamist groups exploit these processes. Islamist groups draw on historical legacies and through doing so, utilize the memories and emotions associated with past injustices. Within this interplay between the past and the present, within self-preservation and self-extermination, narratives and memory become powerful entities. As Allan Young [36, p. 221] notes, memory is the 'struggle over the self's most valued possessions'. In this narrative, injustice and repression become personal experiences. Personal and political grievances lead to perceptions of powerlessness, which positively facilitate the emergence of a group identity and radicalization [37, 38]. Similarly, research by Hamm and Spaaij [39] on 98 US lone wolf terrorists revealed that personal and political grievances contributed to individuals having an affinity with an extremist group. Powerlessness intersects with the pain, anger, vulnerability, and frustration that accompany a reduction of legal rights, experiencing racism and discrimination and/or having a loved one killed [27, 40, 41]. The increase in discrimination positively heightens this identity [26], with research demonstrating how perceived discrimination leads to decreased psychological well-being, anxiety, and depressive symptoms [27, 28]. It is the decrease in psychological well-being and the experiencing of such emotions that, according to John Horgan [5], makes individuals vulnerable to radicalization and is used to recruit individuals [29, 30].

A closer examination of the capacity of social and political structures to impact on beliefs and morals provides a greater insight into the relationship between mental health and radicalization. Research demonstrates how the lack of human rights and the criminalization of freedom and association in the 'War on Terror' have led British Muslims to experience fear, helplessness, risk, vulnerability, and insecurity [25]. As Shamila Ahmed argues, the measures introduced not only violate international human rights law and international humanitarian law, but there is also no recognition of how such violations and their erosion of universal principles of freedom, justice, and fairness impact individuals, their perceptions, their beliefs, and their sense of security in the world [31].

There is an urgent need for approaches that consider the impact of discrimination, a lack of acknowledgment, and so on, on psychological well-being and then assess this relationship in terms of radicalization. However, such an approach also means being non-state centric and thus assessing the impact of states and institutions on mental health. The preoccupation of psychological approaches with establishing pre-existing mental illness and disorders in the quest to find a Lombrosian link between genetics and radicalization pathologizes suspected terrorists. Such narrow approaches deny the capacity of structures to impact beliefs, even though, as will be discussed, there is overwhelming evidence on how structures not only impact beliefs in a 'just world', but also that our experience with them can constitute secondary victimization leading to the existence of trauma and post-traumatic stress disorder (PTSD) [31].

Siding with humanity and adopting a cosmopolitan perspective means suspending prior social ideological constructions and asking questions such as, 'If an individual suffers secondary victimization because their beliefs regarding justice, equality, and so on, are shattered, with such an experience leading to trauma, and we are able to acknowledge the impact of these structural wounds on the person and their psyche, then why is it that when such beliefs are destroyed because of institutions in the "War on Terror", it is difficult to even recognize that these too can create structural wounds that have a capacity to create trauma? The 'War on Terror' is bound by questions of loyalty, where asking questions regarding state methods and the impact of such methods has been constructed as problematic and can lead to being labelled as a threat and as 'one of them'.

The structures prevalent in the 'War on Terror' are capable of affecting one's belief in a 'just world' through fracturing existing beliefs and world views, and, through doing so, they could be interpreted as providing a cognitive emotional opening to radicalization [31]. Such a conceptualization of the relationship between 'structures—mental health—radicalization' acknowledges the capacity for injustice, inequality, victimization, suffering, and so on to impact mental health and, as highlighted later in the chapter, there is overwhelming evidence to support this process.

According to Ellis et al. [32], based on their research with 79 young Somali males, higher levels of trauma were associated with an increased openness towards illegal and violent activism, and this openness was greater for individuals with weak social bonds to both their communities and wider society. As O'Driscoll contends [33], 'trauma can destroy a person's assumptions about themselves and the world around them, which in turn can lead to greater hostility and mistrust that facilitates openness to violent extremism. PTSD symptoms can include a bleak vision of the future and pessimism, which together can lead to the idea of dying for a cause becoming more appealing'. Research on Chechen suicide terrorists via interviews with their family members revealed that trauma changed the course of the suicide terrorists' life, leading Speckhard and Akhmedova to conclude that trauma was the primary motivation in their sample of terrorists [38].

Research demonstrates how institutions affect our beliefs in a 'just world' [39] and there is evidence to demonstrate that, in some cases, our experience of them can constitute secondary victimization and be much more damaging than experiences of primary victimization [40–43]. Through drawing on this research and research on the impact of institutional sexual abuse on secondary victimization, trauma, and PTSD [44, 45], Ahmed [31] highlights how within the 'War on Terror', institutions have betrayed the trust invested in them, diminishing positive beliefs and the possible impact of this process on the experience of trauma and PTSD. To further highlight the relationship between 'structure, mental health (agency–emotions–trauma) and radicalization', Ahmed [31] draws on her research with British Muslims, which reveals how the 'War on Terror' has damaged their beliefs in humanity, taken away fundamental human rights they believed would always exist, challenged their beliefs in justice, and, through doing so, it has taken away their sense of security and safety in the world.

3.4.3 **Moral denial**

Ideas of legitimacy, illegitimacy, justice, and injustice are closely tied to morals. Morton Deutsch [46] contends that although the Universal Declaration of Human Rights does not state that all individuals should be treated identically, it does highlight that systematic disparities should not exist between the social conditions and the rights of people, and therefore all individuals should have the same opportunities. The linkage between resources and justice presented by Jonathan Turner [47, p. 301] demonstrates the importance of subjectivity because, as he argues, 'inequalities generate negative emotions by those who receive less than others, primarily because the former makes justice evaluations that they are not getting their fair share'. Keltner et al. [48] state that concerns over what is just and fair are the glue of social living, with Schwartz and Sagiv [49] highlighting how moral values of fairness and justice are universal and therefore concern all cultures. It is moral mandates that determine how outcomes and procedures are perceived. Where they fail to conform with perceivers' moral mandates, they will be perceived as illegitimate if they are not consistent with perceivers' moral mandates [50]. The 'War on Terror' has had vast implications for understandings of justice, with research by Ahmed [26] demonstrating the negative impact of perceptions of relative deprivation of legal rights for British Muslims attachment and belonging to their British identity.

Moral denial is another mode of denial that Islamist groups seek to destroy, through raising questions of morality and placing a sense of moral duty onto Muslims. As Muhammad Nuruddeen Lemu [27, p. 46] suggests, they incorporate two questions into their narrative;

1. Can a true Muslim choose to do nothing after witnessing all the injustice taking place against Islam and Muslims—discrimination, Islamophobia, violence, misery, humiliation, suffering, human rights abuses, and so on?

2. What will your response be to the suffering of innocent Muslims and the attack on Islam—if indeed you have faith—especially when no peaceful solutions are practical or realistic.

In this way, Islamists use morality to challenge and encourage individuals to destroy existing structures that cause harm, and such a standpoint is based on using individuals' inherent beliefs relating to dignity, recognition, and respect [51–53].

3.4.4 **Active denial**

All the knowledge, the impact on morality, the overwhelming emotions, the purposeful denials, the counter-exposures to document the denials, the shows of horror, atrocities and suffering, the destruction of beliefs, values and human rights, the erosion of safety and security, and the manipulation of the psychological processes that exist to maintain some form of sanity can lead to despair, and the changing of what was once a sound peaceful mind to one that delves into what was, and then crashes into the reality of what is.

The use of Cohen's masterful thesis as the basis of this chapter was entirely fitting because he is right: with what conviction can anyone continuously acknowledge suffering and atrocities and still maintain their sanity? Those that do experience such realities are left with shards of trauma embedded within them and they receive support on how to navigate these new parts that now also define and shape the contours of their psyche. The impetus is on understanding their experience, their narrative, and providing care. As West [54, p. 356] contends, the true therapeutic task 'is to find a way of living that does not deny the horrors that have happened to them, but also that allows them to have some kind of fulfilled life'. However, as this chapter argues, it is the social construction of a particular experience, or set of experiences that determines acknowledgement, compassion, and empathy. In much the same way, the task should also be to assist those that are unsure of how to deal with all the knowledge, the impact on morality, and so on just mentioned, and this involves seeking to understand the relationship between structures and agency.

At present, Islamist groups thrive in providing understanding and being empathetic to this relationship—one that nation states in the 'War on Terror' seem unable to apprehend, leaving an Achilles heel in all counterterrorism strategy and policy. Consider the following quote by Karen Colvard [55, p. 2]: 'people who are willing to use violence in the service of a political idea are usually rather ordinary human beings … not devils or psychopaths but people who may base their actions on morality, commitment, and group loyalty, which in other circumstances we would consider admirable'. Islamist groups portray a viable solution to assist individuals in dealing with their emotions. Research by Speckhard and Akhmedova [38] revealed that 28 out of 34 suicide terrorists were secular Muslims before their experiences of trauma and 27 sought out radical Wahhabi groups in response to their trauma. Trauma can also be linked to the fact that when individuals strongly identify with the trauma of others like them, this increases the likelihood of vicarious trauma. The 'War on Terror' has made suffering a transitional experience and within this context, as the research by Speckhard and Akhmedova [38] found, individuals are likely to seek out those they feel understand them. As RAN [6, p. 4] states, 'ideological extremism can operate as a kind of protective factor, offering a sense of purpose and protection against other mental health problems, while working as a type of "cure" for post-traumatic stress and depression'. Research has also highlighted how membership to a radicalizing group can bring higher social status [56, 57], with individual influence, particularly through a mentor, leading to group membership [58]. Peer pressure can also increase one's vulnerability to being radicalized because it can be experienced as a positive—a way of group bonding [8]. According to Howard Bath [59], the three protective factors for traumatised children who might be at risk of radicalization are trustworthy relationships, establishing safe environments, and providing adequate support to assist and help children to regulate negative emotions. Research therefore suggests that radicalization responds to emotional needs and the need for attachments and bonding. In the absence of public services where individuals feel able to voice their feelings for fear of marginalization or criminalization, where they are taught how to regulate emotions and where they are provided with attachments and belonging, which give them a sense of security, they become susceptible to Islamist narratives and narratives that advocate violence. The boundaries between what Cohen [7] refers to as the triangle of victims, perpetrators, and bystanders become contested and fluid. Victims and bystanders become perpetrators, with terrorism research identifying how perceived injustices have formed a primary motivation for terrorist acts of violence [60], with terrorism also being a by-product of perceived indignities in repressive environments [61, 62].

3.5 **Conclusion**

This chapter has attempted to outline the relationship between 'structure, mental health (agency–emotions–trauma) and radicalization'. In doing so, it has highlighted existing research that demonstrates the validity of this relationship. The lack of extensive evidence relating to mental disorders and radicalization in its broadest sense does not mean that deep psychological processes are not present in the radicalization process, or in specific subgroups; it means that academics, as well as policymakers, have failed to conceptualize this relationship adequately.

In this way, academia can narrow the possibility of understanding through creating fixed, rigid, and predefined frameworks and, through doing so, it can constitute yet another social structure that contributes a further layer of oppression and silences the very voices it seeks to portray. When such narrow and marginalizing frameworks are utilized, these significantly restrict our ability to understand the lived world, the emotions, the motivations, and all the other entities we must know to understand the radicalization process. De-radicalization programmes can only be successful if they engage with the very psychological processes that facilitate radicalization. Just as with other forms of harm that cause suffering and impact beliefs, such as sexual abuse, whereby it has taken decades to bring the structural component into mainstream recognition and, indeed, accept how this structural component compounds beliefs, impacts suffering, trauma, and so on, the same must happen with recognizing and accepting the capacity of structures to cause other forms of harm. Through such an approach it might then be possible to provide services for those that are vulnerable to radicalization and unable to regulate emotions, so they are helped to develop the resilience required.

This chapter has questioned the use of frameworks that dismiss the structural issues associated with radicalization. In terms of policy and research, this means not only developing frameworks that explore the relationship between structure and agency, but it also means recognizing how the use of labels can reinforce binaries. Categories and labels can be imposed simply through advocating that a forensic psychologist is best placed to research and understand radicalization. This can easily lead to and give the impression to vulnerable, at-risk individuals that 'we are the sane ones' and 'they are the insane deviant ones'. Such an approach implies a plethora of instant judgements. From such a standpoint, understanding cannot be achieved because the intersectionality between researchers and participants is replaced with the attribution of labels that signify difference and judgements.

If the true task is to achieve understanding, then there exists a need for conscious awareness of how we risk reproducing labelling mechanisms that marginalize, exclude, and criminalize, rather than produce a safe space where agency, emotions, and experiences can be shared without fear. Although academia has made steps to promote change and challenge harmful state discourses, there still remains a blindness of how, as a power-vested mechanism of knowledge production, it can reproduce harmful social constructions.

One need not be able to recite Foucault's Power-Knowledge to avoid such pitfalls. However, it should be expected that we can deconstruct our decisions and interrogate them to ask questions such as, 'if categories of difference such as "race", those of gender, and so on are accepted as problematic in their evaluation of one binary being superior over the other, then perhaps classifications such as criminal and non-criminal, or those that potentially pathologize, also carry such power and therefore do not represent the best way to understand a deeply personal and immensely complicated process?' Such approaches lead to those that are vulnerable and at risk to question the integrity and true motivations of the researcher. Therefore, the approach taken, and the labels used have immense implications and consequences in the ability to conduct research, to understand deep psychological processes, and the production of knowledge.

References

1. **Martens WH.** The terrorist with antisocial personality disorder. Journal of Forensic Psychology Practice 2004;**4**:45–56.

2. **Dalgaard-Nielsen A.** Studying violent radicalisation in Europe II. Copenhagen: DIIS; 2008.

3. **Ruby CL.** Are terrorists mentally deranged? Analyses of Social Issues and Public Policy 2002;**2**:15–26.

4. **Crenshaw M.** How terrorists think: what psychology can contribute to understanding terrorism. In: **Howard L,** eds. Terrorism: roots, impact, responses. London: Praeger; 1992, pp. 71–80.

5. **Horgan J.** From profiles to pathways and roots to routes: perspectives from psychology on radicalization into terrorism. The Annals of the American Academy of Political and Social Science 2008;**618**:80–94.

6. **RAN.** A mental health approach to understanding violent extremism. Available from: https://ec.europa.eu/home-affairs/sites/homeaffairs/files/what-we-do/networks/radicalisation_awareness_network/about-ran/ran-h-and-sc/docs/ran_hsc_prac_mental_health_03062019_en.pdf. [accessed 10 December 2019].

7. **Cohen S.** States of denial: knowing about atrocities and suffering. Cambridge: Polity Press; 2001.

8. **Prevent Strategy.** Prevent strategy. London: The Stationery Office; 2011.

9. **Gregory D.** The colonial present: Afghanistan, Palestine, Iraq. Oxford: Blackwell; 2004.

10. **Jackson R.** Writing the war on terrorism: language, politics and counterterrorism. Manchester: Manchester University Press; 2005.

11. **Jackson R.** Language, policy and the construction of a torture culture in the War on Terrorism. Review of International Studies 2007;**33**:353–71.

12. **Welch M.** Ordering Iraq: reflections on power, discourse, & neocolonialism. Critical Criminology 2008;**16**:257–69.

13. **Milne S.** Terrorism and counter-terrorism: ethics and liberal democracy. Oxford: Blackwell Publishers; 2009.

14. **Hudson B.** Difference, diversity and criminology: the cosmopolitan vision. Theoretical Criminology 2008;**12**:275–92

15. **Huggings MK, Haritos-Fatouros M, Zimbardo PG.** Violence workers: police torturers and murderers reconstruct Brazilian atrocities. Berkeley, CA: University of California Press; 2002.

16. **Kauzlarich D, Matthews RA, Miller WJ.** Towards a victiminology of state crime. Critical Criminology 2001;**10**:173–94.

17. **Jackson R.** Constructing enemies: 'Islamic terrorism' in political and academic discourse. Government and Opposition 2007;**42**:394–426.

18. **Čehajić, S, Brown R.** Not in my name: a social psychological study of antecedents and consequences of acknowledgment of in-group atrocities. Genocide Studies and Prevention 2008;**3**:195–211.

19. **Asmal K, Asmal L, Roberts RS.** Reconciliation through truth: a reckoning of apartheid's criminal governance. Oxford: James Currey Publishers; 1997.

20. **Hamber B, Nageng D, O'Malley G.** 'Telling it like it is . . .': understanding the truth and reconciliation commission from the perspective of survivors. Psychology in Society 2000;**26**:18–42.

21. **Taylor C.** The politics of recognition. In: **Gutman A**, ed. Multiculturalism and 'the politics of recognition': an essay by Charles Taylor. Princeton, NJ: Princeton University Press; 1992, pp. 25–74.

22. **Halpern J, Weinstein HM.** Rehumanizing the Other: empathy and reconciliation. Human Rights Quarterly 2004;**26**:561–83.

23. **Tutu D.** No future without forgiveness. London: Rider; 1999.

24. **Fridman O.** Breaking states of denial: anti occupation activism in Israel after 2000. Available from: http://citeseerx.ist.psu.edu/viewdoc/download?doi=10.1.1.950.9512&rep=rep1&type=pdf [accessed 10 December 2019].

25. **Ahmed S.** The 'emotionalization of the war on terror': counter terrorism, fear, risk, insecurity and helplessness. An International Journal of Criminology and Criminal Justice 2015;**15**:545–60.

26. **Ahmed S.** Citizenship, belonging and attachment in the 'war on terror'. Critical Criminology 2016;**24**:111–25.

27. **Lemu MN.** Notes on religion and countering violent extremism. In: **Abadi H**, ed. Countering Daesh propaganda: action-oriented research for practical policy outcomes. Atlanta, GA: The Carter Center; 2016, pp. 43–50.

28. **Schomerus M, El Taraboulsi-McCarthy S, Sandhar J.** Countering violent extremism (Topic Guide). Birmingham: GSDRC, University of Birmingham; 2017.

29. **Gavrielides T, Santiago I.** Human Rights and Prevention of Violent Extremism. 18th Informal ASEM Seminar on Human Rights. Available from: https://www.asef.org/images/docs/Background%20Paper%20-%2018th%20Informal%20ASEM%20Seminar%20on%20Human%20Rights.pdf [accessed 10 December 2019].

30. **Kalayjian A, Shahinian SP, Gergerian EL, Saraydarian L.** Coping with Ottoman Turkish genocide: an exploration of the experience of Armenian survivors. Journal of Traumatic Stress 1996;**9**:87–97.

31. **Leyens, JP, Rodríguez-Pérez A, Rodríguez-Torres R, Gaunt R, Paladino MP, Vaes J.** Psychological essentialism and the attribution of uniquely human emotions to ingroups and outgroups. European Journal of Social Psychology 2001;**31**:395–411.

32. **Ahmed S.** A cosmopolitan response to the 'war on terror'. Journal of Theoretical and Philosophical Criminology 2019;**11**:64–78.

33. **Bar-Tal D, Chernyak-Hai L, Schori N, Gundar A.** A sense of self-perceived collective victimhood in intractable conflicts. International Review of the Red Cross 2009;**91**:229–58.

34. **Vollhardt JR.** Collective victimization. In: **Tropp L**, ed. Oxford handbook of intergroup conflict. New York: Oxford University Press; 2012, pp. 136–57.

35 **Silke A.** Holy warriors: exploring the psychological process of jihadi radicalization. European Journal of Criminology 2008;**5**:99–123.

36. **Young A.** The harmony of illusions: inventing post-traumatic stress disorder. Princeton, NJ: Princeton University Press; 1995.

37. **Post JM, Sprinzak E, Denny L.** The terrorists in their own words: interviews with 35 incarcerated Middle Eastern terrorists. Terrorism and Political Violence 2003;**15**:171–84.

38. **Speckhard A, Akhmedova K.** Talking to terrorists. The Journal of Psychohistory 2005;**33**:125–56.

39. **Hamm M, Spaaij R.** Lone wolf terrorism in America: using knowledge of radicalization pathways to forge prevention strategies. Washington, DC: National Institute of Justice; 2015.

40. **Boyns D, Ballard JD.** Developing a sociological theory for the empirical understanding of terrorism. The American Sociologist 2004;**35**:5–25.

41. **Henderson-King D, Henderson-King E, Bolea B, Koches K, Kauffman A.** Seeking understanding or sending bombs: beliefs as predictors of responses to terrorism. Peace and Conflict 2004;**10**:67–84.

27. **Liebkind K, Jasinskaja-Lahti I.** The influence of experiences of discrimination on psychological stress: a comparison of seven immigrant groups. Journal of Community and Applied Social Psychology 2000;**10**:1–16.

28. **Pascoe EA, Richman LS.** Perceived discrimination and health: a meta-analytic review. Psychological Bulletin 2009;**135**:531–54.

29. **Blaker L.** The Islamic State's use of online social media. Military Cyber Affairs 2015;**1**:1–9.

30. **Gould E, Esteban FK.** The long-run effect of 9/11: terrorism, backlash, and the assimilation of Muslim immigrants in the West. The Economic Journal 2016;**126**:2064–114.

31. **Ahmed S.** The 'War on Terror', state crime & radicalization: a constitutive theory of radicalization. London: Palgrave; 2020.

32. **Ellis BH, Abdi SM, Horgan J, Miller AB, Saxe GN, Blood E.** Trauma and openness to legal and illegal activism among Somali refugees. Terrorism and Political Violence 2015;**27**:857–83.

33. **O'Driscoll D.** Violent extremism and mental disorders. Available from: https:// assets.publishing.service.gov.uk/media/5c700673ed915d4a3e8266e7/476_Violent_ Extremism_and_Mental_Disorders.pdf. [accessed 10 December 2019].

39. **Correia I, Vala J, Aguiar P.** The effects of belief in a just world and victim's innocence on secondary victimization, judgements of justice and deservingness. Social Justice Research 2001;**14**:327–42.

40. **Orth U.** Secondary victimization of crime victims by criminal proceedings. Social Justice Research 2002;**15**:313–25.

41. **Skinner T, Taylor H.** "Being shut out in the dark": young survivors' experiences of reporting a sexual offence. Feminist Criminology 2009;**4**:130–50.

42. **Elliott I, Thomas SDM, Ogloff JRP.** Procedural justice in contacts with the police: the perspective of victims of crime. Police Practice and Research 2012;**13**:437–49.

43. **Wemmers JA.** Victims' experiences in the criminal justice system and their recovery from crime. International Review of Victimology 2013;**19**:221–33.

44. **Smith CP, Freyd JJ.** Dangerous safe havens: institutional betrayal exacerbates sexual trauma. Journal of Traumatic Stress 2013;**26**:119–24.

45. **Mcalinden AM.** "Setting 'em up": personal, familial and institutional grooming in the sexual abuse of children. Social and Legal Studies 2006;**15**:339–62.

46. **Deutsch M.** A framework for thinking about oppression and its change. Social Justice Research 2006;**19**:7–41.

47. **Turner J.** Justice and emotions. Social Justice Research 2007;**20**:288–311.

48. **Keltner D, Horberg E, Oveis C.** Emotional intuitions and moral play. Social Justice Research 2006;**19**:208–17.

49. **Schwartz SH, Sagiv L.** Identifying culture-specifics in the content and structure of values. Journal of Cross-Cultural Psychology 1995;**26**:92–116.

50. **Skitka LJ, Mullen E.** Understanding judgments of fairness in a real-world political context: a test of the value protection model of justice reasoning. Personality and Social Psychology Bulletin 2002;**28**:1419–29.

51. **Atran S, Axelrod R.** 'Reframing sacred values'. Negotiation Journal 2008;**24**:221–46.

52. **USAID (US Agency for International Development).** Guide to the drivers of violent extremism. Washington, DC: USAID; 2009.

53. **Botha A, Abdile M.** Radicalisation and al-Shabaab recruitment in Somalia. Paris: Institute for Security Studies; 2014.

54. **West W.** An introduction to the Symposium on Counselling and Armed Conflicts. British Journal of Guidance & Counselling 2003;**31**:355–7. p. 356.

55. **Colvard K.** What we already know about terrorism: violent challenges to the state and state response. Harry Frank Guggenheim Review 2002;**1**:1–5.

56. **USAID.** The development response to violent extremism and insurgency policy. Washington, DC: USAID; 2011.

57. **Ranstorp M.** The root causes of violent extremism (issue paper). Brussels: Radicalisation Awareness Network; 2016.

58. **Mercy Corps.** Motivations and empty promises: Voices of former Boko Haram combatants and Nigerian youth. London: Mercy Corps; 2016.

59. **Bath H.** The three pillars of trauma-informed care. Reclaiming Children and Youth 2008;**17**;17–21.

60. **Hacker FJ, Hacker F.** Crusaders, criminals, crazies: terror and terrorism in our time. New York: Norton; 1976.

61. **Krueger AB, Maleckova J.** Seeking the roots of terrorism. Chronicle of Higher Education. Available from: http://chronicle.com/weekly/v49/139/39b01001.htm [accessed 10 December 2019].

62. **Turk A.** Sociology of terrorism. Annual Review of Sociology 2004;**30**:271–86.

Chapter 4

Terrorism in the context of social capital and community

Edgar Jones

4.1 Introduction

Although a sustained military campaign has almost eradicated the territory controlled by Islamic State (IS), an assessment by the United Nations in February 2019 concluded that, as a global organization, it remains 'by far the most ambitious international terrorist group, and the most likely to conduct a large-scale complex attack' [1]. The coordinated, suicide bombing of churches and hotels in Sri Lanka in April 2019, leading to the death of 253 people, was proposed as an example of this capability, though the proposed link with IS has yet to be substantiated. It is clear, however, that IS had created a message of community and belonging that attracted as many as 40,000 foreign terrorist fighters from across the world [2, pp. 12–13].

Together with ideology and radical politics, the roots of terrorism have been explored within communities. Louise Richardson has argued that terrorism requires a combination of 'an alienated individual, a complicit society, and a legitimizing ideology' [3, pp. 55–6, 216]. Terrorist groups can operate effectively only if they are supported at various levels from sympathizers through to active participants. Communities have been identified as a social driver of radicalization and societies divided by relative deprivation and inequality are said to be at greater risk of being radicalized because recruiters have an opportunity to exploit feelings of alienation and grievance [4]. Further, some studies have found that Internet appeals are effective only if they are supported by offline contact with family or friends who are sympathetic to the radical propaganda [5, pp. 52–3].

Conversely, community has been proposed as a way of neutralizing and even combating the extreme messages of terrorist organizations. The Prevent strand of the UK's Strategy for Countering Terrorism of June 2018 was designed to 'tackle the causes of radicalisation, in communities and online', through engagement with 'civil society organisations, public sector institutions including local authorities, schools and universities' [6, pp. 31–2]. Social capital - a measure of trust and commitment to local networks - is used as a way of assessing whether particular communities are vulnerable to radical messages. This chapter explores the nature of social capital, and the processes of bonding and bridging, to understand how it can appear to serve as an agent of radicalization, while also being considered a protection against terrorist propaganda.

4.2 **Community as a risk factor for terrorism**

The recent rise in terrorist activity has been attributed, in part, to the growth and evolution of the Internet because it has greatly increased the capacity of organizations to offer access to radical messages. However, it has been shown that the impact of social media is greatly diminished without personal contacts to support its message. A recent literature review, supported by 15 interviews, concluded that the Internet alone was not responsible for the adoption of violent radical beliefs. In each case, subjects also had offline contact with family or friends who were sympathetic to an extreme political stance [7]. Further, a study of 1496 individuals drawn from three groups (far left, far right, and radical Islamic), who had been radicalized in the United States and committed ideologically motivated crimes, identified the importance of social networks in legitimizing violent protest [7]. Of the sample, 59% had a friend, 29% a family member, and 27% a significant other so engaged, while those without these links were less likely to participate in violent protest.

The role of the community in terrorist activity is also apparent from recent threat assessments. The European Union Terrorism Situation and Trend Report for 2018 identified five core characteristics of extreme Jihadist attacks within the European Union (EU) [8, p. 5]. They were that the terrorists were 'homegrown'; they had been radicalized in their country of residence without having travelled to join a terrorist organization abroad; they had been born in the EU or lived in the EU for most of their lives; and often they did not have direct links to IS or other extreme political groups. The implication of these findings is that these individuals had been radicalized or motivated to act where they had grown up and established socio-economic roots.

4.3 **Suspect communities**

The risk that communities may be drawn towards radical messages is said to be heightened if they believe that the state regards them with suspicion. 'The Troubles,' or the period from 1968 to 1998, when the Irish Republican Army (IRA) was active in Northern Ireland and the UK mainland, created areas of conflict where citizens and the emergency services had to be vigilant. Bombings and shootings led to 3500 civilian deaths in Northern Ireland and 68 in the UK [9]. In a context of emergency laws devised to address the covert IRA campaign, Paddy Hillyard argued that Irish people in general were treated as a 'suspect community' [10, pp. 257–8]. Counter-measures were predicated on the assumption that terrorists operating in England were living in areas occupied by innocent Irish citizens and using them as cover. While the creation of a suspect community is initiated by state authorities, it is hypothesized that harm is caused by other groups and individuals adopting the categorization, including some from within the community itself leading to stigma and loss of trust. In 2009, Pantazis and Pemberton offered a definition: 'a subgroup of the population that is singled out for state attention as "problematic". Specifically in terms of policing, individuals may be targeted, not necessarily as a result of suspected wrong-doing, but simply because of presumed membership to that sub-group' [11, p. 649].

It has also been argued that the extra protection offered by new antiterrorism legislation may come at the price of increasing the risk of creating suspect communities. Individuals charged under section 57 (possessing an article) or section 58 (collecting or possessing information) of the Terrorism Act 2000 are required to provide a 'reasonable excuse' for their actions, although no statutory guidance was provided as to what this might constitute [12, pp. 6–7] [13]. The Terrorism Acts of 2000 and 2006 include 'precursor offences' and place restrictions imposed on the liberty of individuals suspected of terrorist activity but for whom there is insufficient evidence for a criminal prosecution [11, pp. 651–4] [14]. The precautionary principle has been adopted on the grounds that terrorist activity has created an evident risk of harm in a context of incomplete evidence [15, pp. 1–3]. Pre-emptive strategies are justified by the suggestion that any adverse consequences of forestalling threats are outweighed by the lives or injuries prevented [16, pp. 521–2]. Hence, security forces have been empowered to 'defend further up the field' [17] to allow the arrest of those planning acts of violence before actual attacks have taken place [18]. Training for terrorism, for example, has become an offence, leading to suspicion of legitimate pastimes such as paintballing and martial arts, which have been interpreted by the courts as preparatory acts. The emphasis on precursor offences and restrictions imposed on the liberty of individuals suspected of terrorist activity but for whom there is insufficient evidence for a criminal prosecution have led some academics and lawyers to ask whether antiterrorism legislation is counter-productive [11]. They argue that the creation of a wide net of offending has increased the opportunity for greater cultural and political bias in the application of the new laws. For example, the government focus on al-Qaeda, it is suggested, led to a general suspicion of Muslims who disproportionately attracted the attention of security agencies [19]. In the United States, civil rights groups have raised concerns that Muslims are being disproportionately referred to law enforcement agencies and that Muslim communities are being selected for surveillance, despite government assurances that violent extremism is not exclusive to any ideology [20].

CAGE, an advocacy organization set up in 2003 to resist Islamophobia in civil society, sought to 'become a resistance movement of the suspect community' [21, p. 2]. However, it has found its motives questioned and has been accused of failing to condemn acts of terrorism [22, p. 257]. CAGE argues that this expectation is a product of structural Islamophobia in the sense that white British organizations are not routinely scrutinized over their responses to the violent actions of right-wing extreme groups. The focus on the politics of condemnation has arguably served to divert the debate from the pressing themes of citizenry and social cohesion.

4.4 Community as a protective factor

A functioning democracy does not in itself confer protection against terrorism. Baader-Meinhof, for example, operated effectively in Germany during the 1970s, a nation characterized by regulated and advanced democratic institutions [23]. To be a permanent minority within a democracy can generate a deep sense of injustice, unless the state can provide non-violent but effective means of expressing dissent and addressing grievances [3, p. 50]. Lord John Alderdice has argued that the Troubles arose in 1969 at the point when the Catholic community in Northern Ireland despaired of having legitimate grievances addressed by the majority Protestant assembly and turned to the IRA out of deep frustration [24, pp. 290–1].

Arguably, a community that feels represented by state institutions and engages in a range of democratic processes will see little value in terrorism or its appeals. In his study of democracy in the United States, Alexis de Tocqueville observed that large numbers of public-spirited citizens engaged with municipal bodies where they regularly discussed issues of governance, economics, or issues of diplomacy and trade [25, pp. 82–3]. Widespread participation 'in the local administration,' he argued, 'then affords an unfailing source of profit and interest to a vast number of individuals' [25, p. 84]. De Tocqueville believed that civic associations did more than assist citizens accomplish goals that would be hard to achieve individually; they also taught people to do things together, heightening their sense of civic responsibility for a larger social world. Local groups empowered people in a social contract that served to counterbalance state authority [26, pp. 534–6]. He also observed that in the United States - as in all democracies - the majority rules. As a result, anyone in the minority may find his or her voice drowned out and will have nowhere to turn when they are wronged. Even worse, the opinions and laws of the majority will become so pervasive as to seem like common sense, inhibiting people from critical thinking [27, pp. 158–60].

4.5 **Social capital**

Social capital is defined by the Organisation for Economic Co-operation and Development as 'networks together with shared norms, values and understandings that facilitate co-operation within or among groups' [28, p. 41]. In 1916, L.J. Hanifan had argued that 'an accumulation of social capital' benefitted 'the community as a whole … by co-operation of all its parts, while the individual will find in his associations the advantages of the help, the sympathy and the fellowship of his neighbours' [29, pp. 130–1]. The recognition that people can build trust in their communities through membership of social, sporting, and religious groups led to the idea that social capital is a public good, fostering cooperation in common goals. It is both relational, offering benefits to individuals through social networks, and material, by broadening or deepening the resources to which the person has access [30]. Trust lies at the core of social capital as it underpins the reciprocity and exchange that social networks facilitate.

Two processes operate to increase social capital, and both have to contribute if the community as a whole is to benefit. A distinction is drawn between bonding, whereby trust and reciprocity are fostered within groups, and bridging, which refers to the formation relationships and networks that transcend differences of ethnicity, religion, and socio-economic status [31]. Bridging is said to increase access and resources but sometimes at the expense of community cohesion. Although bonding can promote a shared identity and encourage participation, it can also lead to insularity, alienation from outsiders, and inhibit the formation of links with other groups [32]. If a society is composed of a homogenous majority and little attention is paid to minorities, then bonding will plausibly grant the dominant group material benefits but at the cost of creating an intolerance of difference and fostering tacit demands for obedience to majority norms. As a result, minority groups may experience marginalization, exclusion, or even persecution unless they conform [33]. An overemphasis on bonding is said to inhibit a community's ability to address controversial issues and resolve conflict.

An alienated minority may seek to raise its social capital in a manner that addresses immediate concerns but at the expense of long-term goals. A study of 674 teenage males from three disadvantaged neighbourhoods of Beirut found that those more likely to be involved in physical fights had high scores on bonding elements of social capital: membership of groups; liking living in the area; and trusting most or many in the neighbourhood [34]. Bridging elements of social capital were not significantly associated with this behaviour. The solidarity provided by gang-like bonds may serve to empower young people living in impoverished environments who have limited prospects of personal development [35]. However, the psychological support derived from an emphasis on bonding often relates to a narrow section of the community [36, p. 22]. Hence, the task of building social capital within a diverse society is more challenging than within a homogenous one, although the rewards are potentially greater given the broader range of skills and attributes that can be bridged.

Low social capital is always defined as being harmful to community development. For the individual, it implies isolation, lack of engagement, and low levels of trust in neighbourhood institutions. Putnam argued that progressive civic disengagement in America from the 1960s led to an erosion of trust and informal supportive behaviour [376, p. 73]. Recent studies have shown that low social capital is a risk factor for depression [38], and suicide [39]. Cross-sectional studies conducted in the United States have shown that social capital is inversely associated with rates of homicide and violent crime [40]. However, research found that this relationship functions in both directions. On the one hand, high social capital engenders informal social controls and leads to lower levels of offending, and, on the other, high rates of violent crime, accompanied by greater delinquency, may result in growing mistrust among community members and an erosion of social capital [41].

In relation to radicalization and support for terrorism, social capital has been proposed as both a protective and a facilitating factor [42]. Individuals who actively participate in a range of civic groups are hypothesized as having a legitimate and responsive outlet for political grievances, while also playing a role in sustaining social norms that reject the use of violence against civilians. Conversely, an emphasis on bonding capital may encourage recruitment into terrorist groups and facilitate collective action, while also fostering conditions where political violence serves as a potent signal.

The concept of social capital has been employed to assess risk and protective factors for populations who are considered vulnerable to radical messages. A population study of 608 men and women of Muslim heritage living in East London and Bradford measured sympathies for 16 items of violent protest and terrorism on a seven-point Likert scale [43, pp. 6–7]. The group most sympathetic to radical acts showed higher social capital (as measured by satisfaction, trust, and feelings of safety in the neighbourhood) than those who reported greatest condemnation. The most sympathetic also recorded lower levels of democratic engagement and fewer social contacts. These findings suggest that those potentially vulnerable to radicalization had tighter bonds with a smaller group of people than condemners, and were less likely to engage in bridging activities.

The study also sought to explore whether active involvement in democratic processes may serve to protect against the appeal of radical messages. Activities drawn from the Department of Communities and Local Government Citizenship Survey, including voting in a local election, signing a petition, campaigning for an organization or charity, membership of a political party, and taking part in a demonstration, picket, or march, were included in a measure of sympathies for radicalization [44]. Multivariable analysis of those most condemning of political violence and those most sympathetic to extreme protest found that the latter group had lower levels of political engagement [45]. Therefore, participation in a range of democratic processes appeared to lessen the appeal of extreme messages. Mild depression was also found to be a risk factor for sympathy, whereas three items (death of a close friend or relative, another major life event, and having signed a petition) were all associated with condemnation of violent protest or terrorism. Mediation analysis showed that when all three protective factors were accompanied by depression, the risk of sympathy only increased by a small amount, indicating the importance of political engagement and social connectedness [45]. However, a subsequent study of 618 white British and Pakistani people living in three English locations (Blackburn with Darwen, Bradford, and Luton) found that different levels of political engagement had no significant impact on sympathies for violent protest and terrorism [46].

4.6 **Broadening social capital**

Both radical jihadist and extreme right-wing supporters have been categorized as belonging to marginalized groups in UK society. It appears to be primarily an issue of identity and belonging, rather than socio-economic deprivation. A study of supporters of the English Defence League showed that they were more likely than average to be employed and were politically engaged but felt unrepresented [47, p. 14]. Equally, young Muslims coming before the criminal justice system often describe themselves as 'English' (to reflect where they were born, educated, and have their social networks) but not 'British', which they equate with the government and state systems.[1]

---

[1] Interview with Tayab Ali, 19 December 2016.

The riots in Bradford, Oldham and Burnley in the spring and summer of 2001 prompted both government and academic study of community cohesion. Derek McGhee concluded that white British and Asian working-class communities were characterized by 'excessive bonding capital in a context of insufficient bridging social capital' [48, p. 385]. Others have argued that this interpretation reinforced the idea of Muslim communities as self-segregating and therefore problematic [31]. A qualitative study of 26 Muslim men and women living in Leeds and Bradford explored the impact of counterterrorism measures on their behaviour and social cohesion [49]. The recruitment of community members by intelligence agencies to inform on neighbours was observed to create mistrust in partnerships. Further, being subject to a general environment of surveillance was found to encourage a fear of being monitored, which, in turn, led to people disengaging from some organizations. To address a culture of suspicion, independently funded, locally defined organizations were proposed to serve as a bridge between government agencies and community voices. Their active engagement in policy and projects was proposed not only to result in material changes, but also to give local people a sense of agency and control.

4.7 Conclusion

In a 2019 publication, the Radicalisation Awareness Network argued that 'communities play a central role in the prevention of extremism and radicalisation and their engagement and empowerment needs to be reinforced and supported as a matter of priority' [50, p. 4]. A core challenge in an era of terrorist threat is how to balance the need for intelligence about potential acts of extreme violence, while maintaining a positive relationship with communities that are targeted by recruiters. In the past, community initiatives, such as Prevent, have risked becoming synonymous with surveillance, which erodes trust and cohesion [51]. Population research has demonstrated how vulnerable groups, when feeling threatened or marginalized, tend to bond at the expense of bridging, accentuating divisions, and increasing the likelihood of being labelled as suspect communities. A solution is to foster representative groups to give minorities a voice and establish networks that give them an input into policy and governance. Although the task of building social capital within a diverse society is more challenging than within a homogenous one, the rewards are potentially greater given the broader range of skills and attributes that can be bridged.

References

1. **UN Security Council.** Eighth Report of the Secretary-General on the threat posed by ISIL (Da'esh) to international peace and security and the range of United Nations efforts

in support of Member States in countering the threat. Available from: www.un.org/sc/ctc/wp-content/uploads/2019/02/N1901937_EN.pdf [accessed 28 July 2020].

2. **Barrett R.** Beyond the Caliphate: foreign terrorist fighter and the threat of returnees. New York: Soufan Center; 2017.

3. **Richardson L.** What terrorists want. New York: Random House; 2006.

4. **Smith HJ, Pettigrew TF, Pippin G, Bialosiewicz S.** Relative deprivation: a theoretical and meta-analytic review. Personality and Social Psychology Review 2012;**16**:203–32.

5. **von Behr I, Reding A, Edwards C, Gribbon L.** Radicalisation in the digital era: the use of the internet in 15 cases of terrorism and extremism. Brussels: RAND; 2013.

6. **Home Office.** CONTEST, the UK's strategy for countering terrorism, Cm 9068. London: HMSO; 2018.

7. **Jasko K, LaFree G, Kruglanski A.** Quest for significance and violent extremism: the case of domestic radicalisation. Political Psychology 2016;**38**:815–31.

8. **Europol.** TESAT, European Union terrorism situation and trend report. Europol: The Hague; 2018.

9. **Sutton M.** An index of deaths from the conflict in Northern Ireland 1969–1993. Available from: https://cain.ulster.ac.uk/sutton/ [accessed 28 July 2020].

10. **Hillyard P.** Suspect community: people's experiences of the prevention of terrorism acts in Britain. London: Pluto Press; 1993.

11. **Pantazis C, Pemberton S.** From the 'Old' to the 'New' suspect community. British Journal of Criminology 2009;**49**:646–66.

12. **Walker C.** Briefing on the terrorism act 2000. Terrorism and Political Violence 2000;**12**:1–36.

13. **McCulloch J, Pickering S.** Pre-crime and counter-terrorism: imagining future crime in the 'war on terror'. British Journal of Criminology 2009;**49**:628–45.

14. **Murphy CC.** EU Counter-terrorism law, pre-emption and the rule of law. London: Hart Publishing; 2012.

15. **McCulloch J, Wilson D.** Pre-crime, pre-emption, precaution and the future. Oxford: Routledge; 2016.

16. **Palmer P.** Dealing with the exceptional: pre-crime, anti-terrorism policy and practice. Policing & Society 2012;**22**:519–37, 521–522.

17. **Anderson D.** Shielding the compass: how to fight terrorism without defeating the law. European Human Rights Law Review 2013;233:240.

18. **McCulloch J, Pickering S.** Pre-crime and counter-terrorism, Imagining future crime in the 'war on terror'. British Journal of Criminology 2009;**49**:628–45.

19. **Sentas V.** Traces of terror, counter-terrorism law, policing, and race. Oxford: Oxford University Press; 2014.

20. **Aggarwal NK.** Questioning the current public health approach to countering violent extremism. Global Public Health 2019;**14**:309–17.

21. **Qureshi A.** Fight the power: how CAGE resists from within a 'suspect community'. London: Palgrave Communications; 2017.

22. **Warsi S.** The enemy within: a tale of Muslim Britain. London: Allen Lane; 2017.

23. **Aust S.** Baader-Meinhof: the inside story of the R.A.F. Oxford: Oxford University Press; 2008.

24. **Alderdice JT.** Fundamentalism, radicalization and terrorism. Part 1: terrorism as dissolution in a complex system. Psychoanalytic Psychotherapy 2017;**31**:285–300.

25. **de Tocqueville A.** Democracy in America, Volume One. Reeve H, tr. London: Saunders and Otley; 1835.

26. **Lichtermann P.** Social capital or group style? Rescuing Tocqueville's insights on civic engagement. Theory and Society 2008;**35**:529–63, 534–36.

27. **de Tocqueville A.** Democracy in America, Volume Two. Reeve H, tr. London: Saunders and Otley; 1835.

28. **Organisation for Economic Co-operation and Development (OECD).** The well-being of nations: the role of human and social capital. Paris: OECD; 2001.

29. **Hanifan LJ.** The rural school center. Annals of the American Academy of Political and Social Science. 1916;**67**:130–8.

30. **Hawe P, Schiell A.** Social capital and health promotion: a review. Social Science and Medicine 2000;**51**:871–85.

31. **Alam Y, Husband C.** Islamophobia, community cohesion and counter-terrorism. Patterns of Prejudice 2013;**47**:235–52.

32. **Perkins DD, Hughey J, Speer PW.** Community psychology perspectives on social capital theory and community development practice. Journal of the Community Development Society 2002;**33**:33–52.

33. **McKenzie K, Whitley R, Weich S.** Social capital and mental health. British Journal of Psychiatry 2002;**181**:280–3.

34. **Hajj TE, Afifi RA, Khawaja M, Harpham T.** Violence and social capital among young men in Beirut. Injury Prevention 2011;**17**:401–6.

35. **Ilan J.** Street social capital in the liquid city: a male youth offending group on the socio-economic periphery of Dublin. Ethnography 2013;**14**:3–24.

36. **Putnam R.** Bowling alone: the collapse and revival of American community. New York: Simon and Schuster; 2000.

37. **Putnam RD.** Bowling alone: America's declining social capital. Journal of Democracy 1995;**6**:65–78.

38. **Henderson S, Whiteford H.** Social capital and mental health. Lancet 2003;**362**:505–6.

39. **Patel V.** Building social capital and improving mental health care to prevent suicide. International Journal of Epidemiology 2010;**39**:1411–12.

40. **Kennedy BP, Kawachi I, Prothrow-Stith D, Lochner K, Gupta V.** Social capital, income inequality and firearm violent crime. Social Science and Medicine 1998;**47**:7–17.

41. **Galae S, Karpati A, Kennedy B.** Social capital and violence in the United States, 1974–1993. Social Science and Medicine 2002;**55**:1373–83.

42. **Helfstein S.** Social capital and terrorism. Defence and Peace Economics 2014;**25**:363–80.

43. **Bhui K, Everitt B, Jones E.** Might depressive symptoms, poor health, and psychosocial adversity explain violent radicalization? A cross-sectional population survey of young men and women of Muslim heritage living in two English cities. PLoS One 2014;**9**:e105918, 6–7.

44. **Bhui KS, Warfa N, Jones E.** Is violent radicalisation associated with poverty, migration, poor self-reported health and common mental disorders? PLoS One 2014;**9**:e90718.

45. **Bhui K, Cruz MJ, Topciu RA, Jones E.** Identifying pathways to sympathies for violent protest and terrorism. British Journal of Psychiatry 2016;**209**:483–90.
46. **Bhui K, Otis M, Halvorsrud K, Freestone M, Jones E.** Extremism and common mental illness: a cross-sectional community survey of White British and Pakistani men and women living in England. British Journal of Psychiatry 2019, DOI: 10.1192/bjp.2019.14.
47. **Goodwin M.** The roots of extremism: the English Defence League. London: Chatham House Briefing Paper; 2013.
48. **McGhee D.** Moving to 'our' common ground—a critical examination of community cohesion discourse in twenty-first century Britain. Sociological Review 2003;**51**:376–404.
49. **Abbas M-S.** Producing 'internal suspect bodies': divisive effects of UK counter-terrorism measures on Muslim communities in Leeds and Bradford. British Journal of Sociology 2019;**70**:261–82.
50. **Radicalisation Awareness Network.** Preventing radicalisation to terrorism and violent extremism, community engagement and empowerment. Brussels: European Commission; 2019.
51. **Cherney A, Hartley J.** Community engagement to tackle terrorism and violent extremism: challenges, tensions and pitfalls. Policing and Society 2015;**27**:750–63.

Chapter 5

What attracts people to the English Defence League and who is most vulnerable to recruitment?

Alice Sibley

5.1 Introduction

From April 2017 to March 2018, 18% of 7318 individuals referred to the Prevent programme (a counterterrorism safeguarding strategy that aims to prevent people from getting involved in terrorism) were right-wing extremists. Of the 394 individuals who received support from the Channel programme (the division of the Prevent programme that identifies those that are vulnerable to recruitment into terrorism and gives them support at an early stage), 44% related to right-wing extremism concerns [1], suggesting that there is now a more serious far-right/right-wing extremist threat in the UK. The far-right has long been prevalent in British society. Historically, mergers of far-right groups have created more centralized, significant groups, including The Union Movement, The National Front, and the British National Party (BNP) [2]. Since the growth of the Internet, far-right organizations have become physically more splintered and decentralized (not controlled by a single administrative centre), possibly resulting in physical protests attracting fewer people [3]. However, this does not mean that these groups are less influential than when mergers occurred. The Internet has provided anonymity, where individuals are able to disseminate their views instantly without meeting physically [4], potentially leading to a wider far-right global network.

The English Defence League (EDL) is considered a far-right, counter-jihad movement [5]. A study found that far-right extremism is based on five principles: racism; nationalism; anti-democracy; xenophobia; and the strong state [6]. However, there are differing definitions of the far-right [7], and the individuals within far-right groups are not necessarily homogenous [5]. The term counter-jihad can be defined as a movement that is anti-Muslim/anti-Islam, xenophobic, and anti-immigration [5].

The EDL was created by merging ultra-patriotic, counter-jihadist, and football hooligan groups in the UK [8, 9], and was formed in response to an anti-soldier protest (by a banned Islamist organization called Ahlus Sunnah wal Jamaah) in 2009, during a UK soldiers' homecoming parade in Luton [9, 10]. It is a decentralized social movement and, according to its official public relations campaign, its prime objective is to advocate democracy, human rights, to counter Islamism, to defend English culture, and oppose Sharia law [11]. Fundamentally, the EDL is voicing the concerns of many ordinary British citizens [5]. However, the EDL is different from historical UK far-right organizations in that it claims to support human rights, democracy, lesbian, gay, bisexual, and transsexual (LGBT) rights, and claims not to be racist. The EDL has supported these statements with the creation of their LGBT, Hindu, Jewish, and Sikh divisions [12].

The EDL has connections with international far-right/counter-jihad groups and sees itself as an integral part of the global fight against jihad [9]. The EDL has become an inspiration for other American and European defence leagues [3]. Despite both the leader, Tommy Robinson, and deputy leader, Kevin Carroll, resigning from the EDL in October 2013 [13], regional demonstrations continued to take place under the new leader, Tim Ablitt [14].

The EDL poses new challenges to the UK government owing to its unique online structure. The organization does not have a formal membership joining procedure—they have social media supporters/sympathizers. This makes it hard to establish how many people actively support the EDL and how many are solely social media followers. In 2011, of 1295 individuals who followed the EDL Facebook page, 76% considered themselves to be EDL members [11].

It is argued that the EDL, and the far-right, may begin to pose a more serious threat to the UK. If different far-right groups begin to mobilize under the same cause, it could create a merger. In 2018, Tommy Robinson was arrested for contempt of court [15]. Different far-right groups protested his imprisonment in Leeds and London in June/July 2018 [16, 17]. Research suggests that support for the far-right is not diminishing and new far-right groups, focused on similar grievances and anti-Muslim sentiment, are taking the place of the EDL [18]. Despite Facebook banning the EDL from the social media platform in 2019 [19], the EDL has inspired new counter-jihad/far-right groups to emerge, such as Casuals United [18]. Banned terrorist groups, such as National Action, have also morphed from the BNP (a right-wing political party) and the EDL [20]. In light of the increasing far-right threat in the UK [1], the purpose of this chapter is to provide an understanding of what attracts people to the EDL and who, therefore, based on these variables, is most vulnerable to EDL recruitment.

5.2 **What concerns do supporters of the EDL have in relation to Islam/immigration, identity, and disillusionment?**

A 2011 study of 1295 EDL members found that the three main reasons people supported the EDL were: a perceived threat from Islam and immigration; to protect their cultural identity; and disillusionment with their own lives and the political ruling class [11].

In a study by YouGov (analysed by Matthew Goodwin) of 298 individuals who had heard of the EDL, only 3% stated that they agreed with the methods and values of the EDL. Forty-seven stated that they did not agree with either the methods of values of the EDL and 21% did not agree with their methods but agreed with their values [5].

5.3 **Seeing Islam and immigration as a threat**

The first main threat perceived by the EDL is fear of a foreign force, with specific emphasis on Islam. Although the EDL claims to be a counter-jihad group, research suggests that Muslim immigration generally is actually the major concern of most EDL members [11].

5.3.1 **The perceived threat from Islam**

In the 2011 study by DEMOS (n = 1295), 31% of EDL supporters stated that they joined to oppose radical Islam, but 41% stated that they joined because of their views towards Islam (which manifested in a variety of ways) [11]. Despite the official EDL leaders claiming to distinguish between Muslims and terrorists [8, 21], many leaders and EDL supporters do not separate these two groups. For example, a 2009 predicate analysis by Richardson found that out of 86 news reports posted on the official EDL website there were three main narratives relating to Islam. Firstly, all Muslims were seen by the EDL as posing a threat to British values/the British public. Secondly, the problems that were posed by Muslims were perceived to be related to the religion of Islam generally rather than an extremist interpretation of Islam. Thirdly, EDL members believe that all Muslims are responsible for Islamist terrorist attacks [21].

This fear/hatred of all Muslims by some EDL members may be explained by their concern with mass Muslim immigration and increased Muslim birth rates [5, 22]. This cultural/religious localized change (discussed later in this chapter) may lead some EDL members to feel under threat from Muslims and immigrants. Further, the media is likely to play a role in increasing fear regarding Muslims and the connection with Islamist terrorists. Liz Fekete argues that some British newspapers have been constructing an anti-Muslim narrative for over 20 years, and this dissemination of anti-Muslim sentiment has gone largely unnoticed by experts [23].

The threat of Islam is also heightened through conspiracy theories. A conspiracy theory can be defined as the belief in a false malevolent plot by a group of individuals conspiring together [24]. Conspiracy theories are prevalent in the EDL [3, 9]. According to Hsiao-Hung Pai [25], Tommy Robinson (when talking about the sexual exploitation of young non-Muslim girls) stated '95% of convictions for grooming are Muslims—that's a fact ... It is a Muslim problem' (p. 54). This information is incorrect. In 2012, the Children's Commissioner for England report suggests that perpetrators that come from countries where there is a Muslim majority account for only a minority of child sexual perpetrators in the UK. These figures are only taken from those individuals that disclosed their ethnicity [26]. According to Bartlett and Miller [27], conspiracy theories (such as the notion that Islam encourages the sexual exploitation of young non-Muslim girls [5]) in contexts of extremism can act as a 'radicalizing multiplier', which increases the extremity of group views/behaviour, potentially leading to the justification of violence (p. 4). A YouGov study found that 38% of 298 EDL sympathizers justified violence against extremists, and 72% thought that violence between ethnic/religious groups was inevitable [5].

5.3.2 The perceived threat from immigration

Immigration is a key motivator for EDL recruitment [11]. Therefore, it is important to look at specific geographical locations, such as Luton, where the EDL is most prevalent. The EDL was created in Luton and the ex-leader, Tommy Robinson, and ex-deputy leader, Kevin Carrol, are both from Luton [8, 28, 29]. Owing to the changing cultural and religious make-up of Luton, there have been religious and ethnic tensions [8]. The EDL was borne out of these tensions and it is therefore of interest to look at the ethnic/religious change that occurred from 2001 to 2011.

Research suggests that EDL members are especially suspicious of Asian Muslims [3]. Luton has a high percentage of Muslims. According to Luton Borough Council [30], in 2001, of 204,700 residents, 14.6% were Muslim and in areas such as Dallow (n = 13,154), the Muslim population exceeded the Christian population (51.3% Muslim vs 30.9% Christian) [30]. Further, there was an 85.4% increase from 2001 to 2011 in the Muslim population in Luton, and a 12.5% decrease in the Christian population [31]. Along with the trends in religious representations, immigration levels have been high. In 2001 (n = 204,700), the population of Luton was 65% White British and 18.3% Asian or Asian British [30]. By 2011, 55% were White British and 30% were Asian [31]. These statistics suggest that a sudden localized cultural/religious change occurred in Luton, which may help to explain why some EDL members see Islam and immigration as a threat.

5.4 The perceived threat of loss of identity

The second variable that may attract people to the EDL is the perceived threat to their identity [11]. The central characteristic of far-right extremism is ethnicnationalism, borne from a fear of foreigners [32]. The EDL assumes that immigrants, specifically Muslims, are a threat to its national identity and existence [11, 32]. In the 2011 DEMOS study, 31% of 1295 EDL responders stated that identity-related issues were the reason they joined the EDL [11].

A sense of belonging is important for both physical and mental health. Humans are social creatures who need to feel part of a community [33]. Without a sense of belonging, people can become isolated, leading to mental health issues such as depression [34]. The EDL capitalizes on this need for belonging through a sense of national belonging [35]. For example, group bonding behaviours can be seen during a Leeds EDL protest where the crowd jump and chant 'E, E, EDL' in unison (00:00:30) [36], thereby increasing the coherence of the group. This sense of belonging can also be heightened through a call to war. Certain EDL members believe that an 'Islamic war' has already been declared against the West [8, p. 9]. In addition, some EDL members believe that there is an Islamization conspiracy whereby Muslims, and their allies, are attempting to make Islam the supreme religion in Europe through whatever means they deem necessary [3]. This conspiracy theory furthers the perceived need for war with Islam in the UK.

5.5 Disillusionment with political parties and everyday life

The feeling of disillusionment with their own lives, and the political parties who are supposed to represent them, is the third main reason that people join the EDL [11].

5.5.1 Lack of identification with political parties

Tore Bjørgo [32] states that identification with a legitimate political party is important in feeling that one has a voice. If an individual feels no affiliation to a political party they may feel more inclined to voice their opinions through alternative channels, including far-right extremist channels [32]. The EDL is anti-establishment and believes that modern political parties do not represent ordinary citizens [37]. According to DEMOS (n = 1295), 88% of EDL members said that they do not trust the government versus the national average of 68%, and 21% of respondents 'agreed entirely' that it does not matter who you vote for [11].

5.5.2 The relationship between economic difficulty and the EDL

Economic difficulty and inequality has also been shown to be a factor that attracts people to the EDL [38]. It was reported in 2013 that out of 215 people who donated money to the EDL, 68% came from a UK city/town/village where unemployment was above the national median and 23% lived in areas where jobless rates were among the worst 10% in Wales and England [39]. An example of the relationship between economic difficulty and EDL recruitment is Luton. Luton used to have productive factories and related job opportunities. In 1997, 32% of Luton's economic growth came from manufacturing, but by 2015 this had decreased to 20% [40]. From 2009 to 2012, Luton's gross value (a measure of economic activity produced by the Office of National Statistics) added per head decreased. This was around the same time that the EDL was formed, suggesting that there may be a correlational relationship between economic decline and the rise of the EDL [40].

5.6 Who is most vulnerable to recruitment into the EDL?

At the height of its power in 2011, the EDL had a Facebook membership/following of 85,000 [12]. The EDL has been effective in recruiting individuals who would not historically have been associated with far-right groups [8], and EDL supporters are diverse [5, 11]. Therefore, it is likely that a combination of variables influence an individual to support the EDL.

5.7 Demographics

5.7.1 Gender as a vulnerability factor

Gender plays a significant role in the EDL [25]. Of 85,000 EDL Facebook members, only 1914 were in the Women's Division [12]. In another study, 81% of 1295 Facebook EDL members were male [11]. Therefore, men appear to be the most vulnerable to EDL recruitment. There is a correlation between men and violence [41] and violence is more likely to occur in the presence of other men [42]. Statistics from 2016 suggest that 76% of all violent crimes were committed by men and 42% were committed by people between 25 and 39 years of age [43]. Therefore, for some young men, EDL demonstrations may provide an outlet to express aggression/violence [44]. Despite the EDL claiming that they protest peacefully, nearly all of their protests/marches end in violence [22, 28, 45]. Further, 38% of EDL supporters were more likely than the general public (21%) to believe that violence was justifiable when countering the threat of extremism, and 72% responded that they thought a 'clash of civilizations' was inevitable [5].

5.7.2 Age as a vulnerability factor: 18–29 year olds

Three main pieces of research suggest that the majority of EDL members are under 30 years of age (range 18–29 years) [9, 11, 46]. Based on EDL Facebook data (n = 38,200), DEMOS found that 72% were under the age of 30 years, with 36% of supporters being between 16 and 20 years of age [11]. One factor that may be causing this vulnerability is anxiety-related employment prospects, making both school leavers and university graduates vulnerable [47, 48]. As the EDL typically recruits members through social media, especially Facebook [9, 12], age is an important factor when considering who is most vulnerable to recruitment. Statistics from 2017 suggest that 18–24 year olds are the most active users of Facebook [49]. This may explain why the majority of EDL supporters are between 16 and 20 years of age, according to Bartlett and Littler [11].

5.7.3 Age as a vulnerability factor: 30+ year olds

Research relating to the most common age group for EDL sympathizers is contradictory. Goodwin (n = 298) found that 83% of EDL members were over the age of 30 years [5]. Individuals over the age of 30 years are more likely to read traditional newspapers [50]. Tommy Robinson [8] suggests that people have been encouraged to join the EDL through tabloid newspapers such as the *Daily Star*. Sixty-five per cent (n = 298) of EDL supporters read tabloid newspapers [5], such as the *Sun*, *Sunday Express*, and the *Daily Mirror*, which disseminate anti-immigration/anti-Muslim messages in simplistic, inflammatory language [51]. Therefore, individuals who read tabloid newspapers may be vulnerable to EDL recruitment.

5.8 Identity and disillusionment as a vulnerability factor

The loss of identity and the feeling of disillusionment may also make people more likely to join the EDL. According to Goodwin (n = 298), 52% of EDL supporters claimed that increased Muslim birth rates were a threat to their national identity [5]. There may be an attempt to reclaim this sense of identity through a feeling of belonging and group bonding. This sense of belonging is a key influencer in online EDL activism and at physical rallies [11]. Disillusionment among EDL members is also a contributing vulnerability factor to EDL recruitment. The majority of respondents appeared to be pessimistic about the future of their lives and the UK [11]. Research suggests that 88% of EDL members do not trust the government, 85% do not trust political parties, 85% do not trust the European Union, and 62% were totally dissatisfied with democracy in the UK [5, 11].

5.8.1 Economic situation as a vulnerability factor: education and unemployment

The education level and economic situation of an individual may make them vulnerable to EDL recruitment. Of 804 EDL supporters, 55% stated that school qualifications (GCSEs or A Levels) were their highest qualification [11]. In another study (n = 298), 39% of EDL supporters claimed that GCSEs were their highest academic qualification [5]. In addition, the belief in conspiracy theories may attract people to the EDL [3, 9]. There is a correlation between non-analytical thinkers and the belief in conspiracy theories. Individuals that displayed analytical thinking were less likely to believe in conspiracy theories [52], potentially making less educated people more vulnerable to recruitment. Individuals with lower education levels may be more likely to believe in conspiracy theories than individuals with university-level degrees. This may be owing to the assumption that there is a simple solution and the analytical skills that are developed at higher educational levels [53]. However, a contradictory study by Goodwin (n = 298) found that only 9% of EDL members had no qualifications, which calls into question the stereotype that EDL supporters are less well educated [5].

There is contradictory evidence regarding the role of unemployment and EDL recruitment. Goodwin found that only 3% of 298 EDL sympathizers were unemployed, which was lower than the full-sample (non-EDL supporters) unemployment rate (4%) [5]. However, according to Bartlett and Littler [11], unemployment is a key characteristic of EDL members. Their study (n = 804) found that 28% of EDL members aged 16–24 years were unemployed versus the national average of 20% [11]. Further, 28% of 25–64 year olds were unemployed versus the national average of 6% [11]. Therefore, according to Bartlett and Littler, unemployment may lead to EDL recruitment.

5.9 **Conclusion**

This chapter has attempted to outline what attracts people to the EDL and who is most vulnerable to recruitment. It found that only 3% agreed with both the values and methods of the EDL and that there are different factors that may influence people to join the group. EDL supporters often do not distinguish between Muslims and Islamist terrorists, increasing the perceived threat from Islam generally, which is exacerbated by the groups' belief in conspiracy theories. This perceived fear of Islam/immigration may lead some people to believe that their identity is under threat, which may then lead to disillusionment with both their own lives and the political elite. Some members of the EDL feel no affiliation with any political parties and are struggling economically through unemployment. These issues are likely to attract some individuals to the EDL.

As there are different factors that attract people to the EDL, some individuals are more vulnerable to EDL recruitment than others. Research suggests that a man under 30 years of age, living in an impoverished area with little economic growth is most vulnerable to EDL recruitment. Variables such as a feeling of loss of identity, pessimism about the future, and disillusionment with political parties may increase vulnerability to recruitment. The vulnerable male is likely to have a low level of education, believe in conspiracy theories, and be from an area where there has been a quick and extreme shift in the cultural make-up through mass immigration (especially relating to the Muslim population). It is likely that vulnerability to EDL recruitment is influenced by a combination of these factors and, therefore, a large proportion of the British public could potentially be vulnerable to recruitment into the EDL.

References

1. Home Office. Individuals referred to and supported through the *Prevent* Programme, April 2017 to March 2018. Available from: https://assets.publishing.service.gov.uk/government/uploads/system/uploads/attachment_data/file/763254/individuals-referred-supported-prevent-programme-apr2017-mar2018-hosb3118.pdf [accessed 7 July 2019].
2. **Lowles N.** State of hate: far right terrorism on the rise. Available from: https://www.hopenothate.org.uk/wp-content/uploads/2018/03/State-of-Hate-2018.pdf [accessed 3 August 2018].
3. **Meleagrou-Hitchens A, Brun H.** A neo-nationalist network: the English Defence League and Europe's counter-Jihad movement. Available from: https://icsr.info/wp-content/uploads/2013/03/ICSR-ECJM-Report_Online.pdf [accessed 12 July 2018].
4. **Davenport D.** Anonymity on the Internet: why the price may be too high. Communications of the ACM 2002;**45**:33–5.

5. **Goodwin M.** The roots of extremism: the English Defence League and the counter-jihad challenge. Available from: https://www.chathamhouse.org/sites/default/files/public/Research/Europe/0313bp_goodwin.pdf [accessed 2 March 2018].

6. **Mudde C.** Right-wing extremism analyzed: a comparative analysis of the ideologies of three alleged right-wing extremist parties (NPD, NDP, CP'86). European Journal of Political Research 1995;**27**:203–24.

7. **Rydgren J.** The sociology of the radical right. Annual Review of Sociology 2007;**33**:241–62.

8. **Robinson T.** Enemy of the state. Batley: Press News Limited; 2015.

9. **Copsey N.** The English Defence League: challenging our country and our values of social inclusion, fairness and equality. London: Faith Matters; 2010.

10. **Jackson P, Feldman M.** The EDL: Britain's 'new far right' social movement. Northampton: The University of Northampton; 2011.

11. **Bartlett J, Littler M.** Inside the EDL populist politics in a digital age. Available from: https://www.demos.co.uk/files/Inside_the_edl_WEB.pdf [accessed 22 June 2018].

12. **Allen C.** Opposing Islamification or promoting Islamophobia? Understanding the English defence league. Patterns of Prejudice 2011;**45**:279–94.

13. **Siddique H, Quinn B.** EDL: Tommy Robinson and deputy Kevin Carroll quit far-right group. The Guardian. Available from: https://www.theguardian.com/uk-news/2013/oct/08/tommy-robinson-english-defence-league [accessed 14 August 2019].

14. **English Defence League.** The English Defence League. Available from: https://www.thesun.co.uk/news/11856150/what-is-the-edl/ [accessed 14 July 2018].

15. **Perraudin F.** EDL founder Tommy Robinson jailed for contempt of court. The Guardian. Available from: https://www.theguardian.com/uk-news/2018/may/29/edl-founder-tommy-robinson-jailed-13-months [accessed 29 May 2018].

16. **Johnston, C.** Union leader attacked after counter-protest to Tommy Robinson rally. The Guardian. Available from: https://www.theguardian.com/us-news/2018/jul/14/police-tell-trump-supporters-not-to-gather-at-us-embassy [accessed 18 July 2018].

17. **Daily Express.** Tommy Robinson protest: hundreds march in Leeds for jailed ex-EDL leader. The Express. Available from: https://www.express.co.uk/news/uk/968429/tommy-robinson-protest-edl-leader-jailed-leeds [accessed 14 July 2018].

18. **Alessio D, Meredith K.** Blackshirts for the twenty-first century? Fascism and the English Defence League. Social Identities 2014;**20**:104–18.

19. **Hern A.** Facebook bans far-right groups including BNP, EDL and Britain First. The Guardian Available from: https://www.theguardian.com/technology/2019/apr/18/facebook-bans-far-right-groups-including-bnp-edl-and-britain-first [accessed 12 August 2019].

20. **Collins M.** The collapse of the BNP and EDL has made the far right deadlier. The Guardian. Available from: https://www.theguardian.com/commentisfree/2018/mar/02/collapse-bnp-edl-far-right-terrorists [accessed 2 March 2018].

21. **Kassimeris G, Jackson L.** The ideology and discourse of the English Defence League: "Not racist, not violent, just no longer silent." The British Journal of Politics and International Relations 2015;**17**:171–88.

22. **Busher J.** Grassroots activism in the English Defence League: discourse and public (dis) order. In: **Taylor M, Currie DH**, eds. Extreme right-wing political violence and terrorism. London: Bloomsbury; 2013, pp. 65–83

23. **Fekete L.** The Muslim conspiracy theory and the Oslo massacre. Race & Class 2012;**53**:30–47.

24. **Bale JM.** Political paranoia v. political realism: on distinguishing between bogus conspiracy theories and genuine conspiratorial politics. Patterns of Prejudice 2007;**41**:45–60.

25. **Pai HH.** Angry white people: coming face-to-face with the British far right. London: Zed Books Ltd; 2016.

26. **Children's Commissioner.** "I thought I was the only one. The online one in the world". Available from: https://static.lgfl.net/LgflNet/downloads/online-safety/LGfL-OS-Research-Archive-2012-Childrens-Commissioner-CSE.pdf [accessed 8 July 2018].

27. **Bartlett J, Miller C.** The power of unreason: conspiracy theories, extremism and counter-terrorism. Available from: https://www.demos.co.uk/files/Conspiracy_theories_paper.pdf?1282913891 [accessed 3 June 2018].

28. **Treadwell J, Garland J.** Masculinity, marginalization and violence: a case study of the English Defence League. The British Journal of Criminology 2011;**51**:621–34.

29. **Falkiner D.** London School of Economics: Book review: enemy of the state by Tommy Robinson. Available from https://blogs.lse.ac.uk/lsereviewofbooks/2016/03/02/book-review-enemy-of-the-state-by-tommy-robinson/ [accessed 11 July 2019].

30. **Luton Borough Council.** Demography and ethnicity analysis of 2001 census data for Luton and East of England region. Available from: https://www.luton.gov.uk/Environment/Lists/LutonDocuments/PDF/Planning/Census/Demography%20and%20Ethnicity.pdf [accessed 23 June 2018].

31. **Luton Borough Council.** Luton Borough profile. Available from: https://www.luton.gov.uk/Environment/Lists/LutonDocuments/PDF/Planning/Census/2011%20census%20data/LUTON%20BOROUGH%20PROFILE.pdf [accessed 23 June 2018].

32. **Bjørgo T.** Root causes of terrorism: myths, reality and ways forward. Abingdon: Routledge; 2004.

33. **Flynn CP.** Social creatures: a human and animal studies reader. New York: Lantern Books; 2008.

34. **Kawachi I, Berkman LF.** Social ties and mental health. Journal of Urban Health 2001;**78**:458–67.

35. **Pilkington H.** Loud and proud: passion and politics in the English Defence League. Manchester: Manchester University Press; 2016.

36. **UniteNationale.** EDL LEEDS—against government terrorist and Islamists. Available from: https://www.youtube.com/watch?v=4wkhvIgXzSI&frags=pl%2Cwn [accessed 17 August 2018].

37. **Oaten A.** The cult of the victim: an analysis of the collective identity of the English Defence League. Patterns of Prejudice 2014;**48**:331–49.

38. **Treadwell J.** White Riot: the English Defence League and the 2011 English riots: James Treadwell looks at the public order threat presented by the Far Right and at what fuels disorder. Criminal Justice Matters 2012;**87**:36–7.

39. **Burn-Murdoch J.** What type of place do EDL donors come from? The Guardian. Available from: https://www.theguardian.com/news/datablog/2013/may/31/english-defence-league-edl-white-extremism [accessed 31 May 2018].

40. **Luton Borough Council.** Business intelligence. Available from: https://www.luton.gov.uk/Community_and_living/Lists/LutonDocuments/PDF/Luton%20Gross%20Value%20Added.pdf [accessed 25 June 2018].

41. **Ellis A.** Men, masculinities and violence: an ethnographic study. London: Routledge; 2015.

42. **Hall S.** Daubing the drudges of fury: men, violence and the piety of the 'hegemonic masculinity' thesis. Theoretical Criminology 2002;6:35–61.

43. **Office for National Statistics.** Overview of violent crime and sexual offences. Available from: https://www.ons.gov.uk/peoplepopulationandcommunity/crimeandjustice/compendium/focusonviolentcrimeandsexualoffences/yearendingmarch2016/overviewofviolentcrimeandsexualoffences#profile-of-perpetrators-involved-in-violent-crimes [accessed 22 June 2018].

44. **Lambert R.** Anti-Muslim violence in the UK: extremist nationalist involvement and influence. In: **Taylor M, Currie DH,** eds. Extreme right-wing political violence and terrorism. London: Bloomsbury; 2013, pp. 31–63.

45. **Garland J, Treadwell J.** 'No surrender to the Taliban!' Football hooliganism, Islamophobia and the rise of the English Defence League. Annual British Society of Criminology Conference. Human Rights, Human Wrongs: Dilemmas and Diversity in Criminology, 11 July 2010–14 July 2010, University of Leicester, Leicester; 2010.

46. **Gaston S.** Far-right extremism in the populist age. Available from: https://www.demos.co.uk/wp-content/uploads/2017/06/Demos-Briefing-Paper-Far-Right-Extremism-2017.pdf [accessed 22 March 2018].

47. **Stevkovski L.** The rise of right-wing extremism in European Union. Interdisciplinary Political and Cultural Journal 2015;17:43–57.

48. **Howker E, Malik S.** Jilted generation: how Britain has bankrupted its youth. London: Icon Books; 2013.

49. **Statista.** Facebook penetration among internet users in the United Kingdom from 2017, by age group. Available from: https://www.statista.com/statistics/271304/facebook-user-penetration-in-the-united-kingdom-uk-by-age/ [accessed 21 July 2018].

50. **Statista.** Newspapers: weekly household expenditure in the United Kingdom 2019. Available from: https://www.statista.com/statistics/285720/newspapers-weekly-household-expenditure-in-the-united-kingdom-uk-by-age/ [accessed 4 July 2019].

51. **Moore K, Mason P, Lewis JM.** Images of Islam in the UK: the representation of British Muslims in the national print news media 2000–2008. Available from: http://orca.cf.ac.uk/53005/ [accessed 28 July 2020].

52. **Swami V, Voracek M, Stieger S, Tran US, Furnham A.** Analytic thinking reduces belief in conspiracy theories. Cognition 2014;133:572–85.

53. **van Prooijen JW.** Why education predicts decreased belief in conspiracy theories. Applied Cognitive Psychology 2017;31:50–8.

Chapter 6

The sharing economy and livestreaming of terror: Co-production of terrorism on social media

Yasmin Ibrahim

6.1 Introduction

Today, the circulation of images of terror happens within a sharing economy through social media sites with the notion of human sociality underpinned through audiences relentlessly transacting content through networks. With audiences engaging with social networking sites by constantly sharing messages, reposting, tagging, and re-tweeting, the Internet reiterates the human presence and reciprocity through notions of sociality and exchange online. Within this ambit of human communion and exchange, difficult ethical and moral challenges emerge, particularly with images of violence and terror and how these may be re-mediated through networked communities where content is offered through one's identity in a network and perhaps a sense of belonging to it. This sharing economy is vital for platform capital such as Facebook and Twitter, which thrive by leveraging and monetizing on traffic that is generated on these sites. The distinct dimension of this sharing economy is the role of the human as transmitting messages in this assemblage while coalescing with the machine logic of data capture, profile creation, and commercial data mining. Humans as active agents of traffic and data generation are intrinsically implicated in this economy.

This chapter examines the co-production of terror in the sharing economy and the affordances of new convergent low-cost technologies enabling the broadcasting of terror in real time. Livestreaming as a facility on social media platforms, inviting creators to connect and upload in real time, opens up new ethical frames of enquiry into our modes of consumption of violent images and, more importantly, it also scrutinizes the ways in which real-time terror can be communicated through the vantage point of the perpetrator and its viral duplication through humans as consumers and co-creators. This form of livestreamed 'reality TV' of gratuitous violence raises governance issues in the circulation of terrorist acts when the ability to stop real-time broadcasts, alert mechanisms on social media platforms, and the ability to restrain repostings by online users may be limited despite the proliferation of sophisticated features on social media platforms. This chapter examines these emergent governance and ethical issues through the case study of the New Zealand massacre in a mosque in Christchurch in 2019. This attack was filmed with a GoPro camera and the violence of the xenophobic attack was broadcast live with audiences online commenting and reposting in real time. Originally designed for participants in extreme sports, technologies such as the GoPro enable individuals to film and broadcast from their vantage point. Its appropriation for acts of terrorism renews our anxieties about human trauma and suffering becoming mass entertainment for online communities.

6.2 **Livestreaming of terror**

With intense convergence of technologies we can capture and publish materials on the move through our smartphones. Smartphones, with increasingly new innovative functions and powerful processing capabilities, are portable recording and imaging devices that can connect to high-speed data networks producing an opportunity for people to communicate with large audiences in real time. As such, recording facilities on mobile devices can not only negotiate space, but also time through live broadcasting, creating an immediacy of connection with audiences. The integration of broadcasting, publishing, and livestreaming features on smartphones and mobile devices, and the availability of such features on social networking platforms, enable a sharing economy. The proliferation of user-generated content (UGC) means that we can constantly transact ourselves and environments as content [1].

This seamless integration of our immediate environments with familiar networks and unknown audiences imbues lay people equipped with smart mobile technologies with immense opportunities to not only create social content for sustaining interpersonal relationships, but also to negotiate political events. It is well documented that smartphones and mobile technologies have played a crucial role in disaster and conflict events and in conveying news from the ground, particularly from remote and inaccessible sites to the wider world [2–4]. The convergence of technologies has also recalibrated audiences as creators and producers of content as opposed to just receivers or as part of the consuming public. This is integral to the sharing economy where co-creation and UGC premise on an interactive environment of online content acquiring value through audience comments and endorsements and the ability to go 'viral'.

The ability to broadcast live is also about the remediation of space and temporality through new media technologies, enabling audiences to consume events in real time and in different time zones in distant parts of the world. As such, convergence has produced the screen as a site of new forms of communion and consuming communities and for shared interests. This has invariably raised concerns that the Internet can harbour echo chambers where resonant sentiments and viewpoints can reverberate in niches, as well as among extremist communities seeking to sustain their extremist views online. Livestreaming is becoming increasingly popular with the availability of this feature on apps and platforms such as Instagram Live, Facebook Live, Periscope, Twitch, and YouTube Live. The ability to interact and comment in real time is seen as ever more important for vloggers and celebrities to create an emotional connection with friends, fans, and the general public. Beyond the convening of networks based on shared interest or variants of belonging, social media has been recognized as a space offering the disillusioned, alienated, or the disenfranchised a means to gather and make connections, and for these very reasons it has been used to recruit and radicalize members into ideological agendas [5]. Social media platform like Twitter, through resonant hashtags, also bind networked communities with the political, entwining politics and social events with networks of social relations online.

The ability to broadcast events in real time can be viewed as empowering for citizens and societies in conflict and disaster zones or in a wider quest for social justice. In more quotidian terms, it provides a platform to sustain relationships and everyday interactions. The livestreaming of content is also perceived as offering immense potential for commercial organizations in terms of marketing, public relations, and advertising. On the flip side, the non-stop publishing of content by lay audiences has posed numerous challenges due to the lack of gatekeeping and the appropriation of such technologies for propaganda by terrorist organizations and recruitment by radical, alt-right, and extremist groups. Equally, fake news and half-truths circulated through networks and niche communities can be threats to stable polities. The different phenomena such as the circulation of fake news, gratuitous violence, and the lack of gatekeeping are seen as posing threats to young and vulnerable people, turning the attention back on the governance regimes of digital platforms. The content governance policies of data empires such as Google and Facebook remain areas of renewed scrutiny and concern worldwide, and, equally, the threats these pose to countries and vulnerable populations in their ability to control, order, and manipulate information.

Beyond the growing power of data empires, convergent technologies, their affordability, and the hunger for UGC on image- and video-sharing sites, have enabled terrorist organizations to cross into social networking sites, co-mingling terrorist propaganda and mainstream entertainment. The deployment of convergent mobile technologies by terrorist organizations has been well documented [5–8]. Jason Burke [9] observes that the

> combination of digital cameras, cheap laptops and editing software, and social media has been systematically and massively exploited by the Islamic State (IS) and its sympathizers and to particularly enable small scale attacks by individuals or groups. Their strategy to exploit the capabilities of new technologies to disseminate content on social media has provided an alternative to costly, complex, spectacular attacks that were once the only way terrorists could achieve their messaging aims. The employment of these media tools by IS sympathizers in France and Germany for a series of attacks and attempted attacks has worked to IS's agenda of retaining its terrorist agenda in the headlines despite the declining prowess of the organization.

These media tools have also been appropriated by its various affiliated organizations, such as Boko Haram in Nigeria, and by competing groups in the areas they control [9]. New technologies such as Telegram (an encrypted messaging platform) have become powerful operation tools for organizations like Islamic State (IS) to coordinate, strategize, and publicize attacks, out-doing Al-Qaeda in its endeavour to grab attention with its beheading videos and Hollywood-style productions uploaded from bombed-out cities in Syria [10]. Telegram is a combination of Snapchat and WhatsApp, and it emphasizes security and features a 'secret chat' functionality allowing users to exchange secure messages, as well as to activate a 'self-destruct' timer to delete messages [11]. In view of this, in 2019 the European Union Agency for Law Enforcement Cooperation (Europol) and Telegram acted in concert to delete thousands of IS-related media accounts on the platform. This unexpected purge saw accounts migrating to another site called Riot [10]. As such, ephemerality and security through encrypted messaging have been utilized by terrorist groups to plan and coordinate their activities without leaving explicit, quickly traceable communication trails.

Livestreaming apps are not just exploited by organizations, but also individuals. A French woman used Periscope to film her own suicide [12], while a teenager was jailed for livestreaming the rape of 17-year-old online [13]. In 2015, during a live broadcast, a journalist and a cameraman were shot dead. The killer had used a GoPro camera, forwarded a 23-page manifesto to the ABC news station, and posted a video of the attack on social media [14]. The manifesto revealed that the killings were in retaliation for racial discrimination, particularly triggered by the massacre of nine black churchgoers in Charleston, South Carolina.

In a similar vein, in Christchurch, New Zealand, during Friday prayer, 51 worshippers were massacred at a mosque in March 2019 by a perpetrator who livestreamed the attack, allegedly motivated by white nationalist ideology. The attack was broadcast live on popular video-sharing platforms such as YouTube and Facebook, and on right-wing online forums. The perpetrator had been known to be active in online forums promoting a manifesto outlining his white supremacist worldview. The massacre was seen as a long history of Islamophobic and anti-Semitic attacks in the United States, France, Norway, and Germany.

The livestreaming of terror and violence is not without precedent. Burke [9], using the term 'selfie jihad', refers to the Magnanville terrorist attack in France in 2016 in which a jihadi murdered two police officers in their home and livestreamed the aftermath of the attacks. In this instance, the attacker used Facebook's livestream feature. Livestreaming has also been used in other contexts of violent confrontation. For example, militias on the US–Mexico border incorporate livestreaming into their activities to showcase their confrontations with migrants and refugees, providing a reality TV of violence as entertainment [15].

6.3 **Violence and the 'sharing economy' online**

In the digital age, violence and terror imagery resides within a 'sharing economy'. This sharing economy leverages on users as conveyors and co-creators of content through a networked architecture. In this networked economy an individual's social capital resides in the act of sharing and the expanse of their social networks and connections. Content that piques the interest of the individual and the attendant community is shared, reposted, and attention is gained through the platforms in which content is shared through commentary, emoticons, or endorsements such as 'likes'. As such, the sharing economy equally valorizes the notion of co-creation. The sharing economy is premised through a network of sociality, reciprocity, and the notion of exchange of information as not only a form of online presence, but also social capital [1]. The individual is validated through a community's endorsement and repostings, likes, being pinned, tagged, or being retweeted representing individual and collective engagement with content. Content that flows through these networks is, as such, not static in form with the possibility of acquiring additional material and value through exchange and flows.

The sharing economy of the Internet harbours within it not only the potential for posts and newsfeeds to go viral, but its significance also lies in the trust and proximity to the source that networks can engender. The issue of trust and proximity to the sharing individual may also mediate one's engagement and trust with the content. As such, niche communities with shared interests on platforms can become echo chambers, selecting and distributing news that a community is inclined to endorse and distribute in resonating the sentiments of the community. The sharing economy is an immanent aspect of platform capitalism where sharing sustains networks enabling machines to learn patterns of consumer behaviour, algorithms to push popular content, and the commercial mining of data profiles.

The sharing community, with its stress on sociality and reciprocity, masks the wider primacy of capital where the emotional labour of users not only feeds into content creation, but also the ability to commercialize and leverage on human traffic on different platforms. As such, the idea of sharing takes primacy over veracity. Data giants and platform capitalism exploit virality, or the accumulation of user traffic enabled through 'trending' topics and in designing algorithms to push content that is popular rather than ensuring editorial standards or in weeding out fake news. In addition, as the two-step flow communication theory attests, interpersonal communication can be more influential than that of the media, which then reiterates the role of individuals as opinion leaders and equally networks in how audiences may consume or interpret content [16]. Personal influence, according to this theoretical perspective, can reinforce information from the media and, in applying it to social networks, the remediation of news or content through these can mean news can be received and valued differentially particularly if it accrues from influencers or tight networks where the trust and authority of users is valued.

The sharing economy, with relevance to violent images or terror events, produces more challenges in the age of platform capitalism. Sharing news or outing information fresh from different sources can be seen as social capital, and the sharing economy can keep information or content in circulation through the acts of reposting, re-uploading through different tags, and in binding different sites and communities through signposting of information across sites. Different norms may apply on these sites with regard to violent imagery or terror events, and in niche or alt-right forums gratuitous violence against targeted groups can be endorsed and validated by people with shared extremist views. The sharing economy is made for expanding capital's acquisition of new users, data extraction and leveraging on viral content, and, as such, is not completely attuned to the abuses that can accrue through the sharing of livestreamed violence, as in the case of the NZ massacre. What is worth noting here is that this sharing economy extends the co-production of violence where networks become active in distributing these images and adding commentary to them. The sharing economy, with its emphasis on co-creation, abstracts violence as a form of commodity for exchange where value can accrue from such exchanges for platform capitalism.

In the New Zealand attack the massacre was designed through the theatre of social media and the sharing economy, specifically drawing on its capacity to keep contentious content floating ad infinitum online. It was reported that prior to the mosque massacre the perpetrator had logged onto 8chan, a forum popular with the extreme right. His post read:

> Well lads, it's time to stop shitposting and time to make a real life effort post. I will carry out and [sic] attack against the invaders, and will even live stream the attack via facebook [sic]. By the time you read this I should be going live. I have provided links to my writings below, please do your part spreading my message, making memes and shitposting as you usually do. If I don't survive the attack, goodbye, godbless [sic] and I will see you all in Valhalla! [17]

The links to his writing included a 74-page manifesto setting out his ideology, rationale, and justification for the impending tragedy. A copy of the manifesto was also sent to approximately 70 media outlets. The attack itself had been filmed live through a helmet-mounted GoPro camera and livestreamed online, with the first user report logged 29 minutes after the video started, and 12 minutes after the live broadcast ended. With the video going viral, it was viewed at least 4000 times before Facebook removed it from its site [18].

A whole ecology of platforms became a spectre for this terror in the sharing economy where the intention of the attack was announced on 8chan, livestreamed on Facebook, reposted on YouTube and other sites such as Reddit, and was leaked across multiple sites before data platforms could prohibit its use. According to Facebook, no one reported the video during the live broadcast and it was viewed fewer than 200 times during the live broadcast and about 4000 times after before it was removed from the site [18]. Similarly, other sharing platforms such as YouTube were challenged by this terror event as users sought to circumnavigate the platform's detection system by repackaging and retitling the videos. In fact, more than 800 visually distinct versions of the video were uploaded to YouTube at a rate of one per second in the hours immediately after the shootings [19]. Google sought to discourage the circulation of the video by temporarily disabling several search functions, an unprecedented move for the organization. On '8chan the perpetrator was hailed as a hero who had fought invaders and as a fighter for the extreme right' and users were actively engaged in reposting links to his manifesto and the full-length video of the massacre [20].

The emergence of radical Internet extremism on platforms such as 8chan reasserts the digital era as a space for extremist views and for radicalization. The alt-right 8chan has emerged as a 'go-to resource for violent extremists' and in 2019 alone three mass shootings, including Christchurch and the synagogue shooting in Polway, California, were announced on 8chan in advance, often accompanied by racist writings that seem to be premeditated to go viral on the Internet [18]. Promoted as a free-speech subsidiary to its sister site 4chan, 8chan as an image-based forum is known for its light-touch content moderation and lax restrictions under the ambit of fostering free speech [21]. Such alt-right sites, through the provision of anonymity, use extreme speech and violent language to incite others as a form of hate against liberal politics and become an active site for the accumulation, development, and circulation of extremist views [22].

What is worth noting is that Facebook revealed that 'in the first 24 hours, it removed more than 1.2 million videos of the attack at upload, which were therefore prevented from being seen on its services and an additional 300,000 or so copies were removed after they were posted' [18]. This meant that the video had spread rapidly online and the lack of editorial gatekeeping by human editors meant that it was left to users raising alerts on their system. In this instance, Facebook's explanation was its automatic artificial intelligence (AI) detection system had failed to distinguish between real and visually similar video games, with the organization acknowledging that the immediacy of Facebook Live brings unique challenges [23–25].

The slippages between real and simulated images online bring into sharp focus the promiscuous bind between the two, particularly in the case of the New Zealand attacks. The architecture of the Internet enables simulated environments such as gaming platforms to recreate political events or to re-invent these for digital games, reiterating new forms of victimization of targeted communities online, blurring the lines between the real and the simulated. In direct reference to the New Zealand attacks, the killer was addicted to digital games and his manifesto made references to his favourite games as in-jokes. The New Zealand killer also made references to 'PewDiePie', which is a reference to Felix Kjellberg, a highly popular online gaming personality from Sweden whose YouTube channel has nearly 97 million subscribers [26]. The coalescing of real events with the mimetic violence of video games (and vice versa) and the abject fascination with a reality TV culture redirect the gaze through the vantage point of the perpetrator with livestreaming [27]. If the digital economy can accord terrorists any prowess it is in the ways in which they are exploiting new media technologies and audiences with an insatiable appetite for the unexpected. The visual culture of the Internet embeds the notion of watching and consuming snippets of videos without context, and the notion of instant gratification lies in not only watching, but also in sharing what you have consumed with friends and strangers, or in viewing these in real time with and through the commentary and reaction of others.

The struggles that big data companies and platform giants faced in halting the distribution of the livestreamed video highlighted the difficulties of the sharing economy. David Lyon [28] uses the metaphor of 'leaky containers' (pp. 37–48) to illuminate the power of networked technologies where data is not contained, but can leak through this networked architecture. The term, used by Lyon to underscore the nature of leaking data in the age of surveillance society through technologies, is equally relevant—if not crucial—to the architecture and promiscuity of the sharing economy where nothing is barred from sharing and consumption, with decreasing inhibitions of computer-mediated communications and networks which are sustained through sharing. This relentless leaking between sites and platforms engenders a vulnerable society where terror can be remapped as entertainment for the masses—one in which users seek to outwit the machines' ability to proscribe their possibilities of sharing contentious or objectionable content.

The theatricality of terror through social media and the leaky container of the sharing economy left forums on sites such as Reddit ablaze with anti-Muslim sentiments soon after the Christchurch massacre, prompting Reddit to ban one of the main channels used to disseminate such footage [29–31]. The perpetrator's 'anti-immigration, neo-fascist ideology lamenting the supposed decline of European civilization' [32] was echoed by many others in extreme online environments. In offline society, there were reports of a spike of violence against Muslims. In the UK, Tell Mama, a charity that tracks anti-Muslim hate crimes, reported 95 incidents, both online and offline, between 15 and 21 March 2019, of which 85 (89%) directly referenced the Christchurch attacks [31, 33].

6.4 Regulating the image economy online

The New Zealand massacre and live streaming brought to the fore the limitations in shutting down violent content or live acts of terrorism across the platforms, and that objectionable or violent content can metastasize across the Internet, even when it is prohibited by data giants such as Google and Facebook. More pointedly, it revealed that the governing of violent imagery online has been disparate across the platforms, creating ample opportunity for the video to leak through possible safeguards against objectionable content. The time lag between reporting objectionable content to the time when it is taken down, and the increasing reliance on AI to detect violent images as opposed to human editors, produce a confused image governance economy, particularly in terms of violent images. With regard to the New Zealand attack, platforms such as Facebook and Google were overwhelmed by livestreaming and the speed at which it was being replicated across different sites, highlighting the faults in the existing content governance structures of these organizations. These platforms amass vast amounts of content and data and, in tandem, experiment with human consumption, and the commodification and monetization processes do not necessarily cater to terror events such as the New Zealand attack. Conversely, they provide opportunities for terrorists to leak terror into mainstream culture and consumption.

What is notable is that violent content and hate speech policies are weakly enforced, and their practices for removing graphic videos are inconsistent, at best, across platforms [18]. Today, radical and extreme ideas thrive within this broad commercial agenda where both content and the human can be objectified through the processes of content creation and data assemblage. Over time, many of these companies have faced criticism for their content governance despite their 'claims to be stepping up efforts to use both human employees and artificially intelligent software' [34]. However, the availability of violent videos and radical content remains a concern and these slippages in governance mean that these data giants play a role in harbouring radical and extreme ideas, becoming agents in the spread of ideologies in terms of recruitment to extremist or terrorist causes, particularly when a feed is popular and where algorithms are designed to push popular content. The release of violent and extreme ideas into mainstream platforms through techniques of 'attention hacking' through calculated use of social media, memes, and bots means that extremist and terrorist groups become adept at outsmarting platforms' algorithms to their advantage and using the attention economy online to their advantage [20].

With the Web economy, opportunities for radicalization and terror remain within this vast ecology of niche networked communities fostering echo chambers, leaking content, and constructing the Internet as a space where content can be ineradicable. It is not just the content and the power of suggestion nor the younger generation of audiences who find pleasure and social capital in forwarding links and attachments, but the rhizomatic economy afforded by the World Wide Web that lends to this enterprise of terror. This assemblage makes it difficult to restrict or curb violent or radical content. Terror has found a secure place in popular culture and it is within a complex social economy of social sharing and conversations in networking sites. While news organizations have had to take an ethical stance in deciding to broadcast a video to the public, the dissemination of videos on the Web takes on a life of its own. As such, the videos invariably present an ongoing challenge. One the one hand, there is intense unease about giant data corporations controlling and censoring content or deciding what is objectionable for the world as a whole. On the other hand, violent imagery and horror can be objectified for audiences. Our obsession with this image economy and social sharing has been exploited successfully by radical and extremist groups attuned to the opportunities and the spectacular attention economy these digital platforms offer. With millions of images swimming in in these platforms, and where images attract traffic and the monetization of data, strict editorial oversight with images may not be the preferred option for these data corporations.

Violent videos have remained an area of contention for data giants. One case in point is the circulation of 'beheading videos' by terrorist organizations. Facebook has faced continual criticism for allowing violent and graphic content to remain on the site under the guise of public interest when, in effect, these may often be a means to drive traffic to the sites, particularly when they relate to current news and media events, bearing in mind the site permits videos and images from news reports and documentaries depicting abuse, murders, and terrorist activities [35]. In 2013, Facebook lifted a temporary ban on gory images such as beheadings, arguing that such images are permissible on its site so long as the content posted in a manner is intended for its users to '"condemn" the acts rather than celebrate them' [36]. Nevertheless, Facebook repealed this decision shortly after a public backlash, admitting that its approach was flawed, as hosting such content 'improperly and irresponsibly glorifies violence'. Facebook had briefly experimented with adding a more basic form of warning sign to clips of decapitations in October 2013 after the UK's then Prime Minister David Cameron asserted that 'It's irresponsible of Facebook to post beheading videos, especially without a warning'. Clips showing decapitations taking place were later banned altogether [37].

Facebook's fractured approach to regulating content and its rhetoric of upholding 'community standards' has led to an arbitrary approach. Facebook employs the discourse of 'sharing responsibly'; thus, shifting vetting responsibilities to users preserves its moral position while diverting the onus of the moral guardianship to users. It had in the past banned images of breastfeeding [27], while allowing the posting and sharing of gory images. In 2015 Facebook released new community standards to provide clarification on objectionable content, asserting it will 'remove graphic images when they are shared for sadistic pleasure or to celebrate or glorify violence' [35]. Additionally, it clarified that it would prevent graphic videos and photos from being shown to any user who identified themselves as being under 18 years of age in view of the fact that the social network permits users to sign up for accounts from the age of 13 years. However, users can circumvent age verification to create accounts and video content [35, 37]. The ethics of livestreaming presented an issue for Facebook when the service was launched on its site in 2016 when the death of African American teenager, Philando Castile, was livestreamed. This real-time streaming service positions the company as a live broadcaster without editorial structures and judgement, renewing calls for it to behave like a news organization and to have an ethical responsibility over its content.

6.5 **Conclusion**

Livestreaming of violent imagery within a sharing economy enlarges the co-production and theatricality of terror in unexpected ways. Through the case study of the Christchurch mosque massacre, it became evident that the sharing economy of social media and social networking sites produces a promiscuous and leaky enterprise where terror imagery and new strategies for disseminating radical ideologies emerge as an intrinsic component of this economy. On the one hand, new encrypted apps where messages can be deleted after reading premise ephemerality and, on the other hand, the rhizomatic assemblage of social networking sites enable content such as objectionable matter to float ad infinitum, producing new anxieties about the Internet harbouring and developing sites for extremist and radical views and recruitment strategies that could target the young, vulnerable, or the disenfranchised. With terror imagery and livestreaming of terrorist attacks co-mingling with simulated digital gaming environments that mirror such acts, these blur the boundaries between the real and the reel. The ability to leak prohibited content such as acts of terror and the unrelenting emphasis on sharing by data giants has also repositioned terror as a reality entertainment made for sharing and where these may be downloaded by young or vulnerable audiences without warning on the nature of the content. The narration of terror events from the vantage point of the perpetrator through technologies such as GoPro reconfigure terror into game mode, turning human suffering into a spectacle for the masses.

References

1. **Ibrahim Y.** Production of the "self" in the digital age. Cham: Palgrave Macmillan; 2018.
2. **Alper M.** War on Instagram: framing conflict photojournalism with mobile photography apps. New Media & Society 2014;**16**:1233–48.
3. **Ibrahim Y.** The technological gaze: event construction and the mobile body. M/C Journal 2007;**10**.
4. **Patrikarakos D.** War in 140 characters: how social media is reshaping conflict in the twenty-first century. London: Hachette; 2017.
5. **Thompson R.** Radicalization and the use of social media. Journal of Strategic Security 2011;**4**:167–90.
6. **Bhui K, Ibrahim Y.** Marketing the "radical": symbolic communication and persuasive technologies in jihadist websites. Transcultural Psychiatry 2013;**50**:216–34.

7. **Klausen J.** Tweeting the Jihad: social media networks of Western foreign fighters in Syria and Iraq. Studies in Conflict & Terrorism 2015;**38**:1–22.

8. **Weimann G.** New terrorism and new media. Washington, DC: Commons Lab of the Woodrow Wilson International Center for Scholars; 2014.

9. **Burke J.** The age of selfie jihad: how evolving media technology is changing terrorism. CTC Sentinel 2016;**9**:1.

10. **Taneja K.** Breaking the Islamic State's use of online spaces such as Telegram. Available from: https://www.eurasiareview.com/04122019-breaking-the-islamic-states-use-of-online-spaces-such-as-telegram-analysis/ [accessed 5 December 2019].

11. **Hamberger E.** Why Telegram has become the hottest messaging app in the world. Available from: https://www.theverge.com/2014/2/25/5445864/telegram-messenger-hottest-app-in-the-world [accessed 25 February 2014].

12. **Vasilogambros M.** A live-streamed suicide. Available from: https://www.theatlantic.com/technology/archive/2016/05/france-livestreamed-suicide/482328/ [accessed 11 May 2016].

13. **England C.** Teenager jailed for broadcast of girl's rape on online Periscope app. Available from: https://www.independent.co.uk/news/world/americas/teenager-marina-lonina-livestream-rape-17-year-old-friend-periscope-app-sentence-prison-columbus-a7581196.html [accessed 15 February 2017].

14. **Teague M.** Virginia shooting: how Vester Flanagan forced the world to be his audience. Available from: https://www.theguardian.com/us-news/2015/aug/27/virginia-shooting-in-an-instant-vester-flanagan-broadcast-death-to-the-world [accessed 27 August 2015].

15. **Levin S.** Videos appear to show armed militia detaining migrants at US–Mexico border. Available from: https://www.theguardian.com/us-news/2019/apr/18/new-mexico-migrants-armed-militia-detained [accessed 19 April 2019].

16. **Katz E, Lazarsfeld PF.** Personal influence: the part played by people in the flow of mass communication. Glencoe, IL: Free Press; 1955.

17. **Macklin G.** The Christchurch attacks: livestream terror in the viral video age. Available from: https://ctc.usma.edu/christchurch-attacks-livestream-terror-viral-video-age/ [accessed 29 July 2020].

18. **Rosen K.** 'Shut the site down,' says the creator of 8chan, a megaphone for gunmen. Available from: www.nytimes.com/2019/08/04/technology/8chan-shooting-manifesto.html?searchResultPosition=4 [accessed 4 August 2019].

19. **Dwoskin E, Timberg C.** Christchurch mosque shootings: inside YouTube's struggles to shut down video—and the humans who outsmarted its systems. The Washington Post. 19 March 2019.

20. **Fagnoni F.** Terrorism in the digital era: the dark side of livestreaming, online content and Internet subcultures. Available from: https://mastersofmedia.hum.uva.nl/blog/2019/09/22/terrorism-in-the-digital-era-the-dark-side-of-livestreaming-online-content-and-internet-subcultures/ [accessed 22 September 2019].

21. **Hagen S, Burton A, Wilson J, Tuters M.** Infinity's abyss: an overview of 8chan. Available from: www.oilab.eu/infinitys-abyss-an-overview-of-8chan/ [accessed 8 September 2019].

22. **Marwick A, Lewis R.** Media manipulation and disinformation online. Available from: https://datasociety.net/output/media-manipulation-and-disinfo-online/ [accessed 29 July 2020].

23. **Aldersley M.** Facebook left entire livestream of New Zealand shootings on their site for an HOUR before it was removed, it is revealed, after its AI failed to detect the video. Available from: https://www.dailymail.co.uk/news/article-6833155/The-Latest-New-Zealand-bans-assault-weapons-immediately.html [accessed 29 July 2020].

24. **Guy R.** A further update on New Zealand terrorist attack. Available from: https://about.fb.com/news/2019/03/technical-update-on-new-zealand/ [accessed 29 July 2020].

25. **Taylor R.** New Zealand mosque attack death toll rises to 51. Available from: https://www.wsj.com/articles/death-toll-rises-to-51-in-attacks-on-christchurch-mosques-11556848246 [accessed 2 May 2019].

26. **Cuthbertson A.** 'Subscribe to PewDiePie': what did Christchurch mosque gunman mean in final words before shooting? Available from: https://www.independent.co.uk/life-style/gadgets-and-tech/news/new-zealand-shooting-attack-pewdiepie-subscribe-youtube-mosque-a8825326.html [accessed 29 July 2020].

27. **Ibrahim Y.** Politics of gaze: the image economy online. London: Routledge; 2019.

28. **Lyon D.** Surveillance society, issues in society. Buckingham: Open University; 2001.

29. **Breland A.** Anti-Muslim hate has been rampant on Reddit since the New Zealand shooting. Available from: https://www.motherjones.com/politics/2019/03/reddit-new-zealand-shooting-islamophobia [accessed 29 July 2020].

30. **Hatmaker T.** After Christchurch, Reddit bans communities infamous for sharing graphic videos of death. Tech Crunch. 15 March 2019.

31. **Wakefield J.** Christchurch shootings: social media races to stop attack footage. BBC News. 16 March 2019.

32. **Walden M.** New Zealand mosque attacks: who is Brenton Tarrant? Available from: www.aljazeera.com/news/2019/03/zealand-mosque-attacks-brenton-tarrant-190316093149803.html [accessed 18 March 2019].

33. **Vikram D.** Anti-Muslim hate crimes soar in UK after Christchurch shootings. The Guardian. 22 March 2019.

34. **Greenemeier L.** Social media's stepped-up crackdown on terrorists still falls short. Available from: www.scientificamerican.com/article/social-medias-stepped-up-crackdown-on-terrorists-still-falls-short/ [accessed 24 July 2018].

35. **Gibbs S.** Facebook tackles graphic videos and photos with "are you sure?" warnings. Available from: https://www.theguardian.com/technology/2015/jan/13/facebook-tackles-graphic-videos-and-photos-with-are-you-sure-warnings [accessed 13 January 2015].

36. **Oreskovic A.** Facebook removes beheading video, updates violent images standards. Reuters. 2013, October 22. Available from: http://www.reuters.com/article/net-us-facebook-violenceidUSBRE99K14020131023

37. **Kelion, L.** Facebook restricts violent video clips and photos. Available from: https://www.bbc.co.uk/news/technology-30793702 [accessed 13 January 2015].

Chapter 7

Terrorism: Group dynamic and interdisciplinary aspects

Thomas Wenzel, Reem Alksiri,
and Anthony F. Chen

7.1 Introduction: a question of definitions?

The term terrorism, as demonstrated in other chapters of this book, presently reflects a wide range of concepts depending on political, or professional background, and ethnicity or nationality, as well as the organization of those using the term [1]. One of the commonly cited definitions is Louise Richardson's, which describes terrorism as 'politically motivated violence directed against non-combatants or symbolic targets which is designed to communicate a message to a broader audience' [2–4]. The UN definitions are constantly changing, with a present version given in their Global Counter-Terrorism Strategy [1].[1]

In this chapter, we will use a flexible definition to permit broader discussion of the various factors related to the creation of perpetrators of extreme violence, especially terrorists [5]. This gives us the advantage of drawing on different fields, concepts, and models to discuss specific aspects that are less often considered. The range of definitions in different settings lacks consensus; the many proposed factors contributing to the global rise of terrorism [5] support the idea that there is no comprehensive evidence-based consensus in the field that will fit all possible situations. Political, legal, cultural anthropology, psychology, social sciences, medicine, and human ethology researchers have tried to develop specific models based on their respective disciplines [5, 6] (see other chapters in this book). In addition, there is a wide range of situations, countries, and historical moments where the term has been applied, covering countries such as Turkey, Syria, the United States; organizations such as Islamic State of Iraq and Syria (ISIS) or Euskadi Ta Askatasuna (ETA); and also settings like animal protection [7], abortion clinic-related violence [8], and human rights

---

[1] https://www.un.org/counterterrorism/un-global-counter-terrorism-strategy

groups. This diverse application further underlines that it is risky to explain all aspects of terrorism in a simplified model, especially one based on individual biographies and psychopathology [9].

In this chapter we will respect all models as valuable contributions, to not restrict discourse by excluding any specific concepts. We do not doubt that financial, political, social, religious, historical and cultural factors, and sometimes individual psychopathology of terrorists and terrorist leaders can play a role in shaping different forms of terrorism in specific countries and settings. Authors such as Jerrold Post [10] suggest a historical sequence of different 'waves' of terrorism, from 'labor violence in the United States in the late 19th century; through the Anti-Colonial wave (nationalist-separatist), to the social revolutionary New Left wave (social revolutionary); to the Religious wave'. Each has its own key factors, leading to the present interest in 'lone wolf' Internet-linked terrorists, which we discuss later. In this context, Post has also drawn attention to the increasing importance of right-wing terrorism. The first use of the term terrorism, as a form of state terror during the French Revolution, should be added to this list [11, 12]. Finally, the concept itself has developed a life and discourse of its own, as it is frequently applied as a manipulative allegation, a political tool simply to discredit political opposition [3, 4] and, consequently, justify acts of aggression and violence such as torture, by controlling the dominant discourse, definitions, and application of the term [13].

In this chapter, we do not provide a comprehensive model, but discuss some aspects that can be relevant to the understanding, prevention, and measurement of how people cope with the impact as victims, communities, and societies. This is not to defend or justify the actions, but understanding is necessary to inform prevention. We also do not want to comment on the individual's response to trauma or individual resilience, or disaster preparedness in the medical sense, as these themes are covered by other chapters.

Our personal belief in this context is that terrorism, or more generally violence against civilians and non-combatants, regardless of its labelling as terrorism, antiterrorism ('War on Terror' [14, 15]), or any other derivative, is not justified under any circumstances. The use of such terms must not negate standards of human rights and humanitarian law, which are remarkable achievements of the post-World War II international community [16]. This is a position affirmed in the relevant position statement by the United Nations (UN) High Commissioner of Human Rights and the UN position paper on 'Promoting and protecting human rights and fundamental freedoms while countering terrorism'. These underline that 'The Terrorism Prevention Branch of UNODC [United Nations Office on Drugs and Crime] believes that, to effectively combat terrorism, respecting human rights and fundamental freedoms is not only possible but necessary'.[2]

Despite the larger range of apologetic arguments justifying violence and closely related acts such as torture, or genocide, we believe that protection against violence intending to create terror is a fundamental human right. This argument is based on basic concepts developed before the present international humanitarian law (such as *jus cogens* or 'natural law'). This applies no matter who uses terror as a tool and for what aim, and therefore equally to states [13, 15], non-state actors, and religiously or otherwise motivated wars or [17] 'war on terror' [15]. The control of media and public discourse [18] can give an advantage to autocratic or power-hungry governments and groups such as ISIS.

This chapter will now discuss some of the group dynamic aspects that might be relevant to the development of mass violence, terrorism, and their sequels. Our argument is based on our own background as an interdisciplinary team of psychotherapists, cultural anthropologists, psychiatrists, and lawyers working to support victims of violence from the relatively safe haven of the European country Austria but especially in war and conflict regions such as Syria [19], and in countries with state-sponsored terrorism such as Iran or Turkey.

7.1.1 How to 'create' terrorists and other perpetrators of extreme violence: group- and individual-based factors

Research in recent decades has demonstrated the frightening fact that most perpetrators of severe violence against civilians were initially inconspicuous neighbours who eventually became murderers or sometimes 'book-keepers' of terror, such as Nazi perpetrators [20, 21], or Soviets under the rule of Stalin [22]. This reflects an increasing awareness that the problem cannot be reduced to psychiatric illness or mental health problems, even in the case of suicide bombers [23]. As Piccinni et al. have summarized in a recent review paper, 'no evidence exists that terrorist behavior may be caused either by prior or current psychiatric disorders or psychopathy' [24]. The fact that a normal neighbour could become an accomplice to mass murder indicates that acts of manipulation [25] resulting in a gradual psychological change that eliminates empathy and the respect for life must be required [26]. If this transition is an accurate reflection of the process of radicalization, the process must include, but is not limited to, 'doubling', as described by Robert Lifton in his research on Nazi perpetrators and terrorists (as discussed in [27]); recently this concept has been explored in line with

---

[2] https://www.unodc.org/unodc/en/terrorism/news-and-events/human-rights-while-countering-terrorism.html

adolescent development and the concept of 'heroic' doubling to describe the parallel and apparent contradictory psychological adaptation of terrorists who have no psychiatric history and appear to live normal lives in spite of their willingness to commit atrocities [27].

Again, we do not restrict our observations to a narrow definition of 'terrorism', but look into closely related and overlapping phenomena, especially in regard to the creation of perpetrators [28]. One less commonly considered precondition of violence are the factors required to mobilize a larger group to commit acts of violence against a different group, often a minority. This is especially important in asymmetrical warfare and genocide, as well as in understanding terrorism [29].

Committing violence, especially against non-armed third parties, children, or other vulnerable groups, results, as noted before, from a lowering of the barriers and constraints that normally prevent violence. The earlier attention to individual psychopathology or the psychodynamics of conflict with authority, such as having abusive 'father figures' [30], is now replaced by more evidence of the importance of social and group dynamics [29]. In this age of social and digital media, 'groups' no longer require in-person on-site meetings as in a church, mosque, or other public place, as individuals can be linked over the Internet, resulting in a mechanism to recruit new members and maintain group dynamics [25, 31], as well as an online community that develops a dynamic of its own. Formerly isolated individuals now have a lower barrier to access, and no need for special social skills, resulting in insecure people who feel marginalized gaining a feeling of 'belonging' to a group, even as a 'lone wolf' [10, 32, 33].

Robert Sapolsky draws attention to the structures of the 'primate mind' that guides violence and compassion in humans, and how these structures can be lost through individual or group processes [34]. The building of a 'we' feeling in a tribe of members helps in-group empathy and bonding but at the cost of hate against the 'they' or 'other' out-groups.

Relevant group structures can be small, nuclear groups or large groups based on national, geographical, ethnic, or religious identifiers, with different levels and mechanisms of cohesion. Recently, Spitzmuller and Park [29] have proposed that terrorist teams are 'loosely coupled systems' with very flexible group dynamics that confer cohesion, which makes them more adaptive and fluid in response to different social, legal, and cultural environments.

Vamik Volkan, an experienced American group analyst of Turkish Cypriot origin [35], was frequently invited to apply his concepts in actual political negotiations to promote peace in conflicts (track II diplomacy [36–38]). He proposed that certain manipulations are employed in large groups, potentially with millions of members [39, 40], where group members are persuaded to commit atrocities and create terror among civilians and former neighbours. A joint symbol to represent the identity of the group against 'the other' [41] can emerge from the reactivated or reinvented memory and discourse in regrad to a negative historical event, usually a defeat or perceived injustice experienced in the rather distant past heritage of that group. According to Volkan, this is frequently 'a chosen trauma', or event that is too far removed to be actively creating post-traumatic emotional suffering for members of the group [42]. This symbolic historic defeat or event—key to the identity of the group—is promoted, usually by politicians with their own goals, to strengthen and create a group identity that favours their interests, often to create a common enemy. Focusing on their symbolic event and reliving the trauma is pathological mourning, a form of group narcissism in reaction to a hurt [43], which leads to hatred [44, 45]. Certain objects that are perceived as 'lost' can be 'linked' to this hatred, such as the keys of the last houses occupied by Israel, as perceived by Palestinians [43, 46–49]. Therefore, these objects then carry significant symbolic meaning for the group.

When a symbol associated with that negativity becomes accepted by the group, a predominance of simplified primitive emotional and cognitive processes arises. Psychoanalytically, this is a regression to earlier phases of childhood and group development, which is often related to the loss of critical reasoning. This results in a loss of neutrality, and a biased evaluation of concepts promoted by the group and its leaders, as well as a lowered barrier to committing violence against weaker groups, defined as 'the other' [41].

Volkan analysed in this context the role of reparative leaders [40] and 'strong' politicians to heal narcissistic injuries in recent analyses of flawed leadership [50], and extended the concept of chosen trauma through a complementary model of 'chosen glories'. One example is the (disputed) defeat of the Serb Zar Lazar and his army by the Turkish army under Sultan Murad I in 'Kosovo polje' as a main symbol of Serbian identity [51], instead of an identity based, for example, on leading scientists or artists in the history of the group. Besides the saturation of public media, especially online, physical memorials and monuments serve as a constant reminder of this 800-year-old event and may continuously reinforce the identity of the group. This can be seen as a critical precondition to changing the attitude of previously friendly Serb neighbours—that they were in control of one of the largest military machines of Europe after the collapse of federal multiethnic Yugoslavia—by instilling a belief in their right and duty to protect their own ethnic group against the 'still dangerous' other groups [52]. Volkan observes this as 'time collapse', the dissolution of time in the ubiquitous presence of the long distant past. This can be seen as a key phenomenon in a process that helps to block any reality check on the verbal and visual promotion of terrorism and violent acts by group leaders.

Recently, similar unfoldings have been observed in other countries [52], especially in regions most commonly associated with terrorism. Historically, the former colonial powers of the United States, Great Britain, and France, and their power politics, interfered with local interests and the autonomy of ethnic groups, but the depiction of 'crusaders' [53] invading the Near East is taking up an image from the twelfth and thirteenth centuries. This appears to be a time collapse, and not simply a contemporary take on the intrusive players today. Many terrorist groups have exploited similar time collapses over the last decade [54]. As part of the time collapse, historical, 'noble' leaders such as the Kurdish hero Saladin (سهلاحهدینی ئهییووبی) are cited without critical consideration of the differences between the twelfth and twenty-first century's actual political and economic situations. This mythology was taken up by Jihadist discourse only recently [32, 55], demonstrating a process of historical distortion typical for the creation of chosen traumas and glories by both parties on either side of a conflict.

On the other side, the atrocious 9/11 bombing of the World Trade Center towers has developed into its own emotional reality, which gives a sense of permission or even obligation to perform acts of revenge to people who were themselves removed from the event. Despite not being directly affected, they have been led to abandon respect for human rights, turning to any strategy available, including torture, and accepting collateral killing of non-combatants. Although it could be said that the direct exposure to the event through the video material distributed through American and international media constitutes not a chosen, 'quasi-narcissistic' trauma, but an actual one, the event itself has—in our opinion—developed a symbolic life of its own as a symbolic trauma. It is used to justify violence and create terror, such as the 'shock and awe' military dogma frequently quoted by the US military. It could be argued to be a new category of 'hybrid' chosen trauma, consisting of actual severe emotional group trauma, as well as the later political manipulation and redefinition. In turn, it can be argued to have become a chosen glory used by Jihadist militants to recruit and mobilize persons to become part of a 'we' community. As lone wolves, they might meet first online, then later meet physically and might be trained to abandon critical reality testing and empathy to ultimately create their own atrocities.

Any serious discussion would indicate that groups abolishing the basic rules of humane behaviour, general conventions, human rights, or natural law regardless of who is actually the first to abandon this rules, will affect their own populations: a 'lose–lose' strategy. It would not erase the shame of the historical defeat or help in mourning lost objects, but would instead lead to further defeats, interrupting the healthy mourning process. This can also be seen in the group manipulation employed by Nazi leadership in creating the idea of the ultimate victory (*Endsieg*) and a 'total war' to erase the image of the defeats of the country and necessary mourning in the end phase of World War II [33].

Group manipulation can also be observed in the widespread use of the term 'terrorism' to any political or ethnic minorities in opposition to autocratic governments such as Turkey, or China. This strategy neglects any reality testing. It can become bizarre, such as with Turkish leader Tayyip Erdogan, who mobilized his country's population against all Kurdish groups and against alleged supporters of his former ally Abdullah Gül, who had been instrumental in helping him into power. Logically, this would make Erdogan himself an ally and beneficiary of the support of terrorists. A group dynamic process suspending normal reasoning and the use of critical thinking, described by Volkan as group regression supported by chosen trauma or glories, can be instrumental in the eventual creation of violence, terrorism, and genocide.

The gradual shaping of the 'other', which replaces empathic perception of the neighbour as a fellow human being, is documented in the Holocaust Museum [56–58[that was erected in Rwanda after the Hutu/Tutsi genocide, in which thousands of previously non-violent civilians were mobilized in a very short time to kill more than 100,000 of their neighbours [59, 60]. We see the shaping of 'the other' leading to disregard of any natural empathic barrier, as in the term 'infidel' in religious terrorism [57, 58]. The museum documents how radio, the available social medium in all villages, was used gradually to distort the language used to describe their neighbours. A person who was different was first defined as inferior, then as a non-person, like an animal or plant [61], then dangerous and needing to be 'weeded' out—imagery that was well adapted to their agrarian and animal husbandry lives. This was seen as a duty of Christians who otherwise respected the sanctity of life. Leaders frequently also quoted historical injustices allegedly committed by the other group. Radio has been replaced by the Internet in most countries, with certain sites inheriting the culture of 'hate speech'. The importance of the museum project and its education activities for school children for preventing recurrence, and its contribution to mourning and the healing process [58, 62], has been underlined by the regular respect paid by the Israeli government to the museum [63].

Another situation that could be used to better understand the willingness to commit violence and acts of terror against third parties and neighbours, and the potential rehabilitation later, is that of the child soldiers in Uganda—a key problem region besides Syria and Iraq. Their shaping, socialization, and reintegration afterwards was explored by Klasen et al. [64], Pham et al. [65], and others. Child soldiers often are exposed to abduction [66], torture, and forced 're'socialization as a precondition to become perpetrators and terrorize local communities [64, 65]. Klasen et al. [64] proposes they can be seen as the 'guilt-less guilty', which was similarly proposed by Mika Haritas Fatouros [67].

7.1.2 What comes after terror: group and community aspects

In situations where terror is widespread and has led to a destruction of civil society and rule of law, stability and reconstruction of peaceful frameworks and safety can only be recovered by complex steps that involve the whole society, including both victims and perpetrators. In major postconflict situations, transitional justice (see [68] for an overview) is an important element of rebuilding and healing individuals though the healing of society, or 'therapeutic justice'. It includes a number of important non-legal steps, such as education [62, 69] and the rebuilding of a realistic narrative replacing distorted historical reality [70]. Impunity is usually seen as incompatible with reconciliation [71], but it must be addressed even when practical considerations might lead to a decision to 'shake hands with the devil' and 'reintegrate' or rehabilitate perpetrators of government or non-state-actor terror. International criminal courts can be a decisive step when local courts are dysfunctional and structures of transitional justice do not yet exist, especially for non-state actors such as Joseph Kony's 'Lord's Resistance Army' or ISIS. The limitation of the international courts lies in trying perpetrators in powerful hegemonies such as Russia or the United States.[3]

The role of reintegrating perpetrators in situations of mass violence, conflict, and terrorism as part of transitional justice structures has been widely discussed, especially in regard to child soldiers [72]. Again, we believe that social, community, and group processes in transitional justice [72–74] should be used in situations dominated by group violence, rather than an approach that focuses only on the individual's accountability, imprisonment, or execution [75]. Recent work by medical researchers on returned child soldiers in Uganda has often focused on the treatment of trauma-related disorders, especially post-traumatic stress disorder (PTSD) [76–78], and depression or suicidal ideation [79]. Few authors have addressed the question of trauma and treatment of trauma symptoms in predicting reintegration and the recovery of civil society through justice and reconciliation. Bayer et al. [80] observed that 'Children who showed more PTSD symptoms had significantly less openness to reconciliation (rho = –0.34, $P < .001$) and more feelings of revenge (rho =

---

[3]   https://www.un.org/en/ga/sixth/65/ScopeAppUniJuri_StatesComments/Belgium_E.pdf [accessed 30 December 2019].

0.29, $P < .001$)'. This important finding underlines the importance of processing trauma in both perpetrators and victims of extreme social violence such as terrorism, before rehabilitation and reconciliation can be addressed. Vindevogel et al. [81] documented the importance of postevent community-based support structures in rehabilitation in general. Vindevogel et al. [82, 83] also used qualitative research to identify important subjective reported factors in rehabilitation of child soldiers, listing specifically '(a) to break with former existence as child soldiers, (b) to be able to overcome the challenges in current life, (c) to belong to others and the environment to which they have returned, and (d) to become the person they aspire to be'. It should be noted that we do not believe that earlier traumatic experiences justify committing violence, but that it is important to understand that this factor is a part of the comprehensive strategy to guide rehabilitation and prevention of further violence, including transferred real or chosen trauma between generations [84]. The experience in regions such as Gulu (Uganda) can also be used to—at least partly—give guidance to other situations, such as in the case of ISIS child soldiers, although cultural and situational factors and differences should still be considered.

In transitional justice, especially for developing countries and traditional societies such as South Africa or Nepal (peace and reconciliation commission), Rwanda (Gacatcha courts [85]) or Uganda (Gulu region), traditional courts and models of reintegration like truth and reconciliation commissions have been installed to aid the process but not always with convincing results [85]. This indicates the need for further research and exploration, especially as traditional models of justice did not develop with situations similar to the mass violence and terrorism seen today.

As also noted before, we want to conclude, that the rehabilitation of perpetrators and protection against the desire to be part of a terrorist group cannot be done by focusing on isolating and individually reforming a person, but rather by support of bonding with a positive group. This was used with some success in Uganda and other regions utilizing church services and structures. Owing to the social media factor and Internet-based group identity, it would also be necessary to develop a strong online presence to offer convincing alternatives to the processes that promote the breakdown of empathy, such as replacing symbols that create 'the other' and addressing distorted historical reality like chosen trauma or glories, and re-establish empathy and human rights as fundamental values. In our opinion, this should replace the mythology of a 'war on terror', as that risks the creation of further group dynamics permitting violence and future terrorism, even if not labelled as such. At this point, it should also be mentioned that some authors have drawn attention to the fact that terrorist groups (and also autocratic governments) use the Internet and other media to garner support for their position and justify violent ideals not only in possible recruits, but also with the general audience [86].

A stronger focus on groups and communities might also help victims of violence. This includes many steps, including the necessary correction of historical distortions, like the denial of the Holocaust, that are experienced as continued aggression by the victims, and the clarification of the fate of people who were killed and often disposed of in anonymous mass graves. Indirect victims, like the family members of those killed, have become an increasing focus, not only in regard to 9/11, but also in the case ruling of the Inter-American Court on Human Rights in the Miguel Castro Castro Prison case against Peru, and in the European Court on Human Rights decision in the case of Cyprus versus Turkey.[4] In both cases the needs of the family members as indirect victims of state-sponsored violence and terror were confirmed. The Inter-American Court, using results of focus group research conducted by our group, also acknowledged the need of non-pecuniary redress (measures of reparation) through a symbolic monument to be erected to clarify and correct historical distortions ('in order for Peruvian society to know the truth'). In this case the distortion held that the family members tortured and killed in the Castro Castro prison were criminals (terrorists) and therefore subject to justified violence and execution.[5] The history of the interaction of terrorist (Shining Path, Revolutionary Movement Tupac Amaru (MRTA)) and 'anti-terrorist' violence by governmental forces in Peru on the civilian population is similar to that seen in countries like Nepal [87–89]. The difficult challenges faced in legal and social justice and reconciliation steps obviously require further research. The interaction of the cumulative traumatic impact of sequential governmental and insurgent violence on the civilians creates complex environments, shaped by violence, insecurity, and mutual disrespect for human rights, and cannot be summarized simply by PTSD. These conclusions should also be considered in the interplay of terror and the so-called 'War on Terror'.

7.3 **Conclusion**

In today's world, the label of 'terrorist' in some countries is easily given to alleged members of an ethnic or political opposition group, as mentioned in the case of Turkey. Here, it results in a breakdown of objective rule of law and an increase in

---

[4] https://hudoc.echr.coe.int/eng#{%22itemid%22:[%22001-59454%22]}, May 10. 2ßß1, Application no. 25781/94 [accessed 30 July 2020].

[5] Miguel Castro-Castro Prison v. Peru Judgment of 25 November 2006, http://www.corteidh. or.cr/docs/casos/articulos/seriec_160_ing.pdf [accessed 30 July 2020].

the willingness to commit torture and other forms of state-sponsored violence. The abuse of this term comes not only from asymmetrical relationships, but also the Internet-based creation of hate imagery, images of 'the other', and symbols of chosen trauma or glory. They must be addressed as part of any effective strategy against terror, violence, and the breakdown of respect for human rights and humanitarian law.

Reconstruction of a (more) peaceful civil society and rule of law, to provide healing, recovery, and to prevent further violence, requires an effort by all parties involved and a focus on group processes.

References

1. Arnold JL, Ortenwall P, Birnbaum ML, Sundnes KO, Aggrawal A, Anantharaman V, et al. A proposed universal medical and public health definition of terrorism. Prehospital and Disaster Medicine 2003;**18**:47–52.

2. Richardson L. Terrorists as transnational actors. 1999;**11**:209–19.

3. Ritchie H, Hasell J, Appel C, Roser M. Terrorism. Available at: https://ourworldindata. org/terrorism [accessed 30 July 2020].

4. Martini A, Njoku, E. The challenging of defining terrorism for counter-terrorism policy. In: Romaniuk SN, Grice F, Irrera D, Webb S, eds. The palgrave handbook of global counterterrorism policy. London: Palgrave; 2017, pp. 73–90.

5. Poteliakhoff A, Weerts J, de Leeuw-Korthals Althes M. Terrorism: causes and prevention. Medicine and War 1988;**4**:227–31.

6. Vizioli R. [Psychology and politics. Attempt at a psychopathologic interpretation of terrorism]. Minerva Psichiatrica 1985;**26**:159–66 (in Italian).

7. Collins JG. Terrorism and animal rights. Science 1990;**249**:345.

8. Wilson M, Lynxwiler J. Abortion clinic violence as terrorism. Terrorism 1988;**11**:263–73.

9. Corrado RR. A critique of the mental disorder perspective of political terrorism. International Journal of Law and Psychiatry 1981;**4**:293–309.

10. Post JM. Terrorism and right-wing extremism: the changing face of terrorism and political violence in the 21st century: the virtual community of hatred. International Journal of Group Psychotherapy 2015;**65**:242–71.

11. Schlicht L. [The French revolution as moral shock: on the political dimension of the research and therapy of the human mind, ca. 1792–1806]. NTM 2018;**26**:405–36 (in German).

12. Desan S. Reconstituting the social after the Terror: family, property and the law in popular politics. Past & Present 1999;**164**:81–122.

13. Barbara JS. 'War on terrorism' and deep culture. Medicine, Conflict and Survival 2003;**19**:39–44.

14. Holdstock D. Reacting to terrorism. The response should be through law not war. BMJ 2001;**323**:822.

15. Blakeley R, Raphael S. British torture in the 'war on terror'. European Journal of International Relations 2017;**23**:243–66.

16. **Kaar JF.** The emergence of international terrorism and technological changes: have these changes made the Law of Armed Conflict obsolete? Military Medicine 2007;**172**(12 Suppl.):22–5.

17. **Jones JW.** Why does religion turn violent? A psychoanalytic exploration of religious terrorism. Psychoanalytic Review 2006;**93**:167–90.

18. **Nacos B.** Mass mediated terrorism: the central role of the media in terrorism and counterterrorism. Lanham, MD: Rowman & Littlefield; 2007.

19. **Horton R.** Offline: terrorism and Syria—"a crisis of the world". Lancet 2017;**390**:924.

20. **Haslam SA, Reicher S.** Beyond the banality of evil: three dynamics of an interactionist social psychology of tyranny. Personality and Social Psychology Bulletin 2007;**33**:615–22.

21. **Blass T.** Psychological perspectives on the perpetrators of the Holocaust: the role of situational pressures, personal dispositions, and their interactions. Holocaust and Genocide Studies 1993;**7**:30–50.

22. **Prince C.** A psychological study of Stalin. Journal of Social Psychology 1945;**22**:119–40.

23. **Atran S.** Genesis of suicide terrorism. Science 2003;**299**:1534–9.

24. **Piccinni A, Marazziti D, Veltri A.** Psychopathology of terrorists. CNS Spectrums 2018;**23**:141–4.

25. **Jones E.** The reception of broadcast terrorism: recruitment and radicalisation. International Review of Psychiatry 2017;**29**:320–6.

26. **Lang J.** Questioning dehumanization: intersubjective dimensions of violence in the Nazi concentration and death camps. Holocaust Genocide Studies 2010;**24**:225–46.

27. **Griffin R.** The role of heroic doubling in ideologically motivated state and terrorist violence. International Review of Psychiatry 2017;**29**:355–61.

28. **Horgan JG.** Psychology of terrorism: Introduction to the special issue. American Psychologist 2017;**72**:199–204.

29. **Spitzmuller M, Park G.** Terrorist teams as loosely coupled systems. American Psychologist 2018;**73**:491–503.

30. **Kent I, Nicholls W.** The psychodynamics of terrorism. Mental Health and Society 1978;**4**:1–8.

31. **Kayode-Adedeji T, Oyero O, Aririguzoh S.** Dataset on online mass media engagements on YouTube for terrorism related discussions. Data Brief 2019;**23**:103581.

32. **Horswell M, Phillips J.** Perceptions of the crusades from the nineteenth to the twenty-first century, first edition. ed. London and New York: Routledge/Taylor & Francis; 2018.

33. **Gröper R.** Erhoffter Jubel über den Endsieg: Tagebuch eines Hitlerjungen 1943–1945. Sigmaringen: Thorbecke; 1996.

34. **Sapolsky RM.** Doubled-edged swords in the biology of conflict. Frontiers in Psychology 2018;**9**:2625.

35. **Volkan VD.** In these pages … THE INTERTWINING OF EXTERNAL AND INTERNAL EVENTS IN THE CHANGING WORLD. American Journal of Psychoanalysis 2015;**75**:353–360.

36. **Volkan VD.** Psychological concepts useful in the building of political foundations between nations: Track II diplomacy. Journal of the American Psychoanalytic Association 1987;**35**:903–35.

37. **Volkan VD, Akhtar S.** The seed of madness: constitution, environment, and fantasy in the organization of the psychotic core. London: Karnac Books; 2016.

38. **Volkan V.** Enemies on the couch: a psychopolitical journey through war and peace. Durham, NC: Pitchstone Publishing; 2013.

39. **Volkan VD.** Individual and large-group identity: parallels in development and characteristics in stability and crisis. Croatian Medical Journal 1999;**40**:458–65.

40. **Volkan VD.** Large-group identity, who are we now? Leader-follower relationships and societal-political divisions. American Journal of Psychoanalysis 2019;**79**:139–55.

41. **Volkan VD.** Psychoanalytic thoughts on the European refugee crisis and the other. Psychoanalytic Review 2017;**104**:661–85.

42. **Volkan V.** Killing in the name of identity: a study of bloody conflicts. Durham, NC: Pitchstone Publishing; 2006.

43. **Volkan VD.** Symptom formations and character changes due to upheavals of war: examples from Cyprus. American Journal of Psychotherapy 1979;**33**:239–62.

44. **Victoroff J, Quota S, Adelman JR, Celinska B, Stern N, Wilcox R,** et al. Support for religio-political aggression among teenaged boys in Gaza: part I: psychological findings. Aggressive Behavior 2010;**36**:219–31.

45. **Victoroff J, Quota S, Adelman JR, Celinska B, Stern N, Wilcox R,** et al. Support for religio-political aggression among teenaged boys in Gaza: part II: neuroendocrinological findings. Aggressive Behavior 2011;**37**:121–32.

46. **Volkan VD.** The linking objects of pathological mourners. Archives of General Psychiatry 1972;**27**:215–21.

47. **Volkan VD.** The birds of Cyprus. A psychopolitical observation. American Journal of Psychotherapy 1972;**26**:378–83.

48. **Volkan V, Showalter CR.** Known object loss, disturbance in reality testing, and "re-grief work" as a method of brief psychotherapy. Psychiatric Quarterly. 1968;**42**:358–74.

49. **Volkan VD.** Mourning and adaptation after a war. American Journal of Psychotherapy 1977;**31**:561–9.

50. **Volkan V.** Blind trust: large groups and their leaders in times of crisis and terror. Durham, NC: Pitchstone Publishing; 2014.

51. **Volkan V.** Bloodlines: from ethnic pride to ethnic terrorism. New York: Basic Books; 1998.

52. **Volkan VD.** Bloodlines: from ethnic pride to ethnic terrorism, first edition. New York: Farrar, Straus and Giroux; 1997.

53. **Menache S, Gutwein, D.** Just war, crusade, and jihad: conflicting propaganda strategies during the Gulf crisis. Revue belge de Philologie et d'Histoire 2002;**80**:385–400

54. **Philips J.** Holy warriors: a modern history of the Crusades. London: Random House; 2010.

55. **Phillips J.** Holy warriors: a modern history of the crusades, first edition. New York: Random House; 2010.

56. **Lidman M.** At Rwanda Holocaust tribute, 'Never Again' is a hopeful slogan. The Times of Israel. 14 February 2017.

57. **Sodaro A.** Exhibiting atrocity: memorial museums and the politics of past violence. New Brunswick Camden and Newark, NJ: Rutgers University Press; 2018.

58. **Totten S.** Teaching about genocide: issues, approaches, and resources. Greenwich, CT: Information Age Publishing; 2004.

59. **Jensen O, Szejnmann C-CW.** Ordinary people as mass murderers: perpetrators in comparative perspectives. Houndsmill and New York: Palgrave Macmillan; 2008

60. **Spangenburg R, Moser D.** The crime of genocide: terror against humanity. Berkeley Heights, NJ: Enslow Publishers; 2000.

61. **Smith DL.** Less than human: why we demean, enslave, and exterminate others, first edition. New York: St. Martin's Press; 2011.

62. **Ramirez-Barat C, Schulze M.** Transitional justice and education: engaging young people in peacebuilding and reconciliation. Göttingen: V&R unipress; 2018.

63. **Staff T.** Breaking with West, Israel backs Rwanda in renaming genocide. Available at: https://www.timesofisrael.com/breaking-with-west-israel-backs-rwanda-in-renaming-genocide/ [accessed 30 July 2020].

64. **Klasen F, Schrage J, Post M, Adam H.** [Guiltless guilty—trauma-related guilt and posttraumatic stress disorder in former Ugandan child soldiers]. Praxis Kinderpsychologie Kinderpsychiatrie 2011;**60**:125–42 (in German).

65. **Pham PN, Vinck P, Stover E.** Returning home: forced conscription, reintegration, and mental health status of former abductees of the Lord's Resistance Army in northern Uganda. BMC Psychiatry 2009;**9**:23.

66. **Vindevogel S, Coppens K, Derluyn I, De Schryver M, Loots G, Broekaert E.** Forced conscription of children during armed conflict: experiences of former child soldiers in northern Uganda. Child Abuse & Neglect 2011;**35**:551–62.

67. **Haritos-Fatouros M.** The official torturer: a learning model for obedience to the authority of violence. Journal of Applied Social Psychology 1988;**18**:1107–20.

68. **Brants CH, Hol AM, Siegel D.** Transitional justice: images and memories. Farnham and Burlington, VT: Ashgate Publishing; 2013.

69. **Eltringham N.** Accounting for horror: post-genocide debates in Rwanda. London and Sterling VA: Pluto Press; 2004.

70. **Stier OB, Landres JS.** Religion, violence, memory, and place. Bloomington, IN: Indiana University Press; 2006.

71. **Basoglu M, Livanou M, Crnobaric C, Franciskovic T, Suljic E, Duric D,** et al. Psychiatric and cognitive effects of war in former yugoslavia: association of lack of redress for trauma and posttraumatic stress reactions. JAMA 2005;**294**:580–90.

72. **Corbin JN.** Returning home: resettlement of formerly abducted children in Northern Uganda. Disasters 2008;**32**:316–35.

73. **Ertl V, Pfeiffer A, Schauer E, Elbert T, Neuner F.** Community-implemented trauma therapy for former child soldiers in Northern Uganda: a randomized controlled trial. JAMA 2011;**306**:503–12.

74. **Derluyn I.** Re-member: rehabilitation, reintegration and reconciliation of war-affected children. Cambridge and Portland, OR: Intersentia; 2012.

75. **Sawyer KK.** Grace Akallo and the pursuit of justice for child soldiers, first edition. Greensboro, NC: Morgan Reynolds Publishing; 2015.

76. **Kuruppuarachchi K, Wijeratne LT.** Post-traumatic stress in former Ugandan child soldiers. Lancet 2004;**363**:1648.

77. **Klasen F, Oettingen G, Daniels J, Adam H.** Multiple trauma and mental health in former Ugandan child soldiers. Journal of Traumatic Stress 2010;**23**:573–81.

78. **Ovuga E, Oyok TO, Moro EB.** Post traumatic stress disorder among former child soldiers attending a rehabilitative service and primary school education in northern Uganda. African Health Sciences 2008;**8**:136–41.

79. **Amone-P'Olak K, Lekhutlile TM, Meiser-Stedman R, Ovuga E.** Mediators of the relation between war experiences and suicidal ideation among former child soldiers in Northern Uganda: the WAYS study. BMC Psychiatry 2014;**14**:271.

80. **Bayer CP, Klasen F, Adam H.** Association of trauma and PTSD symptoms with openness to reconciliation and feelings of revenge among former Ugandan and Congolese child soldiers. JAMA 2007;**298**:555–9.

81. **Vindevogel S, Wessells M, De Schryver M, Broekaert E, Derluyn I.** Informal and formal supports for former child soldiers in Northern Uganda. ScientificWorldJournal 2012;**2012**:825028.

82. **Vindevogel S, Broekaert E, Derluyn I.** It helps me transform in my life from the past to the new: the meaning of resources for former child soldiers. Journal of Interpersonal Violence 2013;**28**:2413–36.

83. **Vindevogel S, Wessells M, De Schryver M, Broekaert E, Derluyn I.** Dealing with the consequences of war: resources of formerly recruited and non-recruited youth in northern Uganda. Journal of Adolescent Health 2014;**55**:134–40.

84. **Volkan VD, Ast G, Greer WF.** The Third Reich in the unconscious: transgenerational transmission and its consequences. New York: Brunner-Routledge; 2002.

85. **Rutayisire T, Richters A.** Everyday suffering outside prison walls: a legacy of community justice in post-genocide Rwanda. Social Science & Medicine 2014;**120**:413–20.

86. **Tsfati Y, Weimann G.** www.terrorism.com: terror on the Internet. Studies in Conflict & Terrorism **2002**:317–32.

87. **Kohrt BA, Yang M, Rai S, Bhardwaj A, Tol WA, Jordans MJ.** Recruitment of child soldiers in Nepal: mental health status and risk factors for voluntary participation of youth in armed groups. Peace and Conflict 2016;**22**:208–16.

88. **Williams NE.** How community organizations moderate the effect of armed conflict on migration in Nepal. Population Studies 2013;**67**:353–69.

89. **Ghimire LV, Pun M.** Health effects of Maoist insurgency in Nepal. Lancet 2006;**368**:1494.

Chapter 8

The psychological impact of involvement in the Irish Republican Army during the 'Troubles': Preliminary evidence of moral injury

Eke Bont

8.1 Introduction

While there is a wealth of research available on the psychological effects of terrorism on its victims, little is known about the impact of terrorism on terrorists themselves. Thus far, research has predominantly explored whether psychological illness occurs in terrorists prior to their engagement in terrorism as a potential cause of their involvement. As a result, there is a lack of research on how involvement in terrorism affects the psychological well-being of terrorists either during or after their involvement [1, 2]. Further investigation into this is warranted, given that the terrorist lifestyle involves exposure to stressful, violent, and traumatic situations that may have a lasting impact on psychological well-being [3].

The research that is available on this topic indicates that some terrorists are psychologically affected by their involvement. For example, Kate Barrelle [4] found that former violent extremists may suffer from anxiety, paranoia, trauma, substance abuse, burnout, psychotic breakdown, and emotional breakdowns as a result of their involvement in terrorist groups. Corner and Gill [3] conducted probability-based behavioural sequence analyses on 90 terrorist autobiographies. These analyses indicated that the wide range of risk factors and stressors associated with engagement and disengagement with terrorism impacted on multiple aspects of the lives of less resilient individuals and had long-lasting psychological effects. Additionally, experiences of burnout [4–6] and guilt [7, 8] have been identified in a number of different terrorist groups. Research has also indicated that symptoms of psychological illnesses, such of post-traumatic stress disorder (PTSD), can be experienced by perpetrators of violence and homicide after they commit the offence [9, 10]. This research indicates that involvement in terrorism may have negative psychological consequences on terrorists themselves, and this topic therefore requires greater attention.

8.1.1 The psychological impact of the 'Troubles'

There is currently a mental health crisis in Northern Ireland, as there is indisputable evidence that its population has higher levels of chronic mental illness and substance abuse than other high-income countries [11]. Evidence suggests that the 'Troubles' have contributed directly to these rates [11–13]. The high rates of mental health problems in the general Northern Irish population would suggest that individuals who were directly involved in the 'Troubles' also suffer from resulting negative psychological effects. Former political prisoners of the 'Troubles' will commonly have endured a complex combination of burdens and losses associated with the conflict, including the mourning of deceased friends or loved ones, survivor guilt, fear, regret, anger, and humiliation [14]. They not only perpetrated violence, but often came from the most violent areas of the 'Troubles', suffered many negative experiences during interrogations and imprisonment, and—following the peace process—faced the significant challenges of transitioning from prison or active paramilitary groups [14, 15].

A study by Jamieson et al. [14] not only found indications of resilience and reflectiveness in former political prisoners in Northern Ireland, but also evidence of significant psychological harm as a result of their involvement in the 'Troubles'. For example, 39.9% of former political prisoners had scores indicative of mental health problems, 32.6% were taking prescription medication for anxiety and/or depression, over half reported feeling seriously depressed at some time since their release, and over half reported symptoms characteristic of PTSD. The authors suggested that, as a group, former politically motivated prisoners were substantially more likely than others in Northern Ireland to suffer from some form of psychological distress. Two other studies [16, 17] that interviewed former members of Northern Irish paramilitaries also found expressions of guilt, regret, and psychological distress as a result of their actions during the 'Troubles'. Further investigation is required to elucidate the psychological effects of Irish Republican Army (IRA) involvement. Therefore, this study explored whether former IRA members experienced moral injury.

8.1.2 Moral injury explained

Moral injury has recently received much attention in the field of military psychology, and refers to the lasting psychological and social harm caused by one's own, or another's, actions that transgressed deeply held moral beliefs and expectations in a high-stakes situation [18, 19]. It can occur when one 'perpetrates, fails to prevent, bears witness to, or learns about' such actions [18, p. 700]. While the phenomenon of moral injury appears to be ancient, clinical constructs to describe it are relatively new and developing [20]. Potential sources of moral injury can be divided into ones of personal responsibility (e.g. killing/injuring an enemy in battle, disproportionate violence, and harming civilians and civilian life), or events where others are responsible (e.g. betrayal by trusted others, betrayal by systems, others causing disproportionate violence, or harming civilians and civilian life) [21].

Moral injury can only occur when an individual is or becomes aware of the discrepancy between his/her moral beliefs and the experience, which subsequently creates cognitive dissonance and inner conflict [18]. These individuals are unable to accommodate the experience into pre-existing moral schemas successfully, which results in emotional responses and dysfunctional behaviours. While it is not categorized as a mental illness (22), moral injury can result in significant psychological distress. Its symptoms include guilt, shame, spiritual/existential conflict, loss of trust, depression, anxiety, anger, re-experiencing, intrusive throughs, self-harm, and social problems [18, 23, 24]. Negative self-appraisals of one's self as a result of moral injury may result in one withdrawing socially [18]. The capacity of moral injury to impair trust elevates despair, suicidality, and interpersonal violence because when social trust is destroyed it is replaced with an expectation of harm, exploitation, and humiliation [19]. Lastly, morally injurious experiences are often recalled intrusively and re-experienced, which can lead to psychological distress, avoidance, and emotional numbing [18].

Moral injury can be difficult to separate from other trauma syndromes, especially from PTSD, as they are often associated with one another or comorbid [24–26]. Moral injury and PTSD likely often co-occur given that they both arise after traumatic experiences [23, 24], although PTSD does not directly consider the potential harm produced by perpetration in traumatic contexts [18]. While PTSD arises after a life-threatening event, moral injury develops through a moral conflict of one's actions, or the actions of one's peers or leaders [24]. Moral injury can also occur in the absence of active PTSD symptoms, or with other disorders frequently associated with trauma, such as depression and substance abuse [27]. When moral injury arises in conjunction with mental illnesses, it may make such illnesses more severe or inhibit natural recovery processes.

8.1.3 **Moral injury in former IRA members**

While moral injury has been researched predominantly in the field of military psychology, it has also been applied in several populations other than veterans, and therefore appears not to be an exclusively military-related construct [26]. Contrary to general opinion that terrorists are purposeful and unconflicted in their acts, there are several indicators that moral injury may be experienced by former IRA members.

Members of the IRA during the 'Troubles' often considered themselves as soldiers operating in a military hierarchy, and this conflict as war. Ken Heskin [28] examined political violence in Northern Ireland, and argued that the behaviour in the paramilitaries during the 'Troubles' was, in some respects, similar to other conflict-oriented groups, such as national armed forces who may experience morally injurious events. Additionally, negative judgements about morally injurious events can be appropriate and accurate [18]. Therefore, morally injurious events can be morally unjustified, such as how many individuals would judge civilians being killed by IRA attacks to be. Some other common contextual factors in moral injury include hierarchical organizations, betrayal, and within-rank violence [23]. All of these factors were prevalent in the IRA during the 'Troubles'.

As mentioned previously, individuals involved in terrorism may exhibit psychological distress and guilt as a result of their involvement. Ferguson et al. [16] suggest this guilt may occur in former paramilitary members in Northern Ireland as a result of being 'forced' by paramilitaries to engage in what they perceived as immoral behaviours to bring about political change. This feeling of being 'forced\ to commit violence they later felt guilty about may come as a result of Northern Irish paramilitaries, especially Republican paramilitary members, feeling they had to resort to violence as their grievances could not be addressed through peaceful democratic processes. Therefore, the context of the 'Troubles' in Northern Ireland may have created an environment for moral injury, as some IRA members could have joined to address political grievances but were subsequently in a position where they committed or were associated with acts that they judged to be immoral.

8.2 Analysis of autobiographies

To explore whether former IRA members experienced moral injury, 10 autobiographies [29–38] were qualitatively analysed through interpretative phenomenological analysis (IPA). These autobiographical sources were usually written by the IRA members themselves. When written with or by co-authors, they evidenced a significant contribution to the work by the former IRA members themselves or included a considerable amount of their direct testimony. Autobiographies were chosen as they allowed the former IRA members to reflect on their experiences of membership in-depth, and therefore provided an insight into their personal experiences, perceptions, and insights. In addition, they allowed the individuals to 'speak for themselves', which increases the likelihood that they are reliable, valid, and representative of their experiences [6, 39].

However, there are some limitations associated with these sources that must be considered. This was a very small sample and therefore the results cannot be generalized to the wider population of disengaged IRA members. The sources might be affected by hindsight and retrospective bias, or may be biased as the authors may have been motivated to portray themselves (or the IRA) favourably or to justify previous actions. The findings in this study are only valid provided that the former IRA members offered a truthful account of their experiences. However, the intention of this study was to identify common themes on the psychological effects of involvement in the IRA, and therefore the aim was not to assess the 'truth' of such events, but how these events were represented, constructed into a public narrative, and interpreted by the individuals themselves to assert particular consequences.

8.2.1 **Evidence of morally injurious experiences**

The IPA results revealed there was preliminary evidence of moral injury in five of the autobiographical sources [30, 31, 34, 35, 38]. Despite the different circumstances, in all of these sources there were indications that the former IRA members experienced cognitive dissonance between their moral beliefs and some of the actions that they were affiliated with, witnessed, failed to prevent, or perpetrated themselves.

Some members were exposed to morally injurious experiences when confronted with the reality and consequences of the IRA's campaign of violence, which often resulted in realizations that this violence was morally unjustifiable. IRA members appeared to be at particular risk for moral injury when 'innocent civilians' rather than British targets were killed as a result of their own, or the IRA's, actions.

> This would be the end of my life. I would not be able to live with the guilt of blowing up innocent people. It did not matter that we had given warning by telephone, which was proof that we had not intended to kill or injure innocent people, nor did the collective nature of the effort dilute my own personal sense of guilt. This would be the end of everything. How would I ever rid myself of the guilt of this slaughter? [31, p. 55]

> I was horrified. Here in black and white, was the plainest proof that my use of violence had transformed me from an idealist on high moral ground to an offender with a seemingly endless list of human rights' violations to his name. None of this reeked of justice. I was coming face to face finally with the consequences of my long-distance bombings and I was not happy. There was no justification whatsoever for these injuries, and I was deeply sorry for the selfish and callous disregard I had shown for civilian casualties. [31, p. 157]

Guilt was the most common symptom of the potentially morally injurious experiences, with shame and anger commonly mentioned alongside feelings of guilt when the former IRA members reflected on their resulting affective states. However, depression, psychological distress, nightmares, and intrusive thoughts were also mentioned.

> I felt an extraordinary pain that would not go away. Every now and again I would fall off to sleep, but would wake again after what seemed a few minutes. In my sleep I moved in darkness, but the darkness seemed to have a form; like the mouth of a beast. I was inside the beast. Awake, the images in my mind were worse. I could see Mickey shooting him; see the lunchbox dropping to the ground, see Mickey's English football scarf catching the arc of blood that sprayed the air. I had never felt so empty. I had chosen this way and I could not turn back. I remember touching my wife, kissing her hair and crying silently. I was crying for Hanna, perhaps for his wife and child, but also mostly for myself, for what I had become. [35, p. 118]

A single case of a potentially morally injurious experience was found in Sean O'Callaghan's autobiography, which he experienced as a result of a murder of an informer by the IRA. An informer himself, O'Callaghan had provided persistent warnings to his Garda contact in order to prevent this, but, despite these warnings, the informer was murdered. This experience resulted in symptoms affiliated with moral injury, including lasting psychological distress, anger, exhaustion, and a loss of trust [18, 24].

> His murder haunted and sickened me then and has continued to do so ever since. There is no doubt that it destroyed my desire to continue as an informer. I knew that the work was important but although I could provide the necessary information I was powerless to ensure that people acted upon it. [30, p. 280]

Given that O'Callaghan had turned to informing as a result of his guilt for his actions as an IRA member, his general psychological state and potential moral injury were likely greatly worsened by this experience.

Richard O'Rawe and Brendan Hughes played roles in the hunger strike campaigns: O'Rawe as the provisional IRA press officer in Long Kesh Prison and Hughes as the Officer Commanding during the first hunger strike in 1980. Both individuals were greatly affected by witnessing the hunger strikes. Their moral injury was largely associated with the belief that they should have done more to end the campaign early, especially when the British government offered reasonable proposals.

> I remember almost crying with frustration and feeling that I was letting external influences impact on what I believed was the right thing to do. I hated Long Kesh, I hated the hunger strike, and most of all I hated myself. [38, p. 130]
>
> It was as simple as that, I felt guilty. And I continued feeling that way for many, many years afterwards ... I found it very, very hard to live with myself because I felt that possibly I should have been dead rather than the other ten men. [34, p. 249]

Their experiences led to symptoms of moral injury such as guilt, anger, negative self-appraisals, and despair [18, 23, 24]. To cope with these morally injurious experiences and symptoms, some of the former IRA members resorted to reparative actions such as apologizing, informing, sharing their experiences, and/ or engaging in community work [30, 31, 35, 38]. Reparative actions have been found to be a common response to moral injury, and have been suggested to have a therapeutic role such as by increasing social connectedness and reducing negative self-appraisals [18, 40]. However, it is unclear how much this helped them cope with their moral injury, and it is unlikely to have alleviated it fully. It may also be that the individuals wished to continue to be engaged in the conflict in a non-violent role, a common motivation in former political prisoners in Northern Ireland that aids their reintegration efforts [41].

8.2.2 Evidence of moral disillusionment and protective factors

Terrorists may become disillusioned with terrorism when their expectations are unmet, or when there is incongruence between their fantasies and the reality of terrorism [6, 42]. Disillusionment can occur when they are faced with the 'bitter reality' of perpetrating acts of violence against innocent victims or when 'acceptable' levels of violence are exceeded [6, 42]. Seventy per cent of former IRA members displayed varying levels of this type of disillusionment in their autobiographical sources [30, 31, 33–36, 38]. This experience will be referred to as 'moral disillusionment'. Moral disillusionment often led to them gradually perceiving the IRA's strategy of violence as morally unjustifiable, and sometimes resulted in disengagement from the organization. It evoked feelings of conflictedness, hopelessness, and guilt.

> Surely Belfast had realized how far they were overloading the system, and that twenty warnings could never be dealt with? If they hadn't realized it, they had no business dealing with bombs at all. And if they had ... there was no way their actions could be justified. [36, p. 148]
>
> I had lost so much of what was moral and good in my fight against oppression that I had been left without faith in any defensible aspect of civilization. [35, p. 339]
>
> I was so convinced by my own experience that violence is guaranteed to injure or kill the innocent, that I was being drawn inevitably toward a pacifist position. I could no longer cordon off my attacks on military or political targets as 'legitimate' or 'just'—I felt that only a pacifist position was truly moral, or truly Christlike. I may have been working on the feeling that only a pacifist outlook would guarantee a conscience free from the guilt of having maimed and hurt people. [31, p. 170]

Both moral injury and moral disillusionment occurred most frequently when the IRA condoned acts that resulted in disproportionate violence and 'unnecessary' deaths, including those of civilians, informers, and hunger strikers. This resulted in cognitive dissonance between the individual's involvement in the IRA and their moral beliefs. It is therefore likely that for some individuals, experiences of moral injury interacted with moral disillusionment and led to psychological and/or physical disengagement from the IRA, even if the Republican ideology was still supported. This is in line with suggestions that moral injury in military personnel can cause disenchantment with previously held values and an army's morality [43]. However, there was also evidence that IRA members experienced strategical disillusionment rather than moral disillusionment when they perceived the strategy of violence to be counterproductive to the Republican cause [29, 35–37].

The analysis found that some of the IRA members viewed the IRA's strategy of violence as morally justifiable (either temporarily or consistently). These beliefs are likely to have protected these individuals from moral injury and disillisionment, as they would not have felt conflicted between their actions and moral values. In five of the autobiographies, contextual factors were found to have shaped moral beliefs regarding the justification of violence [29, 31, 32, 35, 38]. Firstly, the culture of romanticization of the Republican cause prevented some individuals from questioning the morality of it.

> But [the romanticization of Republicanism] also inoculated us against the cruelty of our protest and the reality of the situation, and blinded us to the modern world and political events of the day. [38, p. 72]

Violence was normalized, or even seen as exciting, for many of the members who grew up in Northern Ireland during this time. This may have resulted in a gradual disinhibition and perceived legitimization of violence. Additionally, witnessing or experiencing violence caused by British soldiers resulted in some individuals seeking out violence as a form of revenge, which was believed to be justified and legitimized.

There was also evidence of an unquestioning devotion to the Republican cause [29, 30, 35]. Such devotion was commonly found to result in an acceptance of civilian casualties and led to their moral beliefs being dictated by the organization.

> If the IRA told me to shoot somebody, I did, because the IRA was right. [29, p. 154]

Certain personality types were found to be more prone to condoning the use of violence and did not reflect on questions of its morality. Some of these individuals were even found to be enjoying the violence. For example, Eamon Collins stated that a member 'gleefully' described murders he had committed [35, p. 139]. Collins himself attempted to harden himself against his feelings of guilt and doubts but was unsuccessful in this, which eventually resulted in a breakdown. Litz et al. [18] suggest that moral injury is only possible if

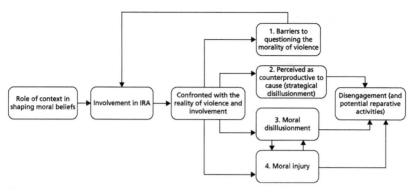

Fig. 8.1 Relationships between the themes relevant to moral injury found in the analysis of the autobiographical sources.

IRA, Irish Republican Army.

an individual has an intact moral belief system. Given that a combination of these different factors would have impaired the IRA members' moral reasoning (either temporarily or consistently), this would have decreased susceptibility to moral injury, as their actions would not conflict with their moral beliefs.

8.3 **Conclusion**

The analysis of the 10 autobiographical sources revealed some preliminary evidence of moral injury in former IRA members, and how these experiences may have contributed to moral disillusionment with the organization. It also demonstrated how specific factors shaped moral belief systems that prevented susceptibility to moral injury. Fig. 8.1 illustrates and summarizes the potential relationships between all of these themes.

However, interviews with former IRA members are required to draw concrete conclusions on the occurrence of moral injury in this population. This would develop an increased understanding of some of the psychological consequences of involvement in violent organizations, such as the IRA. Such an understanding would likely aid disengagement and reintegration efforts. Given the rise in tensions and increase in activity of dissident Republican groups in Northern Ireland in recent years, this research may only prove to be more urgent and necessary.

References

1. **Corner E, Gill P.** The nascent empirical literature on psychopathology and terrorism. World Psychiatry 2018;**17**:147–8.

2. **Horgan JG.** Psychology of terrorism: introduction to the special issue. American Psychologist 2017;**72**:199–204.

3. **Corner E, Gill P.** Psychological distress, terrorist involvement and disengagement from terrorism: a sequence analysis approach. Journal of Quantitative Criminology 2019, DOI: 10.1007/s10940-019-09420-1.

4. **Barrelle K.** Pro-integration: disengagement from and life after extremism. Behavioral Sciences of Terrorism and Political Aggression 2015;**7**:129–42.

5. **Reinares F.** Exit from terrorism: a qualitative empirical study on disengagement and deradicalization among members of ETA. Terrorism and Political Violence 2011;**23**:780–803.

6. **Altier MB, Leonard Boyle E, Shortland ND, Horgan JG.** Why they leave: an analysis of terrorist disengagement events from eighty-seven autobiographical accounts. Security Studies 2017;**26**:305–32.

7. **Horgan J.** Walking away from terrorism: accounts of disengagement from radical and extremist movements. Abingdon and New York: Routledge; 2009.

8. **Kellen K.** On terrorists and terrorism. Available from: https://www.rand.org/pubs/notes/N1942.html [accessed 30 July 2020].

9. **Evans C, Ehlers A, Mezey G, Clark DM.** Intrusive memories in perpetrators of violent crime: emotions and cognitions. Journal of Consulting and Clinical Psychology 2007;**75**:134–44.

10. **Pollock PH.** When the killer suffers: post-traumatic stress reactions following homicide. Legal and Criminological Psychology 1999;**4**:185–202.

11. **O'Neill S, Ferry F, Heenan D.** Mental health disorders in Northern Ireland: the economic imperative. The Lancet Psychiatry 2016;**3**:398–400.

12. **Bunting BP, Murphy SD, O'Neill SM, Ferry FR.** Lifetime prevalence of mental health disorders and delay in treatment following initial onset: evidence from the Northern Ireland Study of Health and Stress. Psychological Medicine 2012;**42**:1727–39.

13. **Ferry F, Bunting B, Murphy S, O'Neill S, Stein D, Koenen K.** Traumatic events and their relative PTSD burden in Northern Ireland: a consideration of the impact of the 'Troubles'. Social Psychiatry and Psychiatric Epidemiology 2014;**49**:435–46.

14. **Jamieson R, Shirlow P, Grounds A.** Ageing and social exclusion among former politically motivated prisoners in Northern Ireland and the border region of Ireland. Belfast: Changing Age Partnership; 2010.

15. **McEvoy K, Shirlow P, McElrath K.** Resistance, transition and exclusion: politically motivated ex-prisoners and conflict transformation in Northern Ireland. Terrorism and Political Violence 2004;**16**:646–70.

16. **Ferguson N, Burgess M, Hollywood I.** Who are the victims? Victimhood experiences in postagreement Northern Ireland. Political Psychology 2010;**31**:857–86.

17. **Burgess M, Ferguson N, Hollywood I.** Rebels' perspectives of the legacy of past violence and of the current peace in post-agreement Northern Ireland: an interpretative phenomenological analysis. Political Psychology 2007;**28**:69–88.

18. **Litz BT, Stein N, Delaney E, Lebowitz L, Nash WP, Silva C, et al.** Moral injury and moral repair in war veterans: a preliminary model and intervention strategy. Clinical Psychology Review 2009;**29**:695–706.

19. **Shay J.** Moral injury. Psychoanalytic Psychology 2014;**31**:182–91.

20. **Nash WP, Carper TLM, Mills MA, Au T, Goldsmith A, Litz BT.** Psychometric evaluation of the Moral Injury Events Scale. Military Medicine 2013;**6**:646–52.

21. **Schorr Y, Stein NR, Maguen S, Barnes JB, Bosch J, Litz BT.** Sources of moral injury among war veterans: a qualitative evaluation. Journal of Clinical Psychology 2018;**74**:2203–18.

22. **Maguen S, Litz BT.** Moral injury in veterans of war. PTSD Research Quarterly 2012;**23**:1–6.

23. **Drescher KD, Foy DW, Kelly C, Leshner A, Schutz K, Litz B.** An exploration of the viability and usefulness of the construct of moral injury in war veterans. Traumatology 2011;**17**:8–13.

24. **Jinkerson JD.** Defining and assessing moral injury: a syndrome perspective. Traumatology 2016;**22**:122–30.

25. **Farnsworth JK, Drescher KD, Evans W, Walser RD.** A functional approach to understanding and treating military-related moral injury. Journal of Contextual Behavioral Science 2017;**6**:391–7.

26. **Griffin BJ, Purcell N, Burkman K, Litz BT, Bryan CJ, Schmitz M, et al.** Moral injury: an integrative review. Journal of Traumatic Stress 2019;**32**:350–62.

27. **Farnsworth JK, Drescher KD, Nieuwsma JA, Walser RB, Currier JM.** The role of moral emotions in military trauma: implications for the study and treatment of moral Injury. Review of General Psychology 2014;**18**:249–62.

28. **Heskin K.** Political violence in Northern Ireland. The Journal of Psychology 1985;**119**:481–94.

29. **Bradley G, Feeney B.** Insider: Gerry Bradley's life in the IRA, second edition. Dublin: The O'Brien Press; 2011.

30. **O'Callaghan S.** The informer. London: Corgi; 1999.

31. **O'Doherty SP.** The volunteer. Durham, CT: Strategic Book Publishing & Rights Agency; 2011.

32. **Doherty T.** The dead beside us: a memoir of growing up in Derry. Cork: The Mercier Press; 2017.

33. **Morrison D.** Then the walls came down: a prison journal. Cork: Mercier Press; 2018.

34. **Moloney E.** Voices from the grave: two men's war in Ireland, paperback edition. London: Faber and Faber; 2011.

35. **Collins E, McGovern M.** Killing rage. New York: Granta Books; 1998.

36. **McGuire M.** To take arms: a year in the Provisional IRA. London: Quartet Books; 1973.

37. **Anderson B, Cahill J.** Joe Cahill: a life in the IRA. Dublin: O'Brien Press; 2004.

38. **O'Rawe R.** Blanketmen: an untold story of the H-Block hunger strike. Dublin: New Island Books; 2016.

39. **Altier MB, Horgan J, Thoroughgood C.** In their own words? Methodological considerations in the analysis of terrorist autobiographies. Journal of Strategic Security 2012;**5**:85–98.

40. **Held P, Klassen BJ, Hall JM, Friese TR, Bertsch-Gout MM, Zalta AK, et al.** 'I knew it was wrong the moment I got the order': a narrative thematic analysis of moral injury in combat veterans. Psychological Trauma 2019;**11**:396–405.

41. **Ferguson N, Burgess M, Hollywood I.** Leaving violence behind: disengaging from politically motivated violence in Northern Ireland. Political Psychology 2015;**36**:199–214.

42. **Horgan J.** The psychology of terrorism, revised and updated second edition. Abingdon: Routledge; 2014.

43. **Molendijk T, Kramer E-H, Verweij D.** Moral aspects of 'moral injury': analyzing conceptualizations on the role of morality in military trauma. Journal of Military Ethics 2018;**17**:36–53.

Chapter 9

Terrorism and radicalization: Social factors—a narrative review

Donato Favale and Antonio Ventriglio

9.1 Introduction

Over the history of humanity, people have killed themselves for all kinds of reasons, some of which are personal and some are more social. On occasion, those killing themselves have decided to take others with them, either as an act of vengeance or simply as a political statement in order to achieve some specified or unspecified goal. Acts of terrorism and underlying causes are not recent phenomena, but the practice and reasons may have changed. It has been traditionally argued that wars are often for reasons of land grab, property, or imposing ideologies on others. Acts of terrorism frighten people, but equally importantly they often create a counterterror response, which must be firm and can be subtle and tailored, or aggressive and perhaps disproportionate. Those who commit terrorist acts or atrocities may reach that decision for a number of reasons because of a number of personality traits or external social or societal factors. In this chapter we provide a brief historic overview and then develop reasons for why people ascribe to radicalisation and terrorism. Social factors and social determinants play a major role in influencing social cohesion or alienation, which may contribute to radicalization. We illustrate these by using examples from Italy.

9.2 Brief history

In ancient Rome, rates of suicide and suicidal attempts were high among slaves. Individuals who feel trapped can use suicide as an act of freedom from entrapment and to gain a sense of control. In ancient Rome, slaves used suicide to punish their owners for the cruelty that had been bestowed upon them. Such acts of suicide also caused economic damage to the owners [1]. Consequently laws were brought in to make acts of suicide or attempts illegal, thereby reducing the rates dramatically. Although such laws are in place in many countries, even now their failure to control suicides indicates that certain behaviours and reactions to oppression will continue, irrespective of societal expectations. Control of certain behaviours by social constraints and societal expectations can, in turn, lead to further simmering resentment and rebellion.

However, one of the early examples is the movement spearheaded by the Zealots in first century BC. The Zealots were Jewish nationalists who encouraged mass insurrection by the poor against the emperor by refusing to pay taxes. There were mass suicides because they felt unable to defeat their enemies in other ways [2]. Almost a millennium later, in 1090, Hasan-i-Sabbah founded the sect of Muslim assassins who used hashish before killing people in crowded places for political and religious reasons [3–5]. The underlying philosophy was that it was better to die in a battle than to survive a lost battle. Similar concepts were described in kamikaze pilots in the Second World War. These were pilots who died in the process killing others as a result of their actions. They were often young and their acts were strongly culturally influenced in that they were sacrificing themselves for their Emperor and country.

Terrorism has been used as term to ascribe an activity that, in theory, focuses on attacking other individuals or groups for the purpose of obtaining certain rights and freedom, but the reality is often quite different. It has been argued that one man's terrorist is another man's freedom fighter. François-Noël Baboeuf (1760–1797) suggested that, in order to defeat an oppressor, every possible way was legitimate. Similar sentiments were expressed by others, such as Karl Heinzen (1809–1880). Others, for example in Russia, saw terrorism as a humanitarian activity. When Spain invaded the Philippines and imposed religious conversion to Roman Catholicism, the native population could resist it only by using suicide attacks [1].

The scenarios are complex and show variations that are difficult to generalize. We use biographies to illustrate some of the factors that play a role in developing radicalization. The following biographies show a diversity of terrorist threats, individual circumstances, religious histories, and preoccupations; we have only presented a few and propose that there are many more typologies that could be presented. Indeed, each convicted terrorist or those under suspicion appear to present with unique features, making it difficult to generalize. Thus, in the chapter, although we seek to present overarching theories that are historically contextualized, the challenges in so doing are great and we urge the readers not to adopt a formulaic approach.

Usman Khan, aged 25 years, used a knife to hack at and kill people in a crowded place near London Bridge in November 2019. He had a past history of being involved in terrorist offences when he was 15 years, and had been released from prison; thus, he is not the usual terrorist/jihadist. Osama bin Laden was a well-known terrorist of his generation who came from a reasonably well-to-do family from Saudi Arabia. He worked in Afghanistan with American support against Russian invaders, and then turned against the United States by plotting major terrorist attacks. The third example is Steven Chand from Canada. He was born of Fijian Hindu parents but converted to Islam. Under the influence of an extremist Imam, he became involved in terrorist activities. These three individuals offer very different views about terrorism and their radicalization. In this chapter, we illustrate some of the influencing factors using these examples. These are not meant to be psycho-biographies waiting to be analysed, but simple indicators. For example, as in the case of Usman Khan, the Madrid bombers Alleka Lamari and Jamal Ahmidan were deeply indoctrinated in prisons, which may have a very provocative way of seeking revenge if not on the target, but on someone else representing that target.

9.3 **Social dynamics**

The main aim of terrorist activity is to use indiscriminate violence in order to scare people to take them away from their usual activity and frighten them in a way to perpetrate acts that carry a political, religious, or ideological aim to create change [2]. The target of such extreme political ideologies is not only to subvert, but also to bring about social, political, racial, religious, and economic change and supremacy. The term radicalization is used to describe a degree of change in a vulnerable individual that alters their worldview and thinking to deliver their political, ideological, or religious aims. Research interest in this field has grown since the 9/11 attacks in New York in order to understand why, how, and at what point people like bin Laden get radicalized and carry young people with them.

Radicalization should be seen as a process by which a group or an individual develops interest in and then carries out a violent action, which is connected to an extremist ideology and challenges the established cultural, social, or political order. As in all the biographies illustrated above, it is the violent nature of the act that is worrying, as well as frightening. Doosje et al. [11] created a three-level model after analysing risk factors of radicalization in European youth. These three levels were macroenvironmental factors, microenvironmental factors, and individual factors. In this model, macroenvironmental factors were represented by geopolitics, societal polarization, and religiosity, while microenvironmental factors were friendship with radicalized individuals and dysfunction in the family, thus creating a sense of isolation and alienation. These combine with other factors at an individual level such as personal uncertainty, perceived injustice, psychological vulnerability, experiences of vulnerability, and abandonment to contribute to a move towards radicalization. Therefore, an interaction between the radical system and the subject may contribute to a sense of acceptance and acknowledgement. These changes at an individual level can be linked with microenvironmental factors, which, combined with the use of dehumanization, make the use of violence legitimate and then analogous with sectarian communities or groups, which then interact with the macroenvironmental level and lead to the proposal of a new societal model [2]. With modern technologies, especially the immediacy and perpetual nature of social media, connections are rapid, as is the sharing of disgruntlement, leading to rapid transmission of ideologies that can make violent acts more likely in the right circumstances.

9.3.1 Social media

Social media has a major role in communication, in providing support, and in managing responses. According to Sageman [53], the increasing use of the Internet by jihadist movements since the 2000s has modified terrorist organizations. Consequently, today's radical groups are less centralized than previous hierarchical institutions such as Al-Qaeda. In this new organization the groups are younger, more discrete, smaller, and may well have more fragile persons. In Europe, it seems difficult to integrate the second- and the third-generation children of immigrants from both a social and economic and cultural point of view, so many young people of Muslim heritage find themselves in precarious positions trying to balance religious heritage and the secular West. It is argued that this conflict and ambivalence of identity is a vulnerability factor for extremism. But not everyone in such a position is lured to crime or terrorism, so we need more research on what additional factors are at play, rather than overly emphasizing more evident group characteristics as if these alone account for such rare and complex phenomenon.

9.3.2 Re-radicalization and social factors

Another model proposes that the radicalization process is constituted by four distinct steps: pre-radicalization, self-identification, indoctrination, and jihadization [3]. Some argue that pre-radicalization involves internalization and exposure to extremist and more fundamental religious ideologies, such as jihadi Salafism. In this phase an individual reconsiders their world—religion, lifestyle, neighbourhood, and social status—before the commitment to a process of radicalization. People involved in terrorist activities appear to have little contact with the criminal justice system and come from ordinary backgrounds, although even this apparent finding is inconsistent. In the self-identification stage people are conditioned by external and internal factors, and individuals begin to investigate more extremist movements. External factors are represented by social and economic marginalization, the abuse of the security forces and the state, the failure of governance, and human rights violation. Other internal factors are relevant such as frustration, lack of opportunity, or unemployment [4]. Generally, there are some crises that start in this phase that are especially political, economic, social, and personal, and lead people to 'religious seeking'. Furthermore, in this stage, the Internet can play a very important role because through it people can virtually meet and so share and discuss, for example, Salafi-jihadi messages that selectively advocate violence as a solution. In the indoctrination stage an individual internalizes jihadi principles. That action is militant jihad. At the end, in the jihadization stage, members feel dutybound to sacrifice themselves as holy warriors. In this phase the group prepares the terrorist attack. In this stage reinforcement plays an important role to progress their decision to die. The reinforcements include extremist websites and jihadist videos that exalt death by jihad as a true hero's destination. For some, seeking religious justification often represents a sacred cause and suicidal trigger, while for others seeking action is more to fight for a particular cause and to become a mujahedeen [3].

As detailed earlier, other external factors can be social and economic, among others, and each of these factors can play a role and sometimes there may be a cumulative effect.

9.3.3 Sympathy for the cause

Sympathy for a cause and a degree of belief in it can lead to a sense of purpose and belonging. This can be one of the many determining social and personal factors. Links with the family and their perceptions also play a major role in determining how individuals deal with alienation, which can contribute to believing in a cause. Believing in a cause does not always lead to action or response.

In a survey from 2019, 618 White British and Pakistani living in London aged 18–45 years were recruited in three different localities [5] Different variables were measured: ethnicity, mental disorder, social capital, SyfoR (16-item inventory of radicalization), age, discrimination, and mental status. The study showed that 61% of respondents condemned terrorist actions and violent protest, while only 13% had sympathy for violent protest and terrorism (SVPT). SVPT was more frequent in persons with a criminal history, heavy alcohol users, drug users, and those with a history of trauma. There was no association with personality disorder or autism. SVPT was positively associated with a diagnosis of dysthymia, major depression, anxiety disorders, and post-traumatic stress disorder. SVPTs were most often expressed by people born in the UK, those who spoke English at home, and those who were single, younger, and with a higher income and full-time education than those born outside the UK, older, married, and divorced. Extremist sympathies were less prevalent in Pakistani people than White British, suggesting a focus on Muslim populations may be mistaken, if right-wing extremism is more important and prevalent. Other studies suggest the link between extremist attitudes and mental illness are weaker in group-based terrorism than in lone actors [5, 6]. Unemployment, poverty, discrimination, cultural marginalization, and political isolation led to complaints, which, in turn, predisposed to political violence [7].

The experiencing of a serious problem with a close friend, relative, or neighbour, or another major event can cause depression. Generally, depression has been shown to be associated with suicidal behaviour and impulsivity and these, in turn, can be connected to a risk of violence [8, 9]. It is possible that poor political engagement and preventing the development of depressive responses to adverse life events might lower the risk of SVPT. Low levels of socio-economic and educational backgrounds were not found to be typical of terrorists [10]. Doosje et al. [11] found that perceived injustice predisposes to perceived societal disconnectedness and this increases violent attitudes. Perceiving collective deprivation induces emotional uncertainty, which, in turn, predicts in-group superiority (the members of the in-group evaluate themselves to be superior to all other groups). This feeling predisposes to violence. When self-uncertainty becomes pervasive, people are very attracted to extremist groups, because they provide a clear example for how one should think, behave toward out-group members, and feel in every situation [12]. Albert Ellis [13] identified some absolutist questions that terrorists might have. These include the position that Americans must absolutely not hinder their standpoint; they had to punish America (self-questions); and the world should be fair and just (world demands) [13]. These absolutist questions determine two categories of irrational beliefs: global evaluation of human worth (ego disturbance beliefs) and low frustration tolerance beliefs (discomfort disturbance beliefs). Thus, it is entirely possible that individuals who act in terrorist ways may well become envious and vengeful, and are conditioned by extremist propaganda, which claims that Western countries (or another perceived oppressor) are unfaithful. They may feel envy for Western countries' affluence and power.

Terrorism can be seen as a truly scary and powerful form of persuasion that makes political gains and causes fear by sustaining infectious and dangerous ideas [14]; however, these actions are strongly influenced by social dynamics. Stares and Yacubian see this as an infection [15, 16]. In their model, militant ideologies are the infectious agents, terrorist organizations are similar to a vulnerable host, and settings such as the Internet and prison act as vehicles or vectors for transmission. Hence, their presumptive observation is that by strengthening individuals and eliminating social stressors, radicalization may be limited.

9.4 **Alienation**

As already mentioned, alienation is important, but it cannot be seen as a separate characteristic and ought to be recognized as related to identity (individual and group) and acculturation. There is little doubt that migrants as individuals and as a group go through the process of acculturation and one of the potential consequences is alienation. This has been described in various ways, and here we describe some of the steps.

Quintan Wiktorowicz [17] introduced the notion of 'cognitive opening', which is the moment when a person who faces political repression, socio-economic crisis, and discrimination is trying to understand life events and suddenly their previous beliefs shake and they become vulnerable and sympathetic to the new radical ideology. Although concepts of individual self may change across cultures, the degree of belonging to a community or to a group is very important and allows acculturation. As Gezentsvey Lamy et al. [18] suggest, small groups might meet uncertainty about their existence so ethnocultural continuity is indispensable for emotional survival. Cultural continuity means consideration of connections between future and the past, as well as cultural and symbolic heritage [18]. John Berry [19] affirms that intercultural contacts are very important and that cultural identity is a sense of commitment or attachment to a cultural group. According to Berry, acculturation and cultural identity are both a psychological and cultural phenomenon, which is in opposition to the position of Theodore Graves [20], who states that acculturation is only psychological. Berry et al. [21] explained that acculturative stress might affect social, somatic, and psychological aspects of an individual's functioning. Bhui et al. [22] say that some of the risk factors for radicalization (causative) may be changed by increasing social capital, improving well-being, and managing depression. Violent radicalization might reflect inequalities in health or social status, and is not a new phenomenon. Poor education, discrimination, and unsatisfactory employment can play a role. Religious conversion, a sense of alienation, and poor political engagement induce vulnerability to many adverse health outcomes and social isolation [23].

Alienation is an individual's feeling of discomfort or unease, reflecting their self-exclusion or exclusion from cultural and social participation [24]. Poor acculturation and consequent violent radicalization may be provoked by alienation emerging from a failed search for belonging and identity. A sense of alienation may be sparked by many factors and can be worsened by culture conflict; it causes delinquency and deviance, while radicalization provides individuals with a sense of belonging. Factors that are very close or similar between two cultures may support and enable acculturation—such as shared language, and diet and lifestyle preferences—and reduce alienation. Whereas differences such as religious values and practice may increase the sense of alienation and isolation. The sense of primary non-belonging will cause belonging to a subgroup or a gang with its own cultural taboos and nuances. It has also been observed that religious fervour and malignant narcissism may conduct to radicalization [25]. Of the three biographies, bin Laden certainly was not a migrant to the West where he needed acculturation, whereas other three did. bin Laden moved from Saudi Arabia to Afghanistan and other places, but his alienation was of a different kind.

9.5 **Lone actors**

Behavioural differences were analysed between lone actors with and without mental illness [6]. Lone actors without a history of mental illness were 18.07 times less likely to have a partner involved in a wider movement than lone actors who were mentally ill. Those with a mental illness were more likely to have experienced chronic and proximate stress, to have been a recent victim of prejudice, and to have a proximate upcoming life. The attempts to understand such behaviours have included psychoanalytic, developmental, and behavioural theories. For example, throughout the 1980s terrorists were defined from a psychoanalytical point of view as emotionally damaged youths who were rejected by their families, which delayed their attainment of adult identity, and not as aggressive psychopaths [26].

Gill and Deckert [27] analysed the antecedent behaviours and sociodemographic network characteristics of 119 lone-actor terrorists in Europe and the United States. The authors observed that the vast majority (96.6%) of the sample were male and the age of the offenders ranged from 15 to 69 years (mean 33 years). Gender remains an important factor. Half of the sample was made up of single individuals who had never married, although one-quarter (24%) were married and over one-fifth (22%) were separated. Over half (52.9%) of the sample was socially isolated. At the time of their terrorist event or arrest, 40.2% were unemployed. The three most prevalent ideologies identified in the members of the sample were single issue (environmentalism, antiabortion, and animal rights), right-wing, and al-Qaeda-related ideologies. -inspired represented one-third of the total sample. The average age of al-Qaeda-related lone actors was 10 years younger than that of either the single-issue or the right-wing cohorts, and the members had more culture and sought legitimization from social, political, and religious leaders. Compared to al-Qaeda-inspired offenders and single-issue ones, right-wing lone-actor terrorists did not have a university education and were unemployed. Single-issue lone actors were more likely to be in relationships than the other two groups and more often had been previously imprisoned and had previous criminal convictions. Successful lone-actor terrorists were more often socially isolated, with a university education, a history of mental illness, and had been previously rejected from a wider movement or group.

9.5.1 Terrorism and psychiatric disorders

Psychiatric disorders have been identified as one of the factors contributing to the acts by lone actors, as shown in the case of Usman Khan detailed earlier. These are worth exploring in detail as appropriate and adequate treatments should help reduce the incidents and potential for damage. A key question for debate is whether these individuals have various kinds of personality disorders or not.

Mental illnesses (including a range of conditions but not clinically diagnosed), were 13 times more likely to occur in lone actors than in group-based terrorists, especially psychoses rather than depression [6, 27]. It would appear that autism spectrum, delusional disorder, and schizophrenia might be more common in lone actors, as is the likelihood of affective and schizophrenia-spectrum disorders. However, it has been noted that terrorism groups have refused to recruit people with a history of mental illness [28]. As mentioned earlier, the development of extreme beliefs might be related to certain personality traits, such as the need for group identification, identity fusion, low levels of empathy, cognitive complexity, uncertainty, rational decision-making, and morbid transcendence [29–32]. Radicalization has also been shown to be connected with higher scores on schizotypal personality disorder and paranoid personality disorder. A recent systematic review revealed that radical involvement among European youths might be encouraged by personal uncertainty, family dysfunction, perceived injustice, early experiences of abandonment, social changes, and friendship with radicalized individuals [2]. Thus, vulnerable personality traits and micro- and macroenvironmental factors interact together to create a purpose that may well lead to or follow radicalization.

Analysis of the difference between lone actors with and without mental illness indicated that successful lone actors terrorists were more often isolated, with a history of mental illness, and rejected from a group or wider movement. It is important to understand the interaction of various factors, and we turn to French sociologist Emile Durkheim. Durkheim studied the rates of and possible explanations for variations in rates of suicide.

9.6 **Durkheim's anomie**

Durkheim explained anomie as one of the contributing factors in rates of suicide. We correlate anomie with religious fundamentalism and experiences related to migration. One of the major types of suicidal acts is that of terrorism in which people die while trying to kill others. Durkheim described anomie as state of normlessness in society. Hence, he argued, anomic suicide occurs in a society where an individual has a sense of anxiety and feelings of separation or rejection from groups or society, and a perception that no certain goals exist [33]. Durkheim described two types of anomie. The first is inappropriate procedural rules to control complementary relationships among the interdependent and specialized parts of a complex social system. The second is having insufficient moral norms of social control. It is well recognized that rates of suicide tend to go up in times of financial and industrial crises. Although such an increase of suicide is not caused by poverty but by 'crises of prosperity' (periods of prosperity and economic growth). The type of society (whether it is egocentric or sociocentric) has a moral power over the person through control of human desires and needs. Crises can induce the society to become incapable of exercising control over individuals. This itself can lead to a sense of normlessness and anomie. Suicide bombs and suicide attacks reflect the confusion in the society caused by social changes, as the needs and the values of both the individual and society—particularly of alienated people—may suddenly change.

To explain the external and internal variation in rates of suicide, Durkheim used concepts of moral regulation and social integration. He postulated a relationship between degree of social integration and suicide rates. His four types of suicide—altruistic, egoistic, fatalistic, and anomic—are all related to the integration and cohesion of the social group. Both religious suicide bombing and apocalyptic suicide represent a final cosmic war in which violence is sanctioned to rid the world of evil forces [34]. This may be seen as a vulnerable and radicalized individual trying to take control back in their life even if it leads to the destruction of their own life which can be seen as ultimate control. Therefore, that the act of self-destruction may take others with them is an acceptable scenario. Terrorist attacks are about asserting a degree of control in their own lives.

9.7 **Religious fundamentalism**

We do not plan to cover the role or definitions of religion in this chapter. Suffice it to say that all religions—but especially the monotheistic ones—expect a certain amount of ritualistic behaviour from the individual. Consequently, if these rituals are not followed, they can be overtly or covertly excluded from the community. As mentioned earlier, part of the acculturation process is related to identity, which will include religion as a microidentity and thus second- and third-generation migrants may try harder to hang on to their identity by embracing religion in a more rigid and ritualistic manner.

It is possible to consider religious fundamentalism as a defence mechanism against anxiety, which will be seen as protective, especially when an individual is performing religious rituals. Four coping strategies described in the literature include, firstly, that religious fundamentalism gives a sense of coherence and meaning to life. Secondly, fundamentalists are isolationists but follow clear rules. Thirdly, extreme religious integralism and the resulting behaviour are seen as a purification from sins. Lastly, it is about coping without involving God [23, 35, 36]. Violent radicalization is both the consequence of religious fundamentalism and its cause in creating a sense of purpose and belonging. It can be argued that this phenomenon has led to discrimination of migrants and particularly people of Muslim heritage who are born and brought up and born in the West but still face daily Islamophobia. Generally, the first generation attempts to assimilate two cultures, while in the second generation the risk of a culture conflict increases. The third generation may feel further isolated, not having a sense of belonging and in search for an identity [37]. We postulate that these identities and acculturative strategies will vary whether individuals are first-generation or second- or third-generation migrants, and this needs to be explored and studied in future research.

Different dimensions have been suggested for religious fundamentalism. Various authors have introduced the 'three-B' classification of religious belief, behaviour (praxis), and belonging (group identification). It has been observed that these three aspects have conflicting and different effects [38, 39]. It is possible that child-rearing practices may inculcate various ideas of religious fundamentalism in children and young people, but research in the Netherlands, Denmark, and the UK has demonstrated that that there is no clear relation between radicalization and child-raising practices in Muslim families [40].

As part of the acculturation process and in spite of culture conflict, all generations carry cultural norms that respond to processes of assimilation. It is, indeed, inevitable that in many settings and cultures, intergenerational struggles occur very often where young Muslims opposed the culturally influenced practices and beliefs of their parents [41, 42]. Not every radicalized individual has been to religious schools, and some individuals like Usman Khan and Steven Chand mentioned earlier converted to Islam late in life, indicating that perhaps something was missing, which they were trying to find [43–45]. There is no doubt that some of these vulnerable individuals are susceptible to the charms of charismatic leaders.

Max Weber points out that the leader of the group influences other members and induces them to perform actions according to the leader's will. Lynne Lamberg, studying authoritarianism, notes that the leader holds total control over the group [46], while others have described charisma as being a contagious pathology [47]. These types of leadership are associated with group fragility and under those circumstances these leaders can persuade their followers to commit mass suicide [48]. In Freudian theory the passivity of the crowd is interpreted as a return to archaic patterns in which the leader represents the superego of each follower. Other explanations have been offered by Géza Róheim [49], who sees these acts as an attempt to find a state of childhood happiness, and Georges Devereux, who attributes these to the 'infantilised leader alone' [50].

9.7.1 **Role of migration**

Migration has been happening for millennia, but the question remains of whether those who are vulnerable to psychiatric disorders or terrorist acts are more likely to migrate, or whether something changes in them or their circumstances after migration that contributes to their acts. Following an analysis of a number of terrorist attacks in 145 countries carried out between 1970 and 2000, it was noted that migrants who migrate from terror-prone states are more likely to spread these acts [51]. This contradicts other studies that have shown migrants to be less likely to be involved in terrorist acts, and it is the second and third generation—so called 'home grown'—that become terrorists. There is no doubt that any migrant inflows could constitute a connection between states, leading to the spread of ideologies and subsequent behaviours. In January 2015, the then Italian Minister of Foreign Affairs Paolo Gentiloni affirmed that there was a risk that terrorists could come among the thousands of migrants who arrive in Italy from North Africa every year [52]. However, not all migrants are terrorists, and political ideologies and anti-immigrant feelings in recent times in many countries have led to nationalism and xenophobia. The important thing to remember is that what happens to migrants after they have reached the new country, their acceptance and welcome, racism, and attitudes to them will all play a role in acculturation and settlement. As mentioned earlier, theoretically, it is likely that others charismatic leaders may act as recruiters among migrants for membership of terrorist groups [43, 53]. Of course, the immigration laws and welcome will facilitate the settling down of individuals and organizations who may act as terrorist supporters [51, 54]. It has been shown that those who are unable to seek work outside the house, have a disability, or are less politically engaged are less prone to radicalization [55–57].

9.8 **Managing terrorism**

Given the challenge, we argue that it is critical to follow a combined criminal justice and public health model in helping develop resistance and in getting rid of, or minimizing, the causative factors and inoculating vulnerable individuals against terrorist thinking. It has been shown that there are three different strategies employed to manage terrorism: disengagement, de-radicalization, and counter-radicalization. Disengagement and de-radicalization pertain more to the intervention programmes. Disengagement determines changes in behaviours by not using violence and by abandoning the association with violent groups [58]. De-radicalization entails a change in the cognitive framework of radicalized individuals to help, support, and engage them to reintegrate into society and to discourage their involvement in violence [59, 60]. Counter-radicalization processes include educational prevention, and political, legal and social programmes designed to discourage perhaps already radicalized people from becoming terrorists [59]. In general, disengagement in radicalized behaviour is connected with the de-radicalization of beliefs, but it is well recognized that changed beliefs may not always lead to altered behaviours, so both of these need to be tackled, whereas in some settings radical behaviour can be blocked without moderation of radical beliefs [61].

9.9 **Conclusion**

Terrorism is considered to be the use of indiscriminate violence to create terror or fear, in order to achieve ideological, political, and religious aims. In history and literature there are many examples of people who have sacrificed their own life to kill other people. These cases can be considered antecedents of terrorism, but the phenomenon of suicide bombers is very different today. Terrorism and radicalization are interrelated and strongly influenced by a number of factors—a majority of which are social or psychological. There is often an attempt to denigrate migrants as the distinction between migrant terrorist and home grown terrorist is often used by politicians for serving their political ideologies. The relationship between acculturation and migration and between migration and terrorism needs to be teased out carefully in future research, which can then go on to feed into policy. The models for tacking radicalization and consequently preventing terror attacks need to be multifaceted, and a range of approaches using a range of stakeholders are required. Understanding reasons and potential vulnerabilities is the first step in this journey.

References

1. **Salvatori S, Marazziti D.** To die to kill: suicide as a weapon. Some historical antecedents of suicide terrorism. In: **Marazziti D, Stahl SM,** eds. Evil, terrorism and psychiatry. Cambridge: Cambridge University Press; 2019, pp. 1–11.

2. **Campelo N, Oppetit A, Neau F, Cohen D, Bronsard G.** Who are the European youths willing to engage in radicalisation? A multidisciplinary review of their psychological and social profiles. European Psychiatry 2018;52:1–14.

3. **Bhatt A, Silber MD.** Radicalization in the West: the homegrown threat. New York: New York City Police Department; 2007.

4. **Stoppini L.** New perspectives in the fight against radicalisation: which preventive responses? Available from: https://issat.dcaf.ch/Share/Blogs/ISSAT-Blog/New-perspectives-in-the-fight-against-radicalisation-which-preventive-responses [accessed 3 August 2020].

5. **Bhui K, Otis M, Silva MJ, Halvorsrud K, Freestone M, Jones E.** Extremism and common mental illness: cross-sectional community survey of White British and Pakistani men and women living in England. The British Journal of Psychiatry 2019, DOI: 10.1192/bjp.2019.14.

6. **Corner E, Gill P.** A false dichotomy? Mental illness and lone-actor terrorism. Law and Human Behavior 2015;39:23–34.

7. Home Affairs **Committee.** The roots of violent radicalisation. Available from: https://publications.parliament.uk/pa/cm201012/cmselect/cmhaff/1446/1446.pdf [accessed 3 August 2020].

8. **Witt K, Hawton K, Fazel S.** The relationship between suicide and violence in schizophrenia: analysis of the Clinical Antipsychotic Trials of Intervention Effectiveness (CATIE) dataset. Schizophrenia Research 2014;154:61–7.

9. **Apter A, Plutchik R, van Praag HM.** Anxiety, impulsivity and depressed mood in relation to suicidal and violent behavior. Acta Psychiatrica Scandinavica 1993;87:1–5.

10. **Krueger AB. Malečková J.** Education, poverty and terrorism: is there a casual connection? Journal of Economic Perspectives 2003;17:119–44.

11. **Doosje B, Loseman A, van den Bos K.** Determinants of radicalization of Islamic youth in the Netherlands: personal uncertainty, perceived injustice and perceived group threat. Journal of Social Issues 2013;69:586–604.

12. **Hogg MA, Wagoner JA.** Uncertainty-Identity Theory. In: **Kim YY,** ed. The International Encyclopedia of Intercultural Communication; 2017, DOI: 10.1002/9781118783665. ieicc0177.

13. **Ellis A.** Anger. How to live with and without it. New York: Citadel Press Books; 2003.

14. **O'Shaughnessy NJ, Baines PR.** Selling terror: the symbolization and positioning of jihad. Marketing Theory 2009;9:227–41.

15. **Stares PB, Yacoubian M.** Terrorism as a disease: an epidemiological model for countering Islamist extremism. Pittsburgh, PA: Mathew B Ridgeway Centre for International Security Studies; 2007.

16. **Stares PB, Yacoubian M.** Rethinking the War on Terror: new approaches to conflict prevention and management in the post 9/11 world. In: **Magnusson Bruce ZZ,** ed. Contagion, health, fear, sovereignty. Washington, DC; 2008, pp. 425–36.

17. **Wiktorowicz Q.** Radical Islam rising: Muslim extremism in the West. Lanham, MD: Rowman & Littlefield Publishers; 2005.

18. **Gezentsvey Lamy MA, Ward C, Liu JH.** Motivation for ethno-cultural continuity. Cross-Cultural Psychology 2013;**44**:1047–66.

19. **Berry J.** Acculturation and identity. In: **Bhugra D, Bhui K,** eds. Textbook of cultural psychiatry. Cambridge: Cambridge University Press; 2018, pp. 185–93.

20. **Graves T.** Acculturation, access, and alcohol in a tri-ethnic community. American Anthropologist 1967;**69**:306–21.

21. **Berry J, Kim U, Minde T, Mok D.** Comparative stresses of acculturative stress. International migration review. Transcultural Psychiatry 1987;**21**:491–511.

22. **Bhui K, Everitt B, Jones E.** Might depression, psychosocial adversity, and limited social assets explain vulnerability to and resistance against violent radicalisation? PLoS One 2014;**9**:e105918.

23. **Bhugra D, Ventriglio A,** Bhui K. Acculturation, violent radicalisation and religious fundamentalism. The Lancet 2017;**4**:179–81.

24. **Jan H.** Alienation and integration of student intellectuals. American Sociological Review 1961;**26**:758–77.

25. **Manne A.** Narcissism and terrorism: how the personality disorder leads to deadly violence. Available from: https://www.theguardian.com/world/2015/jun/08/narcissism-terrorism-violence-monis-breivik-lubitz-jihadi-john [accessed 3 August 2020].

26. **Victoroff J.** The mind of the terrorist: a review and critique of psychological approaches. Journal of Conflict Resolution 2005;**49**:3–42.

27. **Gill P, Horgan J, Deckert P.** Bombing alone: tracing the motivations and antecedent behaviors of lone-actor terrorists. Journal of Forensic Sciences 2014;**59**:425–35.

28. **Dom G, Schouler-Ocak M, Bhui K, Demunter H, Kuey L, Raballo A,** et al. Mass violence, radicalization and terrorism: A role for psychiatric profession? European Psychiatry 2018;**49**:78–80.

29. **Besta T, Szulc M, Jaskiewicz M.** Political extremism, group membership and personality traits: who accepts violence? International Journal of Social Psychology 2015;**30**:563–85.

30. **Feddes AR, Mann L, Doosje B.** Increasing self-esteem and empathy to prevent violent radicalization: a longitudinal quantitative evaluation of a resilience training focused on adolescents with a dual identity. Journal of Applied Social Psychology 2015;**45**:400–11.

31. **Laor N, Yanay-Shani A, Wolmer L, Khoury O.** A trauma-like model of political extremism: psycho-political fault lines in Israel. Annals of the New York Academy of Sciences 2010;**1208**:24–31.

32. **Soliman A, Bellaj T, Khelifa Maher.** An integrative psychological model for radicalism: evidence from structural equation modelling. Personality and Individual Differences 2016;**95**:127–33.

33. **Durkheim E.** On suicide. Glencoe, IL: Free Press; 1897/1951.

34. **Dein S, Littlewood R.** Apocalyptic suicide: from a pathological to an eschatological interpretation. International Journal of Social Psychiatry 2005;**51**:198–210.

35. **Zafar ZA, Herriot P.** Religious fundamentalism and social identity. Journal of Muslim Mental Health 2007;**3**:117–19.

36. **Hood RW, Jr, Hill PC, Williamson WP.** The psychology of religious fundamentalism. New York: Guilford Press; 2005.

37. **Ventriglio A, Bhugra D.** Identity, alienation, and violent radicalization. In: **Marazziti D, Stahl SM,** eds. Evil, terrorism & psychiatry. Cambridge: Cambridge University Press; 2019, pp. 17–29.

38. **Ben-Nun Bloom P, Arikan G.** A two-edged sword: the differential effect of religious belief and religious social context on attitudes towards democracy. Political Behaviour 2012;**34**:249–76.

39. **Nunn CZ, Crockett HJ, Williams JA.** Tolerance for nonconformity. San Francisco, CA: Jossey-Bass Publishers; 1978.

40. **Sieckelinck S, Van San M, Sikkens E.** Formers and families: Transitional journeys in and out of extremism in the United Kingdom, Denmark and The Netherlands. The Hague: National Coordinator for Security and Counterterrorism Ministry of Security and Justice; 2015.

41. **Lewis P.** Young, British and Muslim, annotated edition. London: Continuum;2007.

42. **Vertovec SR, Rogers A.** Introduction. In: **Vertovec SR, Rogers A,** eds. Muslim European youth: reproducing ethnicity, religion, culture (research in ethnic relations). Aldershot: Ashgate Publishing; 1998, pp. 1–24.

43. **Marc S.** Understanding terror networks. Philadelphia, PA: University of Pennsylvania Press; 2004.

44. **Milena U.** European converts to terrorism. Middle East Quarterly 2008;**15**:31–7.

45. **Maykel V.** Religious fundamentalism and radicalization among Muslim minority youth in Europe. European Psychologist 2018;**23**:21–31.

46. **Lamberg L.** A psychiatrist explores apocalyptic violence in Heaven's Gate and Aum Shinriyko cults. JAMA 1997;**278**:191–3.

47. **Weston LB.** The ghost dance: the origins of religion, first edition. Maidstone: Crescent Moon Publishing; 1970.

48. **Gerth HH, Wright Mills C.** From Max Weber: essays in sociology, first edition. London; 2014.

49. **Géza Róheim.** 'The Garden of Eden.' Psychoanalytic Review, 1940, Vol. XXVII, Nos. 1 and 2, pp. 1–26 and 177–199.

50. **Devereux Georges.** Charismatic leadership and crisis. New York: International Universities Press; 1955.

51. **Bove V, Böhmelt T.** Does immigration induce terrorism? The Journal of Politics 2016;**78:572–88**.

52. **Ansa.it.** Gentiloni says risk terrorists among migrants. Available from: https://www.ansa.it/english/news/2015/01/22/gentiloni-says-risk-terrorists-among-migrants-update-2_06c48d8f-7d3b-4b99-90bd-009941aa54b1.html [accessed 3 August 2020].

53. **Sageman M.** Leaderless jihad: terror networks in the twenty-first century. Philadelphia, PA: University of Pennsylvania Press; 2011.

54. **Zimmermann D, Rosenau W, Whine M, Bell S, Cesari J, Menkhaus K.** The radicalization of diasporas and terrorism. Zurich: Center for Security Studies; 2009.

55. **Alcala HE, Sharif MZ, Samari G.** Social determinants of health, violent radicalization, and terrorism: a public health perspective. Health Equity 2017;**1**:87–95.

56. **McGilloway A, Ghosh P, Bhui K.** A systematic review of pathways to and processes associated with radicalization and extremism amongst Muslims in Western societies. International Review of Psychiatry 2015;**27**:39–50.

57. **Misiak B, Samochowiec J, Bhui K, Schouler-Ocak M, Demunter H, Kuey L,** et al. A systematic review on the relationship between mental health, radicalization and mass violence. European Psychiatry 2019;**56**:51–9.

58. **Butt R, Tuck H.** Tackling extremism: de-radicalisation and disengagement. Copenhagen: Institute for Strategic Dialogue; 2012.

59. **CounterTerrorism Implementation Task Force.** First report of the working group on radicalisation and extremism that lead to terrorism: inventory of State programmes. Available from: https://data2.unhcr.org/en/documents/download/44297 [accessed 3 August 2020].

60. Schmid **AP.** Radicalisation, de-radicalisation, counter radicalisation: a conceptual discussion and literature review. Available from: http://www.icct.nl/download/file/ ICCT-Schmid-Radicalisation-De-Radicalisation-Counter-Radicalisation-March-2013. pdf [accessed 3 August 2020].

61. **Demant E, Slootman, M, Bujis F,** and **Tillie, J.** Decline and disengagement: an analysis of processes of de-radicalisation. Available from: https://dare.uva.nl/ search?identifier=4f819bfb-4ea9-4196-a7fd-3c107594205f [accessed 3 August 2020] (in Dutch).

Chapter 10

The equifinality and multifinality of violent radicalization and mental health

Paul Gill, Frank Farnham, and
Caitlin Clemmow

10.1 Introduction

In its early decades, terrorism studies fixated on the idea of developing a terrorist profile. To that end, researchers theoretically posited a series of mono-
causal explanations such as psychopathy, narcissism, or sociodemographic
traits [1]. The current lack of a distinguishable terrorist profile is not because
of a lack of effort. Instead, the lack of a terrorist profile should be seen as a distinct empirical finding [2]. The field now largely agrees on two principles [3].
Firstly, there are multiple pathways into violent extremism. Typically, multiple
factors contribute to a single individual's pathway. These factors and their relative causal weight differ between individuals who become violent extremists.
Individuals with very different initial states can experience different processes
and still end at the same end outcome of violent extremism. In parallel research
fields, this is known as the principle of equifinality. Secondly, different people
with similar initial states may produce different outcomes. Additionally, the
impact of experiencing a single factor may impact upon an individual's development in very different ways. In parallel research fields, this is known as the
principle of multifinality [3].

This chapter's purpose is to elaborate upon the principles of equifinality and
multifinality with respect to violent radicalization and mental health. For equifinality, we synthesize the evidence base regarding pathways into violent radicalization and the varying roles of mental health problems within these pathways.
For multifinality, we demonstrate that the starting point of poor mental health
problems can lead to multiple end outcomes, of which violent radicalization
is a low base rate phenomenon, compared to the others. To do so, we draw on

the evidence base from various systematic reviews and meta-analyses of other public/personal harms.

10.2 **The equifinality of violent radicalization and mental health problems**

The study of how individuals become radicalized and join terrorist groups has developed rapidly in the past 15 years. There is a consensus that there is no single variable that can explain these phenomena. Instead, it has repeatedly been demonstrated that radicalization and terrorist engagement should be viewed as a process. The multiple pathways into violent radicalization have been eloquently depicted in both theoretical frameworks and empirical (qualitative and quantitative) approaches.

There are multiple influential theoretical frameworks and models depicting many different processes leading to the same outcome. This section touches upon nine such theoretical pathways and highlights the role, if any, mental health problems are said to play.

Five of these theoretical frameworks do not mention mental health problems or parallel processes. For example, Randy Borum's 'Terrorist Mind-Set Model' demonstrates a progression from the development of a grievance, to a sense of injustice, the identification of a target, and a process of dehumanization [4]. Quintan Wiktorowicz's model involves a cognitive opening, religious seeking and frame alignment, and finally, socialization and joining an extremist group [5]. Fathali Moghaddam's model moves from a perception of injustice and unfairness to searching for perceived options to fight unfair treatment to displacement of aggression, then moral engagement, solidification of categorical thinking, seeing the legitimacy of the terrorist group, and, finally, sidestepping inhibitory mechanisms for terrorist engagement [6]. Marc Sageman's model promotes the importance of moral outrage, cognitive frame alignment, resonance with personal experience, and situational dynamics [7]. McCauley and Moskalenko's mechanisms of individual political radicalization account for personal victimization, political grievance, tests of commitment and trust, and development of social connections with other group members [8].

Four theoretical models implicitly account for some form of mental health problem being potentially important. Thomas Precht developed a four-phase model of homegrown terrorism and Islamic extremism in Europe [9]. The phases consist of (1) pre-radicalization; (2) conversion and identification; (3) conviction and indoctrination; and (4) action. Precht characterizes experiencing personal traumas as one of five contributory background factors in the pre-radicalization phase that increase an individual's propensity for radicalization.

Similarly, Silber and Bhatt also propose a four-phase model of radicalization based on analysis of five homegrown terrorist incidents in Northern America and Western Europe. The first phase is the pre-radicalization stage [10]. During this stage, Silber and Bhatt argue that the nature of a person's environment prior to exposure to an extremist ideology may make them more vulnerable to the extremist narrative. Social, demographic, and psychological factors interact with physical spaces and individual differences, resulting in an individual being vulnerable to radicalization. Taylor and Horgan's conceptual framework incorporates issues related to cognitive factors such as reduced social contact, which may sit parallel to mental health problems [11]. Other factors within their framework account for family and early experiences, socialization processes, dissatisfaction, personal contacts with other extremists, risk taking, sense of purpose, ideology, and pre-existing skills and interests. Taylor and Horgan describe involvement in terrorism as a process that moves along a trajectory as such factors interact. At the first stages of involvement, setting events and personal involvement are key. What distinguishes those who pursue terrorist goals and those who do not may be the style of interaction among their personal context, setting events, and the social/political/organizational context. In the latter stages of involvement, they argue that social/political/organizational context plays a more significant role. Finally, Loo Seng Neo's online radicalization model proposes five phases: (1) the Reflection phase; (2) the Exploration phase; (3) the Connection phase; (4) the Resolution phase; and (5) the Operational phase [12]. Stage 1 is characterized by vulnerabilities that make an individual susceptible to radical influence. Personality, individual-level vulnerabilities and personal environment interact to increase a person's propensity for radicalization. In these pertinent theoretical models, the mechanism through which mental health problems impact on violent radicalization is that they increase individual vulnerabilities.

Empiricism within terrorism studies has grown rapidly in the last decade. Many of these studies focus upon the sociodemographic and antecedent behaviours experienced by violent extremists. The results reassert this principle of equifinality in a number of ways.

Firstly, empirical studies typically reflect the diversity in backgrounds and experiences within a single sample. No terrorist profile exists. For example, studies have measured the prevalence rate of reported clinical diagnosed mental health disorders at 4.5% in a sample of European jihadists (n = 242); 7.6% US far-right-inspired group members who had committed at least one murder (n = 92); 11.9% in a diverse ideological sample of terrorist group members (n = 97); 12.9% of Palestinian lone-actor terrorists (n = 62); 25.6% of US ideological active shooters (n = 40); 31.9% of lone-actor terrorists (n = 119);

32.7% of lone-actor terrorists (n = 49); 40.4% of far-right inspired lone actors who had committed at least one murder (n = 47); 43.7% of US extremists (n = 284); and 57% of white supremacists (n = 44) [13–21].

Secondly, although four studies have found an elevated presence of mental disorder in lone-actor terrorists versus group terrorists, the rates of mental disorders in these lone-actor samples never exceeded 45% [14, 15, 22, 23]. Even in those samples, where diagnosed disorders were at the higher end of the spectrum, these individuals were also significantly more likely to experience other recent stressors than their non-mentally disordered counterparts [15]. Similarly, in the study by Soliman et al. [24] of activism-radicalism intentions in 662 Egyptian adults, the results only became significant when psychopathological, cognitive, and psychosocial indicators were treated collectively rather than individually. Rarely are mental health problems the sole problem. Sometimes mental health problems may compound other problems. Sometimes other problems may compound the mental health problems.

Thirdly, even in those studies reporting relatively high rates of diagnosable mental disorder, the diagnoses themselves vary greatly. Anton Weenink studied the police files of 140 Dutch individuals who became foreign fighters [25]. Six per cent had reported clinically diagnosed disorders. These disorders included psychosis, narcissism, attention-deficit–hyperactivity disorder (ADHD), schizophrenia, autism spectrum disorder (ASD), and post-traumatic stress disorder (PTSD). In Corner et al.'s universe of 153 Western-based lone-actor terrorists, 1.3% experienced traumatic brain injury, 0.7% drug dependence, 8.5% schizophrenia, 0.7% schizoaffective disorder, 2.0% delusional disorder, 0.7% other psychotic disorder, 7.2% depression, 3.9% bipolar disorder, 1.3% unspecified anxiety disorder, 0.7% dissociative disorder, 1.3% obsessive compulsive disorder, 3.3% PTSD, 0.7% unspecified sleep disorder, 6.5% unspecified personality disorder, and 3.3% ASD [23]. Ariel Merari's study of suicide bombers found 60% had avoidant-dependent personality disorder [26]. Gill et al.'s closed-source study of 49 UK lone-actor terrorists found that 12.2% experienced a mood disorder, 10.2% schizophrenia, 4.1% intellectual disabilities, and 2% an assortment of personality disorders [19]. In Knight et al.'s study of 24 UK-based violent extremists [27], some individuals had Asperger syndrome, personality disorder, and schizophrenia. The closed source study by van Leyenhorst and Andreas of 26 Dutch terrorist suspects demonstrated single cases of ADHD, psychotic disorder, borderline personality disorder, or post-traumatic stress symptoms [28].

Fourthly, while some studies found elevated rates of certain diagnoses versus the societal base rate, they still largely occurred in <50% of the terrorist sample. These studies include schizophrenia and psychosis in Dutch foreign fighters

[25]; schizophrenia, autism, and delusional disorder in lone-actor terrorists [23]; and subscale measures of psychopathic, paranoid, depressive, schizophrenic, and hypomanic tendencies in Palestinian and Israeli terrorists [29]. Other studies found lower rates of personality disorders and psychiatric illness versys non-ideologically inspired murderers [30]. Clearly, multiple other factors are contributing towards others' violent radicalization within these samples.

10.3 The multifinality of violent radicalization and mental health problems

Research also heavily supports the principle of multifinality in a number of ways.

Firstly, even for those who become violently radicalized and who also suffer from mental health problems, the role the latter plays differs from case to case. Empirical studies demonstrate that (unlike the suggestion of the theoretical models) mental disorders do not solely increase individual vulnerabilities. They may, in certain circumstances, have other impacts. For example, sequence analyses of lone-actor terrorist data demonstrate that during radicalization 'mental health problems appear to be a precursor to, and consequence of, criminal behaviours, which are themselves markers of lack of commitment to prosocial moral rules (moral susceptibility) and/or markers of selection into criminogenic settings, some of which may be radicalising (including prison)' [31]. In other contexts, research shows how extremist propaganda provided extremists with an explanation for their negative personal experiences, including experiences of trauma and mental health problems [21]. Mental health problems (or markers thereof), in certain circumstances, may also be attractive to particular recruiters for particular tasks and functions within an extremist network [21].

A single specific disorder may also play different roles for different people. For example, research on ASD and violence highlights four routes through which those with autism may be more inclined toward aggressive behaviour:

> (a) Their increased social naiveté may leave people with ASD open to manipulation by others (b) A disruption of routines, or over-rigid adherence to rules, might lead people with ASD to becoming aggressive (c) A lack of understanding of social situations (and poor negotiating skills) might lead to people with ASD becoming aggressive and (d) An obsessional interest might lead someone to committing an offence in the pursuit of that interest, perhaps exacerbated by a failure to recognise the implications of his/her behaviour for him/herself and others' [32].

Secondly, the factors associated with developing an attitudinal affinity with a cause (e.g. radicalization) may not associate with violence on behalf of that cause (e.g. violent radicalization). Take depression, for example. Bhui et al. [33,

34] conducted a survey of 608 members of the general public. The results demonstrated a positive linear association between those who score highly on a radicalization scale and those who score highly for depression. They therefore found a strong link between some facets of radicalization and depression within that sample. However, the study by Corner et al. [23] of those who conducted lone-actor terrorism found the diagnosed rates of depression to be much lower than in the general population. So, while depression might contribute to radicalization more often than one would expect, it might also inhibit the violent expressions of this radicalization in certain cases.

Thirdly, the same factors may be highly associated with multiple end outcomes. For example, in a survey of more than 400 Hezbollah fighters, Ayla Schbley found a strong statistical relationship between 'some self-reported criteria of intermittent explosive, psychotic, and oppositional personality disorders and a person's absolutist tendency, affinity for martyrdom, susceptibility to the culting process, psychotic depression, and acts of terrorism and self-immolation' [35, pp. 115–16]. The comparison of 24 violent extremists and 16 non-violent extremists by Knight et al. [27] showed no difference in the prevalence of Asperger syndrome, depression, suicidal ideation, personality disorder, schizophrenia, fanaticism/narcissism, obsessiveness, paranoia, grandiosity, irrationality, or delusional thinking. Similarly, Michele Groppi's study found no relationship between traumatic experiences and support for Jihadist violence in a sample of 440 Italians [36].

In many ways the empirical results outlined in the previous section are just a mirror reflection of the wider criminological literature. For example, results consistently showed higher rates of mental disorders among lone actors than in group/networked offenders. However, research also demonstrates that this may be typical of offending in general, and not just terrorism. For example, Roscoe et al. [37] examined >5000 homicide offenders in the UK. Lone perpetrators were significantly more likely to have suffered mental illness in their lifetime (37% vs 16%), in the 12 months prior to the homicide (20% vs 11%), and have diagnoses of schizophrenia (14% vs 3%), and affective disorder (13% vs 6%). Similarly, systematic reviews and meta-analyses point toward the increased rate of psychotic illnesses within prison populations, and bipolar disorder among violent offenders [38, 39]. The systematic review of Yu et al. [40] of personality disorders, violence, and antisocial behaviour synthesized the results of 14 studies and found there was a 'substantially increased risk of violent outcomes in studies with all PDs [personality disorders]' [40]. Studies of serial killers, mass murderers, mass shooting perpetrators, arsonists, and other forms of violent crime find a greater presence of autism diagnoses than is found in the general population [41–46]. King and Murphy's systematic review of people with ASD and the criminal justice system found seven studies that examined the prevalence of the disorder in offender populations [47]. Each of the prevalence rates were higher than the 1% base rate of the general population and ranged from 3% to 27%. King and Murphy additionally found six studies that incorporated a comparison group of individuals without ASD and found rates of offending behaviour to be the same or lower than in the comparison groups. It is typically the co-occurring risk factors such as poor parental control, family environment, criminality, bullying, or untreated/undetected psychosis that drives violence [48]. A focus on mental health problems alone cannot tell us why some went down the terrorism route, whereas others went down the criminality route.

Additionally, those with severe mental illness are also—depending on the study—between 2.3 and 140.4 times more likely to be criminally victimized than those in the general population. This is particularly the case when alcohol or illicit drug use/abuse, homelessness, severe symptomatology, and engagement with criminal activity are also present [49]. This section strongly suggests a focus on mental health problems alone is insufficient and requires a system-level approach [50]

10.4 **Conclusion**

The emergent research demonstrating both equifinality and multifinality has a number of implications for future research and practice in the area of psychopathology and violent extremism.

Firstly, the principles suggest we adopt approaches that take account of the constellation of multiple factors that interact with (and sometimes enable or disable one another) rather than solely focusing upon single disorders. In terms of equifinality, violent extremists may display similar risky and adverse behaviours, yet emerge from multiple pathways, some of which may involve mental health problems. Treating them as a homogeneous group because of their presenting behaviours (e.g. reading extremist propaganda) and instituting a single intervention (e.g. counternarrative work) is insufficient. People may be engaging in such behaviours because of curiosity, peer pressure, identity seeking, fixation, social isolation, and other factors related or unrelated to mental health problems. In terms of multifinality, many individuals display similar mental health problems, where only a few go on to engage in terrorism. Risk assessments should therefore focus on the whole of an individual's life circumstances.

Secondly, preventing individuals with mental health problems from becoming radicalized or going on to engage in violent extremism may necessitate tailored, rather than broad, generalized policies. If multiple trajectories into violent extremism exist, there should be multiple policies to encourage prevention. Not all policies will have relevance to all individuals presenting with the same mental health problems, as their constellation of other risk and protective factors likely differs.

Thirdly, the vast majority of empirical research on mental disorders and violent extremism takes the nomothetic route. Typically, the route taken has been to count the prevalence of mental health disorders within large(ish) samples of terrorists and those with attitudinal affinity with a terrorist cause. Such approaches leave us with various 'counts', within-group comparisons, and across-group comparisons. They leave us with a sense of how prevalent mental health disorders are. In some cases, they identify common relationships between variables within the whole sample. Such studies, however, are, to a large degree, difficult to apply to a single case, which needs assessing and managing in the here and now. We need more than an understanding of 'presence', we need an understanding of 'relevance'. For a risk factor to be meaningful, we need to understand the mechanisms through which it impacts upon violent extremism, and why the risk factor does not impact on each individual equally. To this end, much more work is needed from the idiographic perspective. This could help untangle the *relevance* of mental health disorders in particular individuals who became violent extremists at particular moments in their life. Control groups of individuals who presented with similar problems but did not engage in violent extremism may help us understand the mechanisms and mediators through which a distal risk factor like a mental health disorder may be linked to violent extremism.

Fourthly, there are further strides to be taken in nomothetic approaches, both in terms of the populations they examine and the methods they adopt. For the latter, recent uses of sequence analyses help untangle the myriad pathways into violent extremism and where mental health disorders and psychological crises typically occur within them [15, 31]. With further refinement, such approaches may provide insight into individual cases, the trajectory they appear to be on, and the pinch points that could maximize impactful interventions. Other future analytical approaches could include finer-grained sequence analyses, including T-pattern analysis (if temporal data are sufficiently exact) [51, 52]. Such temporally focused analyses could demonstrate how the relationship between mental health disorders and violent extremism develops differentially over time for different people. Deductive methods, such as cluster analysis, may help identify subsets of fairly homogeneous constellations within larger datasets [53]. Other approaches, such as network modelling (see psychometric network analysis) may help uncover the causal structure of complex constructs, such as radicalization, or engagement in violent extremism, and as such the multi- and equifinality of mental health problems within these complex systems.

Finally, there is a lot of potential for studying multifinality into holding violent extremist beliefs prospectively (rather than the more usual retrospective approach). For example, multiple life-course criminological studies exist where the same participants are surveyed on a range of measures every few years (e.g. the Peterborough Adolescent and Young Adolescent Study). One such study, The Zurich Project on the Social Development from Childhood to Adulthood (Z-Proso), has measured extremist attitudes of 1400 youths in its last couple of data collection waves. Although it is unlikely that any will transition into actual engagement in violent extremism, these sorts of approaches hold promise, especially if deployed consistently in areas where conflict reoccurs frequently (e.g. Northern Ireland) or are said to have a radicalization problem (e.g. Molenbeek).

References

1. **Gill P, Corner E.** There and back again: the study of mental disorder and terrorist involvement. American Psychologist 2017;**72**:231.
2. **Horgan JG.** The psychology of terrorism. New York: Routledge; 2004.
3. **Borum R.** Radicalization into violent extremism II: a review of conceptual models and empirical research. Journal of Strategic Security 2011;**4**:37–62.
4. **Borum R.** Understanding the terrorist mind-set. FBI Law Enforcement Bulletin 2003;**72**:7.
5. **Wiktorowicz Q**, ed. Islamic activism: a social movement theory approach. Bloomington, IN: Indiana University Press; 2004.
6. **Moghaddam FM.** The staircase to terrorism: a psychological exploration. American Psychologist 2005;**60**:161.
7. **Sageman M.** A strategy for fighting international Islamist terrorists. The Annals of the American Academy of Political and Social Science 2008;**618**:223–31.
8. **McCauley C, Moskalenko S.** Mechanisms of political radicalization: pathways toward terrorism. Terrorism and Political Violence 2008;**20**:415–33.
9. **Precht T.** Home grown terrorism and Islamist radicalisation in Europe. Available from: https://www.kennisplein.be/Documents/Home_grown_terrorism_and_Islamist_radicalisation_in_Europe_-_an_assessment_of_influencing_factors__2_.pdf [accessed 11 December 2007].
10. **Silber MD, Bhatt A, Analysts SI.** Radicalization in the West: the homegrown threat. New York: Police Department; 2007.
11. **Taylor M, Horgan J.** A conceptual framework for addressing psychological process in the development of the terrorist. Terrorism and Political Violence 2006;**18**:585–601.
12. **Neo LS.** An Internet-mediated pathway for online radicalisation: RECRO. In: Information Resources Management Association (USA), ed. Violent extremism: breakthroughs in research and practice. Hershey, PA: IGI Global; 2019, pp. 62–89.
13. **Bakker E.** Jihadi terrorists in Europe. Den Haag: Netherlands Institute of International Relations; 2006.

14. **Gruenewald J, Chermak S, Freilich JD.** Distinguishing "loner" attacks from other domestic extremist violence: a comparison of far-right homicide incident and offender characteristics. Criminology & Public Policy 2013;**12**:65–91.

15. **Corner E, Gill P.** Psychological distress, terrorist involvement and disengagement from terrorism: a sequence analysis approach. Journal of Quantitative Criminology 2019, DOI: 10.1007/s10940-019-09420-1.

16. **Perry S, Hasisi B, Perry G.** Who is the lone terrorist? A study of vehicle-borne attackers in Israel and the West Bank. Studies in Conflict & Terrorism 2018;**41**:899–913.

17. **Capellan JA.** Lone wolf terrorist or deranged shooter? A study of ideological active shooter events in the United States, 1970–2014. Studies in Conflict & Terrorism 2015;**38**:395–413.

18. **Gill P, Horgan J, Deckert P.** Bombing alone: tracing the motivations and antecedent behaviors of lone-actor terrorists. Journal of Forensic Sciences 2014;**59**:425–35.

19. **Gill P, Corner E, McKee A, Hitchen P, Betley P.** What do closed source data tell us about lone actor terrorist behavior? A research note. Terrorism and Political Violence 2019, DOI: 10.1080/09546553.2019.1668781.

20. **LaFree G, Jensen MA, James PA, Safer-Lichtenstein A.** Correlates of violent political extremism in the United States. Criminology 2018;**56**: 233–268.

21. **Bubolz BF, Simi P.** The problem of overgeneralization: the case of mental health problems and US violent white supremacists. American Behavioral Scientist 2019, DOI: 10.1177/0002764219831746.

22. **Hewitt C.** Understanding terrorism in America. New York: Routledge; 2003.

23. **Corner E, Gill P, Mason O.** Mental health disorders and the terrorist: A research note probing selection effects and disorder prevalence. Studies in Conflict & Terrorism 2016;**39**:560–8.

24. **Soliman A, Bellaj T, Khelifa M.** An integrative psychological model for radicalism: evidence from structural equation modeling. Personality and Individual Differences 2016;**95**:127–33.

25. **Weenink AW.** Behavioral problems and disorders among radicals in police files. Perspectives on Terrorism 2015;**9**(2):68–76.

26. **Merari A.** Driven to death: psychological and social aspects of suicide terrorism. Oxford: Oxford University Press; 2010.

27. **Knight S, Woodward K, Lancaster GL.** Violent versus nonviolent actors: an empirical study of different types of extremism. Journal of Threat Assessment and Management 2017;**4**:230.

28. **van Leyenhorst M, Andreas A.** Dutch suspects of terrorist activity: a study of their biographical backgrounds based on primary sources. Journal for Deradicalization **2017**;12:309–44.

29. **Gottschalk M, Gottschalk S.** Authoritarianism and pathological hatred: a social psychological profile of the Middle Eastern terrorist. The American Sociologist 2004;**35**:38–59.

30. **Lyons HA, Harbinson HJ.** A comparison of political and non-political murderers in Northern Ireland, 1974–84. Medicine, Science and the Law 1986;**26**:193–8.

31. **Corner E, Bouhana N, Gill P.** The multifinality of vulnerability indicators in lone-actor terrorism. Psychology, Crime & Law 2019;**25**:111–32.

32. **Howlin P.** Autism and Asperger syndrome: preparing for adulthood. New York: Routledge; 2004.

33. **Bhui K, Everitt B, Jones E.** Might depression, psychosocial adversity, and limited social assets explain vulnerability to and resistance against violent radicalisation?. PLoS One 2014;**9**:e105918.

34. **Bhui K, Silva MJ, Topciu RA, Jones E.** Pathways to sympathies for violent protest and terrorism. The British Journal of Psychiatry 2016;**209**:483–90.

35. **Schbley A.** Defining religious terrorism: a causal and anthological profile. Studies in Conflict and Terrorism 2003;**26**:105–34.

36. **Groppi M.** An Empirical analysis of causes of Islamist radicalisation: Italian case study. Perspectives on Terrorism 2017;**11**(1).

37. **Roscoe A, Rahman MS, Mehta H, While D, Appleby L, Shaw J.** Comparison of a national sample of homicides committed by lone and multiple perpetrators. Journal of Forensic Psychiatry & Psychology 2012;**23**:510–21.

38. **Fazel S, Seewald K.** Severe mental illness in 33 588 prisoners worldwide: systematic review and meta-regression analysis. The British Journal of Psychiatry 2012;**200**:364–73.

39. **Fazel S, Lichtenstein P, Grann M, Goodwin GM, Långström N.** Bipolar disorder and violent crime: new evidence from population-based longitudinal studies and systematic review. Archives of General Psychiatry 2010;**67**:931–8.

40. **Yu R, Geddes JR, Fazel S.** Personality disorders, violence, and antisocial behavior: a systematic review and meta-regression analysis. Journal of Personality Disorders 2012;**26**:775–92.

41. **Allely CS, Minnis H, Thompson L, Wilson P, Gillberg C.** Neurodevelopmental and psychosocial risk factors in serial killers and mass murderers. Aggression and Violent Behavior 2014;**19**:288–301.

42. **Allely CS, Wilson P, Minnis H, Thompson L, Yaksic E, Gillberg C.** Violence is rare in autism: when it does occur, is it sometimes extreme? The Journal of Psychology 2017;**151**:49–68.

43. **Tantam D.** Asperger's syndrome. Journal of Child Psychology and Psychiatry 1988;**29**:245–55.

44. **Långström N, Grann M, Ruchkin V, Sjöstedt G, Fazel S.** Risk factors for violent offending in autism spectrum disorder: a national study of hospitalized individuals. Journal of Interpersonal Violence 2009;**24**:1358–70.

45. **Mouridsen SE, Brønnum-Hansen H, Rich B, Isager T.** Mortality and causes of death in autism spectrum disorders: an update. Autism 2008;**12**:403–14.

46. **Hodgins S.** Violent behaviour among people with schizophrenia: a framework for investigations of causes, and effective treatment, and prevention. Philosophical Transactions of the Royal Society B: Biological Sciences 2008;**363**:2505–18.

47. **King C, Murphy GH.** A systematic review of people with autism spectrum disorder and the criminal justice system. Journal of Autism and Developmental Disorders 2014;**44**:2717–33.

48. **Del Pozzo J, Roché MW, Silverstein SM.** Violent behavior in autism spectrum disorders: Who's at risk? Aggression and Violent Behavior 2018;**39**:53–60.

49. **Maniglio R.** Severe mental illness and criminal victimization: a systematic review. Acta Psychiatrica Scandinavica 2009;**119**:180–91.

50. **Bouhana N.** The moral ecology of extremism: a systemic perspective. UK Commission for Countering Extremism. Available from: https://assets.publishing.service.gov.uk/government/uploads/system/uploads/attachment_data/file/834354/Bouhana-The-moral-ecology-of-extremism.pdf [accessed 3 August 2020].

51. **Quinn-Evans L, Keatley DA, Arntfield M, Sheridan L.** A behavior sequence analysis of victims' accounts of stalking behaviors. Journal of Interpersonal Violence 2019, DOI: 10.1177/0886260519831389.

52. **Keatley D.** Pathways in crime: an introduction to behaviour sequence analysis. New York: Springer; 2018.

53. **Clemmow C, Bouhana N, Gill P.** Analyzing person-exposure patterns in lone-actor terrorism: implications for threat assessment and intelligence gathering. Criminology & Public Policy 2020;**19**:451–82.

54. For access to all used instruments in the latter study—see https://www.jacobscenter.uzh.ch/en/research/zproso/aboutus/inst_erheb/inst_summ.html

Section 3

Prevention, evaluation, and intervention: New paradigms of research for policy and practice

Chapter 11

Police–community relations and cultural competency: Important means of countering violent extremism

Myrna Lashley, Ghayda Hassan,
Sara Thompson, Michael Chartrand,
and Serge Touzin

11.1 Introduction

Cultural competency may be helpful to police in fighting violent extremism. Recent years have seen concern over the diffusion of terrorist ideology and entities. These events prompted security agencies in many nations, including Canada, to anticipate the possibility of similar attacks by persons radicalized to violence. To cite two examples: March 2016 saw a Canadian soldier injured by a knife attack at a Canadian Armed Forces recruitment centre; and in August of the same year, a Daesh supporter was killed by Canadian police when attempting to detonate a homemade device [1]. These incidents speak to phenomena involving individuals born or raised in Western nations, who become radicalized and involved in terrorist acts at home or abroad [2]. Thus, today's security agencies must grapple with two distinct forms of terrorist violence: transnational and homegrown [2].

Identifying those who may be radicalized to violence is, however, difficult. Research consistently indicates that there is no terrorist 'profile' [3–7], and that the characteristics of those who radicalize to violence are varied and complex, as are the motivations underpinning this violence [3, 4, 8]. Research also demonstrates that counterterrorism strategies that disproportionately rely on heavy handedness can come with significant backlash, which may serve to increase the risk of radicalization to violence [5, 9, 10, 11]. For these and other reasons, including the trend toward the 'localization of national security' [12–14], growing numbers of police services in Canada (and elsewhere) are adopting programmes and initiatives aimed at cultivating better relationships with communities in their jurisdictional areas. The rationale behind this approach is simple: as radicalization processes generally occur in relatively private settings [15–18], detection by police and intelligence services is greatly reduced. Given the foregoing, police often need to rely upon cooperation and information provided by citizens in order to gather information that may result in successful outcomes and create good police–citizen relationships [19, 20]. However, for this cooperation to fully materialize, the quality of police–citizen interaction must demonstrate trust, mutual understanding, and respect. One way for this to occur is for members of police and security services to display behaviours indicative of cultural competency, which is being operationalized as a set of skills and associated knowledge that improve interactions in culturally diverse contexts. These skills include openness to diversity; non-judgemental and antiracist attitudes; acceptance of the other; empathy and sensitivity to the effects of society on persons; and respectful co-construction of solutions with the individual or community.

The importance of cultural competency has been expressed by scholars from various disciplines who are concerned with interactions taking place between individuals as they engage in their professional lives. For example, Ow and Nur [21] discuss the need for social workers working with Malay Muslims to develop an understanding of the role of Islam in the cultural and religious aspects of clients' lives as it relates to help-seeking behaviours. Similarly, Rew et al. [22] emphasize the necessity for nurses to be skilled in cultural competency in order to provide sensitive and acceptable care. In discussing the importance of globalization on world economies, an editorial in the *International Journal of Hospitality Management* identifies cultural competency as a major skill needed to interact with people of different cultures. Finally, Sarah Florini [23] discusses the manner in which black people display their cultural knowledge and competency while interacting with others on Black Twitter—a skill not accessible to those 'not in the know'. Despite lacking a single definition of the concept, there is a consensus regarding three basic elements: recognizing and understanding how one's heritage shapes one's behaviour; the ability to use that knowledge and understanding to maximize one's interactions with the 'other'; and internalizing the knowledge and understanding such that it can be applied to different communities of people [24]. These skills and knowledge will be of importance as police, security officials, and other governmental personnel work with communities to deter individuals, particularly youth, from engaging in conduct leading to violence extremism. Accordingly, Mills and Miller [25] highlighted the necessity for personnel in homeland security, emergency management, and other security professions, to be culturally competent in order to interact with cultures other than their own, in ways that do not escalate situations that may already be tense. This reflects findings that military advisors working with foreign security forces must be cognizant of cultural norms and employ cultural competency in order to build fruitful relationships as they battle the 'war on terror' [26].

11.2 **Rationale and objectives**

Perceived cultural competency of security officers may have a direct effect upon the response of citizens, especially those from vulnerable communities, as they interact with officers carrying out official duties; engaging in community policing; and outreach activities—especially when communities are perceived to be, or perceive themselves as being viewed as, problematic relative to the security of Canada. Such perceptions and interactions are of paramount significance when one considers that Statistics Canada projects that, by 2031, between 29% and 32% of the Canadian population will be represented by visible minorities [27]. How well integrated the immigrant perceives him/herself to be will be a function of many variables, not the least of which will be the perceptions that security officers hold of the 'other'. Therefore, not only must officers be trained in cultural competency, but such training must also provide the skills necessary to focus on Canada's security, without adding to feelings of alienation by citizens.

As there are several definitions of the concept, consistency in citizens' determination of police cultural competency will be elusive. Citizens can, however, determine the quality of interaction and behaviour of officers with whom they engage. Therefore, by analysing these components, identification of the perceptions of citizens regarding the cultural competency of officers can be ascertained.

If citizens perceive they are viewed as equal partners in protecting Canada's safety and their race, ethnicity, religion, and other characteristics are respected [28], not only will this lead to greater community resilience, but citizens will also be more likely to engage with, and request the support of, security officers when problematic communal situations arise. Conversely, as suggested by Davis and Henderson [29], if citizens perceive the opposite to be true, they are more likely to view security officers as an impediment to their security and be less inclined to seek assistance from, or share crucial information with, them. Thus, this study sought to examine how and whether cultural competency training could lead to increased experiences of trust from diverse communities towards security officers; and to identify how, in the view of those communities, cultural competency is exercised during officer–citizen interactions.

Table 11.1 Comparison of survey sample VS

Representativity of sample*

Cultural groups	Survey (%)	Canada (%)
Caucasians	60.3	80.9
Muslim	8.7	3.2
Black	8.4	2.9
Asian	9.0	5.0
South Asian	9.6	4.8

*Data for Canada taken from the National Household Survey (2011).

Source: The source for the National Household Survey of Statistics Canada is: https://www12.statcan.gc.ca/nhs-enm/2011/dp-pd/prof/details/page.cfm?Lang=E&Geo1=PR&Code1=01&Data=Count&SearchText=Canada&SearchType=Begins&SearchPR=01&A1=All&B1=All&Custom=&TABID=1

This chapter presents the findings of research on cultural competency in police. We present a description of the research methods employed and the findings, based on answers to questions posed in the online survey. The results of discussions with focus groups included their explanations for responses provided by survey respondents, and recommendations to improve police–citizen relationships. Finally, an overall synthesis of the findings is provided followed by some suggestions to improve police–citizen relationships.

11.3 **Methods**

11.3.1 **Community-based survey and focus group participants**

11.3.1.1 Sample

Seven hundred participants from both Toronto and Montreal, and 500 from Saskatoon (n = 1900) acted as our base group. Our ethnic subgroup oversampling (Muslims, Black Canadians, and Asians/South Asians) was composed of 100 of each group in Toronto and Montreal, and 50 of each in Saskatoon (n = 750), giving a total sample size of 3387 (see Table 11.1).[1]

Demographics for the sample are shown in Table 11.2.

General population samples (n = 3387) achieved representivity within accepted norms for sampling precision (i.e. margins of sampling error ±3.7% for Toronto and Montreal, ±4.4% for Saskatoon, all at the 95% confidence level). The sample sizes for the ethnic subgroups are the largest possible within the

---

[1] Because the survey firm split the Asians/South Asians group and because general population quotas were overfilled, we ended up with a total of 3387 respondents.

Table 11.2 Comparison of average age, education, and income between cultural groups

Education scale	Income scale
01—Some high school or less	01—Under $40,000
02—Completed high school	02—$40,001–$60,000
03—Some university/college or technical school	03—$60,001–$80,000
04—Completed college/technical school	04—$80,001–$100,000
05—Undergraduate or university degree	05—$100,001–$150,000
06—Postgraduate or higher	06—More than $150,000

available budget, given the high cost of identifying eligible respondents within the population using representative sample selection methods. The samples provided sufficient scope to conduct a full analysis both by city (all ethnic groups; n = 250 in each city (margin of sampling error of ±6.2% at the 95% confidence level)), or by ethnic group across cities (also 250 for each ethnic group, also ±6.2% at the 95% confidence level).

These support full analysis of subgroups demographically (e.g. gender, age cohorts, and broad household income brackets), and partial analysis for smaller-sized subgroups. These samples exceed what is normally used for similar-type sample surveys in major Canadian cities (which typically range from 300 to 600) [30].

Focus groups consisted of 15 adults from each city, based on ethnicity and interest (i.e. n = 45).

11.3.1.2 Recruitment

Online participants were recruited by the polling firm Environics from a bank of paid individuals, aged ≥18 years, registered with Ethnic Voice, from which the firm procures participants. Focus groups were recruited through advertising and snow-balling techniques.

11.3.1.3 Instrument

To explore communities' views of their interactions with security officials, Environics Institute, in concert with the researchers, constructed an online, primarily quantitative, survey focusing on community quality of life; community relations and discrimination; perceptions of local police; experience with local police; police surveillance and profiling; and circumstances under which one would involve police. The survey—consisting of 41 Likert-type items and 10 focusing on demographics—took 15–20 minutes to complete. Qualitative elements requested explanations of some responses.

11.3.1.4 Validation

Representatives of the entire sample were asked, by the researchers, to complete the questionnaire and identify what was being measured, as well as the appropriateness of language. None had registered to be a part of Environics or any of its affiliates. Therefore, it was impossible for them to answer using the online version. Feedback was also solicited from mental health professionals and police officers.[2] Based on the feedback, necessary changes were made. Ethnocultural categories were those used by Statistics Canada.

11.3.1.5 Procedure

Approval to conduct the study was gained from the ethics committees of the four academic institutions. Environics Institute also conducted its validation and translated the document into French. The researchers viewed the online beta version, rating it on ease of completion and comprehension. Environics administered the surveys in both French and English, compiled the data, and sent them to the researchers for analysis. This arm's length strategy by the researchers was to reduce community members' concern that a project funded by the government may introduce bias into researchers' interactions with them.

11.4 **Findings**

11.4.1 **Community-based survey**

Participants were first asked about their experiences with, and perceptions of, police. They then responded to similar questions in the context of national security. The findings were then presented to focus groups in each of the three cities to contextualize and better understand them. Presented in this section are some of the most important findings from the survey.

11.4.2 **Experience with police**

11.4.2.1 Citizens' perceptions of police

Participants' opinions concerning police contingents servicing their communities were solicited. The results indicated that, with some cultural variations, perceptions are 'generally positive'.

---

[2] These officers were never involved in any part of the study.

11.4.2.2 Police community relationships

Relationships between community residents and police, as well as those between police and one's own ethnic group, were 'generally positive'.

11.4.2.3 Direct experience with police

Survey respondents were asked about direct contact they, or their family members, had with police over the previous five years. Results indicate that most 'did not have any contact'. Those answering affirmatively were asked about the quality of the exchange(s). Most indicated being 'treated fairly' with police acting 'professionally'. Of those reporting negative interactions, Muslims, Black Canadians, and South Asians felt their treatment was 'likely' attributable to their religion or ethnicity.

Participants were asked to rate perceived surveillance practices of local police. Most opined police 'likely' keep watch on certain individuals in their neighbourhoods. However, the preponderance of responses suggests that participants do not perceive that they, or family members, were being surveilled.

11.4.2.4 Surveillance by security and customs officials.

Most responded 'likely no' when asked whether security and customs officials treated them differently from other Canadians because of ethnic or religious backgrounds. However, both Black Canadians and Muslims believe that when they were treated differently, it was because of ethnicity or religion.

11.5 **Perceptions in the context of national security**

11.5.1 **Ability of police services to protect communities**

While no group identified violent extremism in the community as a concern, most viewed local police as being 'very' and 'somewhat important' in protecting communities and declared themselves 'somewhat confident' in their abilities. Participants who thought local police either 'not very important' or 'not at all important' in this regard, questioned their mandate and preparedness to undertake this role. Most respondents' perceptions of Canada's federal police service (Royal Canadian Mounted Police [RCMP]) is not only that they are 'very important', but respondents are 'somewhat' or 'definitely' confident in RCMP's capacity to provide protection.

11.5.1.3 Likelihood of contacting the police in the event of potential extremist activities

The likelihood of contacting local police, or the RCMP, should participants become aware of potential violent extremism in their community[3] was measured. The majority stated they would 'definitely' contact local and/or federal police. It was also shown that the more positive police–citizen interaction, the higher the perception of police cultural competency.

11.6 **Focus groups**

Focus group discussions in the three cities centred on police–citizen interactions, perceived police cultural competency, and general national security.

11.6.1 **Police–citizen interactions**

Despite the mostly positive survey findings, focus group participants suggested those results might overshadow tensions between police and ethnic minorities that stem from historical contexts and experiences that are not always personal. Furthermore, it was stated that one good police–citizen interaction will not change negative opinions. Illustratively, one participant revealed that, despite never having had an experience with police, historical relationships have led to personal dislike. Moreover, as police should 'act properly', a positive interaction would not lead to a change of opinion.

Although none expressed surprise that some, especially Black Canadians, perceive police less positively, all were surprised Muslims were not more negative. That the majority suggested positive perceptions of police by survey respondents was probably because only local police, and not the RCMP, were considered—which could have resulted in more negativity, especially among Muslims as they are often viewed as 'suspect communities'. Others recalled secondary inspection at borders based on officers' opinions that individuals 'fit the profile of a terrorist'. Some spoke of their distrust of intelligence agents,

---

[3] A scale of participants' perception of police cultural competency was developed by performing Cronbach's alpha on the following statements: 'I trust the local police to protect the safety of all citizens in my community'; 'Local police do not really care about my community's concerns about safety and security'; 'Local police consistently act in a professional manner'; 'Local police treat citizens the same regardless of their ethnic or religious background'; 'Local police are properly trained to understand people from different ethnic and religious backgrounds'; and 'Local police rely too much on physical force to deal with issues in my community'. Alpha was 0.840. Principal component analysis verified the Cronbach's alpha, producing a single factor.

declaring them 'worse than local police'. By contrast, most perceived local police to be doing 'a decent job' in serving their communities.

11.6.2 Police cultural competency training

There was agreement that while the concept of 'cultural competency' was meaningless to participants, they could address behaviours of, and manners in which, police treat citizens. There was consensus that officers must be culturally competent if they are to safeguard Canada. However, it was also stated that they cannot be considered to have achieved such competency, as they have not established trust with communities. One Muslim participant related a situation in which a government intelligence agent came to his home to interrogate him, apparently without reason. He invited the agent to share a meal with him and expressed his aggrievement at being profiled, resulting in he and the agent reaching a mutual understanding and respect.

Saskatoon is a middle-sized city with an expanding ethnocultural demographic. Participants were concerned that police do not seem to have internalized this reality. Thus, participants opined that officers' concept of diversity needs to be more expanded and inclusive, as it still mostly refers only to indigenous groups.

11.6.3 National security issues

Torontonian group members were surprised that survey participants placed such importance on the role of local police in national security. Members were initially unsure whom they would call and, finally, decided that it would likely be the RCMP. They were astonished when they were advised that their local police service also had a counterterrorism portfolio. This information also surprised those in Montreal.

While acknowledging differences in definitions of 'terrorism', Muslim participants spoke of a religious duty to identify those who would cause harm and, thus, community members stand ready to identify 'danger' elements in the community. However, the community and the RCMP need to establish trust as the service is viewed—in contrast to local police—as following a political agenda that is used against the community to increase negative stereotypes, resulting in the RCMP being viewed as culturally incompetent, untrustworthy, and acting with impunity. One individual stated: 'We don't want District 12 or Hunger Games right?'

11.7 Focus group suggestions for police

Most of the suggestions for police centred around the concept of trust, especially as it pertains to the RCMP. It was suggested that if the RCMP or intelligent agents want to gain a community's trust, they must not only help empower them, but must view such trust as a shared responsibility between communities and officers. Moreover, accountability for officers' behaviours must be demonstrated. According to one individual: 'No accountability equals no trust because of the constant fear of abuse.' In addition, police need to learn more about the cultures of people they are policing, including participating in their cultural activities.

Schools were also cited as possible institutions that could assist police to develop better partnerships with communities. For instance, it was suggested that police could visit schools and provide information to students of the consequences of bad behaviour, making poor social decisions, and so forth. It was further suggested that police could assist educational institutions with programmes teaching people about cultures and religions, hopefully leading to the appreciation of different diversities and nationalities, and better impressions of police.

11.8 **Discussion**

There appears to be good relationships between citizens in communities across the three cities, suggesting that communities possess a base from which to implement common strategies to address challenges and exercise resilience. However, the fact that respondents fear certain groups are being watched could prove problematic and lead to common mistrust between those being 'watched' and those who are of the opinion that there are those who 'should' be watched. Therefore, government and its representatives need to be attentive to messages they send and reduce the possibility of creating an 'other' against whom one must be guarded.

There was focus group consensus that survey respondents' 'good' perceptions of police are based on views of municipal police and not the RCMP. It should be mentioned that citizens are more likely to be visited by the RCMP and agents of intelligent services if individuals are suspected of national security breaches. Furthermore, it would most likely be these security agents who would attempt to enlist them as confidential informants in the 'war against terror'. Therefore, how these agents are perceived to have interacted with citizens will influence citizens' sentiment towards the service.

Focus groups highlighted the fact that Muslims surveyed were not as negative in their views of police and their cultural competency as focus group members. This disparity is easily explained when one considers that in responding to surveys, individuals are 'forced' to choose a category with little possibility of clarification. However, in focus groups, participants can expand on their responses and provide personal reflections—indeed, it is expected. Thus, the quality of information gleaned from focus groups tend to be more nuanced and richer than that measured with quantitative scales.

It should be borne in mind that although the term 'cultural competency' has meaning for academics, it means little for people in their day-to-day lives as neither survey nor focus group respondents emphasized the concept. However, both stressed the behaviours that comprised the construct, indicating that the actions measured in this study are of importance to both groups. Thus, in the focus group and survey participants, there is a strong relationship between quality of citizen–police interaction and perceptions of police cultural competency. It should be noted that not only do Black Canadians and Muslims find discrimination with police and other intelligence systems problematic owing to race and religion, but most discriminatory practices were identified by the four ethnoracial and religious groups, while very few were identified by those who self-identified as white.

Focus groups want police to display less-biased behaviours and demonstrate cultural competency. Furthermore, they stated that without exhibiting such competency, officers will have difficulty gaining the confidence of ethnocultural communities, despite Muslims stating a belief in the moral responsibility to identify those who would harm the country. Clearly then, when individuals feel targeted, misunderstood, and racially profiled, the stress engendered is not conducive to motivating trust toward authority figures.

Nonetheless, most survey respondents stated that they would contact local police or the RCMP if the country were threatened, suggesting citizens would put the safety of the country before their own anger and pain. However, government and its agencies should not take this for granted and should do what is necessary to assist all individuals to feel included in the body politic [28–30]. In other words, when communities feel included and empowered, they are more likely to become involved not only in their community's security, but in that of Canada's.

None of the above negates efforts being made by police and other governments agencies to reach out to communities. For example, Saskatoon's Violent Threat Risk Assessment; Montreal's Plan d'action; Toronto's Hate Crime Unit (part of Intelligence Services), and the Threat Assessment Section are all in place. While it could be assumed that portions of the 'good' responses concerning local police may be a result of these efforts, without data a definitive statement cannot be made. Moreover, citizens may view these programmes as more concerned with 'police work' than with interacting with citizens. Regardless, based on respondent's responses, more work is needed to bolster police legitimacy in the public eye—particularly within racialized communities.

That so many question the role of local police in national security is troubling, especially as this is the first line of defence and the service that should be contacted in an emergency. Additionally, the existence and role of Integrated National Security Enforcement Teams[4] seems to be unknown in Montreal and Toronto—two cities in which the programme exists. Although most are not overly concerned about possible acts of violent extremism occurring in their neighbourhood, citizens should, nonetheless, be provided with information concerning available resources.

11.9 **Conclusion**

Given the foregoing, police should meet with the communities they serve, in order to develop cooperative strategies aimed at creating better police–citizen relationships. Furthermore, strategies should be developed to provide opportunities for police and citizens to interact in non-judicial situations, in order to develop trust and practice cultural competency skills.

References

1. **Public Safety Canada**. Public report on the terrorism threat to Canada. Available from: https://www.publicsafety.gc.ca/cnt/rsrcs/pblctns/pblc-rprt-trrrsm-thrt-cnd-2018/index-en.aspx#s11 [accessed 4 August 2020].

2. **King M, Taylor DM.** The radicalization of homegrown jihadists: a review of theoretical models and social psychological evidence. Terrorism and Political Violence 2011;23:602–22.

3. **Hudson RA.** The sociology and psychology of terrorism: who becomes a terrorist and why? Available from: https://www.loc.gov/rr/frd/pdf-files/Soc_Psych_of_Terrorism.pdf [accessed 4 August 2020].

4. **Gill P, Young JK.** Comparing role-specific terrorist profiles. Available from: https://ssrn.com/abstract=1782008 or http://dx.doi.org/10.2139/ssrn.1782008 [accessed 4 August 2020].

5. **Bhui K, Hicks M, Lashley M, Jones E.** A public health approach to understanding and preventing violent radicalization. BMC Medicine 2012;10:1–8.

6. **Rae JA.** Will it ever be possible to profile the terrorist? Journal of Terrorism Research 2012;3:64–74.

7. **Okemi M.** Boko Haram: a religious sect or terrorist organization. Global Journal of Politics and Law Research 2013;1:1–9.

8. **Borum R.** Radicalization into violent extremism II: a review of conceptual models and empirical research. Journal of Strategic Security 2011;4:37–62.

----

[4] Programme consisting of federal, provincial, and municipal agencies to address threats from groups or individuals.

9. **Bruton B.** Somalia a new approach. Council on Foreign Relations, Center for Preventive Action: New York; 2010.
10. **Al Dajani A.** The War on Terror: a survey of counter-terrorism strategies. Available from: https://ssrn.com/abstract=2769882 [accessed 4 August 2020].
11. **Haigh C.** The political discourse of the 'new age of terror: an historical examination of the United Kingdom's approach to counter-terrorism post-9/11 with a critical discourse analysis observing how counter-terrorism strategies are framed to present a specific narrative for the 'new age of terror'. Available from: http://uu.diva-portal.org/smash/get/diva2:1257457/FULLTEXT01.pdf [accessed 4 August 2020].
12. **Sloan S.** Meeting the terrorist threat: the localization of counter terrorism. Police Practice and Research 2002;**3**:337–45.
13. **Capie D.** Localization as resistance: the contested diffusion of small arms norms in Southeast Asia. Security Dialogue 2008;**39**:637–58.
14. **Hocking B.** Patrolling the 'frontier': globalization, localization and the 'actorness' of non-central governments. Regional & Federal Studies 1999;**9**:17–39.
15. **Boucek C.** The Sakinah Campaign and Internet counterradicalization in Saudi Arabia. Available from: https://carnegieendowment.org/2008/08/25/sakinah-campaign-and-internet-counter-radicalization-in-saudi-arabia-pub-20423 [accessed 4 August 2020].
16. **Koehler D.** The radical online: individual radicalization processes and the role of the Internet. Journal for Deradicalization 2014;**1**:116–34.
17. **Berger JM.** Tailored online interventions: the Islamic State's recruitment strategy. Available from: https://ctc.usma.edu/app/uploads/2015/10/CTCSentinel-Vol8Iss1036.pdf [accessed 4 August 2020].
18. **Holt T, Freilich JD, Chermak S, McCauley C.** Political radicalization on the Internet: Extremist content, government control, and the power of victim and jihad videos. Dynamics of Asymmetric Conflict 2015;**8**:107–20.
19. **Weitzer R. Tuch SA.** Determinants of public satisfaction with the police. Police Quarterly 2005;**8**:279–97.
20. **Mazerolle LE, Antrobus E, Bennett S, Tyler TR.** Shaping citizen perceptions of police legitimacy: a randomized field trial of procedural justice. Criminology 2013;**51**:33–63.
21. **Ow R, Nur HBS.** Malay Muslim worldviews: some thoughts for social work practice in Singapore. Journal of Religion & Spirituality in Social Work: Social Thought 2014;**33**:73–94.
22. **Rew L. Becker, B, Chontichachalalauk J, Lee HY.** Cultural diversity among nursing students: reanalysis of the cultural awareness scale. Journal of Nursing Education 2014;**53**:71–6.
23. **Florini S.** Tweets, tweeps, and signifyin': communication and cultural performance on 'Black Twitter'. Television & New Media 2014;**15**:223–37.
24. **Whaley AL, Davis KE.** Cultural competency and evidence-based practice in mental health services. American Psychologist 2007;**62**:563–74.
25. **Mills JT, Miller DS.** Educating the next generation of emergency management and Homeland Security professionals: promoting racial and ethnic understanding via cultural competency and critical race theory. Journal of Applied Security Research 2015;**10**:466–80.

26. **Hajjar RM.** Military warriors as peacekeeper–diplomats: building productive relationships with foreign counterparts in the contemporary military advising mission. Armed Forces & Society 2013;**40**:647–72.

27. **Malenfant, MC, Lebel A, Martel L.** Projections of the diversity of the Canadian population, 2006 to 2031. Available from: https://www150.statcan.gc.ca/n1/pub/91-551-x/91-551-x2010001-eng.htm#archived [accessed 4 August 2020].

28. **Mazerolle LBS, Antrobus E, Eggins E.** Procedural justice, routine encounters and citizen perceptions of police: main findings from the Queensland Community Engagement Trial (QCET). Journal of Experimental Criminology 2012;**8**:343–67.

29. **Davis RC, Henderson NJ.** Willingness to report crimes: the role of ethnic group membership and community efficacy. Crime & Delinquency 2003;**49**:564–80.

30. **Statistics Canada.** Survey methods and practices 2010. Available from: https://www150.statcan.gc.ca/n1/en/pub/12-587-x/12-587-x2003001-eng.pdf?st=P8ZpPcm3 [accessed 4 August 2020].

Chapter 12

Clinical intervention to address violent radicalization: The Quebec model

Cécile Rousseau, Christian Savard,
Anna Bonnel, Richard Horne,
Anousheh Machouf, and
Marie-Hélène Rivest

12.1 Introduction

The place of clinical medical or health professional interventions in addressing violent radicalization is a topic of ongoing debate [1–3]. Firstly, there remains significant uncertainty about the claimed over-representation of mental health disorders in radicalized perpetrators, and the relative importance of psychological factors as determinants of violent radicalization is also disputed. Although there is general consensus about the fact that violent radicalization is a social phenomenon with psychological dimensions, research over the past decades has shown an absence of over-representation of psychiatric disorders in terrorists; this raises doubts about the pertinence of clinical medical- or health professional-related services for tackling violent radicalization [4]. At the same time, the high prevalence of mental health 'issues', and past psychiatric diagnosis in lone actors [5, 6], suggests that the population of at-risk individuals and perpetrators is diverse. Therefore, it may be useful to distinguish socialized actors who have strong ties to structured extremist organizations from relatively socially isolated actors who act alone but claim and even boast about virtual affiliation to extremist groups.

Secondly, considerable harm can be done through clinical intervention in cases of radicalization. The literature highlights the risk of profiling and stigmatization of minorities and patients with mental health issues, where mental illness is associated with violence and extremism [7]. Also, there are numerous historical accounts of pathologizing social dissent and resistance [8]. However, an analysis of the personal trajectories of lone actors shows that many of them were struggling with psychological distress and mental illness, and that a number of them had asked for, but never obtained, medical or psychological help. This raises an important question on the capacity of health services to implement effective secondary and tertiary prevention with at-risk individuals and with those who are already known to the justice system.

There is presently no definite empirical consensus on these debates, which is a strong reminder of both the importance of critically reflecting on the potentially harmful impact of clinical intervention for violent radicalization, and the need to redefine our roles as clinicians. This includes examining the way clinical knowledge may support vulnerable individuals and prevent escalation of at-risk behaviours and attitudes toward extremist violence.

Until the effectiveness of clinical interventions in reducing radical violence is improved through evaluative research, exchanges about existing clinical models can only serve to support practitioners in the field and provide initial insights about good and potentially harmful practices.

This chapter has two objectives. The first is to present a model of service provision for cases of radicalization in the province of Quebec (Canada) and to illustrate some of the clinical and institutional challenges associated with the implementation of service delivery and partnership with security agencies in this field. The second, based on a discussion of this experience, is to outline some of the possible implications in terms of broad assessment, treatment orientations, and service models for the clinicians, their institutions, and their partners. Initially, we will explain the premise of the Quebec model and describe its structure and functioning. A profile of the clientele served over the last three years will then be presented. To conclude, we will discuss the treatment principles that have shown promise to date, in addition to establishing parallels and contrasts between the Quebec experience and other international clinical experiences.

12.2 The Quebec model of clinical services to address violent radicalization

In July of 2016, following recommendations from the 2015–18 Quebec governmental action plan, a network of specialized clinical services was commissioned to target radicalization potentially leading to violence. A multidisciplinary team of experts attached to a mental health and primary care institution (*Centre Intégré Universitaire de Santé et Services Sociaux du Centre-Ouest-de l'Ile de Montral*) was developed to offer consultation services to various partners across the province. An ecosystemic, intersectorial, and interdisciplinary intervention model was developed to maximize outreach, and develop specialized clinical and community services.

The Quebec model is based on Alex Schmid's definition of *radicalization* as intrinsically intertwined with a given social, cultural, historical, and political context [4]. This individual and collective phenomenon is usually linked to a context of political polarization, in which attempts at dialogue and negotiation among various parties have been terminated by one or both parties, resulting in escalating conflict. This definition is based on a systemic, bidirectional outlook on radicalization, emphasizing the dynamics of interaction between the opposing parties at hand. We consider this systemic perspective to be crucial in pinpointing solutions, however partial, to the present context of social polarization in Quebec. This involves tensions between the majority and minorities, defined around ethnic, racial, religious, or gender identity or orientation identities [9]. The service model is structured around three pillars: multiple access points to facilitate outreach and decrease stigma; specialized teams to assess and formulate treatment plans based on existing best practices in forensic, social, and cultural psychiatry; and collaborative involvement with primary care services such as community mental health, educational, and youth protection institutions, which are in charge of social integration and long-term management.

12.3 **Multiple access points**

Specialized services can be accessed through different channels to offer rapid, non-stigmatizing access points that facilitate outreach and collaboration between relevant partners (individuals, families, and communities, as well as health, education, and security institutions). These entry points consist of two modalities: the first—*Info-Social (811)*—is a free and confidential province-wide telephone consultation service, which provides the general public with 24-hour-a-day advice, support, and orientation in relation to a wide range of psychosocial issues, including violent radicalization, for which respondents have received special training. The second is a specialized *Partner Consultation Line*, operated by the Montreal Polarization Team, which is available seven days a week from 8am to 10pm. Calls received on this line are specifically related to issues of radicalization and are answered within two hours. An in-person assessment is proposed in the following week if required. The *Partner Consultation Line* number is known to crisis centres, health and education professionals, and security agency staff. It is also available to clients and families who are followed by the team, ensuring a rapid response in case of emergency. A joint decision algorithm has also been developed with the Hate Crimes and Incidents Unit of the Montreal Police to assist schools in assessing risk and taking steps in situations related to radicalization involving students.

12.4 **Specialized clinics**

Specialized consultation and supervision clinical teams have been developed in five regional areas (Montreal, Laval, Quebec City, Sherbrooke, and Gatineau). Team members, which include experts in psychology and forensic psychiatry, are invited to discuss cases via monthly videoconferences. The Montreal team consists of eight senior clinicians (psychiatrists, child psychiatrists, social workers, and psychologists) from various ethnic, cultural, clinical, and theoretical backgrounds working under the Ministry of Health Mental Health and Primary Care Services as well as from various external agencies.

The clinical team's consultation model is inspired by the Cultural Consultation model developed and validated by the McGill Division of Social and Cultural Psychiatry [10]. The team offers clinical consultation to its partners as needed and provides mostly short-term follow-up to clients. However, in cases involving high risk, the team will remain involved while supporting a progressive involvement of primary care services with a wrap-around approach. With client consent, clinical progress can be reviewed on a regular basis with the various professionals involved, if required.

In cases where a client does not consent to personal clinical information being shared between professionals, confidentiality is maintained in line with the Canadian professional codes of ethics, with the exception of cases where risk is deemed to be high and imminent. It is important to note that unless there is an imminent risk to human life, sensitive information is also kept confidential and not shared with security agencies. The relevant agencies are aware of this and understand the importance of clinicians developing a trust-based alliance with individuals, families, and communities.

12.4.1 **The central role of primary care services**

While initial assessment, psychotherapy and/or psychiatric services can be offered by the Polarization Team, the Quebec clinical model makes it a priority to provide clients with primary care services in institutions such as frontline mental health, education, and youth protection organizations. Such services include intensive mental health follow-up in local community-based clinics and intervention by *readaptation* centres for clients with intellectual delay or autism. Public, community, and religious organizations can offer such services as employment and education support, as well as mentorship, and are highly equipped to foster clients' social integration and life-skill development [11].

Artistic programmes offer a semi-structured, non-judgemental environment, fostering self-expression and creativity. These are offered in partnership with the Montreal Museum of Fine Arts. A multimedia pilot programme involving young artists has shown to provide youth with alternative means of expressing their dissent. These programmes are particularly useful in reaching out to those socially isolated young people at risk of radicalization that may be more reticent to using healthcare-related institutions.

12.5 **Profile of the clientele**

Over the first three years of operation (2016–2019), the demographic and diagnostic profile of the clientele serviced by the Polarization Team has changed drastically. In general, clients tend to be older, present with more severe psychopathology than previously, and are at greater risk of suicidal and homicidal acting out. The type of prominent radical ideology has also shifted from more religious radicalization toward masculinist and far-right ideologies. These changes appear to be associated with local and national social transformations, as well as media coverage of international events such as the Christchurch and Pittsburgh shootings. Overall, three factors appear to play a role in the transformation of referral patterns: changes in social context; perception of the relative importance of these changes; and the continuing development of partnerships and alliances by the clinical team. However, it is not possible to determine the exact contribution of each of them in the observed shifts.

12.5.1 **Sources of references and partnerships**

The number of referrals to the team has grown owing to the increasing awareness of its existence in security, health, social service, and education sectors, to the national and international sociopolitical climate, and to the growing trust in the team's services.

In 2015 and 2016, following the widely publicized departure of Montreal college and high-school students to take part in the war in Syria, colleges and health and social service professionals became highly vigilant of potentially radicalized individuals. For example, for a number of youth or families, religious beliefs, and practices which diverged from mainstream norms, or behavioural or family difficulties, were often misinterpreted as signs of radicalization because of cultural misunderstandings and internalized stereotypes [12]. During this period, a considerable number of referrals were due to the implicit radicalization of the majority, expressed through Islamophobia. In Quebec, like in other parts of North America and Europe, fear and anger

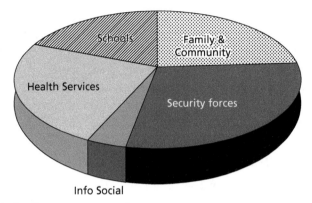

Fig. 12.1 Referral sources.

triggered by social uncertainty was projected onto the Other [13]. Although rather minimized in 2015–16, with time, it became more evident from public opinion, and also from the education and health sectors, that the upsurge in extreme right discourse, associated with anti-Semitic, xenophobic, and masculinist rhetoric, was equally concerning, if not more so. The types of referrals coming from these institutions began to shift. Simultaneously, the development of strong partnerships with federal and provincial security agencies resulted in a sharp increase in referrals of cases involving national security issues and/or actual hate crimes and incidents. Recently, the team started receiving referrals from the provincial detention network and is providing a safety net for individuals who have been convicted and, because of mental health issues, are considered to be high risk. Fig. 12.1 illustrates the main sources of referrals.

12.5.2 **Categories of referral and their evolution**

The Polarization Team receives three major types of referral: radicalized individuals (most often with a lone actor profile), with a suspected or proven risk of violence; families and significant others of radical individuals; and other persons or groups affected in one way or another by social polarization. The latter group is heterogeneous and includes individuals or families who have been targeted as 'radicals' because of prejudice and associated religious or racial profiling. In 2016 and 2017 the two last categories were predominant; however, since 2018, clients with a lone actor risk profile, adhering to an ideology or consuming different forms of extremist violence (from mass killing videos to Daesh propaganda), have accounted for more than half of the team's requests.

12.5.3 **Radicalized individuals**

Radicalized individuals represent 55% of the team's clientele, with 90% being male and 10% female. The mean age is 24.7 years, the overall age range 13–68 years, with the vast majority of clients being between 15 and 25 years of age. In terms of ideology type, 35% adhere to extreme right and/or nationalistic ideologies, with or without anti-Semitic and xenophobic beliefs. Thirty per cent of our clientele holds religious ideologies (mostly of the Muslim and Christian faith, but including other belief systems as well). A growing category (15%) can be considered masculinist in their views and this includes individuals involved in the Incel (i.e. involuntary celibates) movement. Extreme-left ideologies are present in only 5% of referrals. Finally, another 15% of our clientele tends to be more attracted to scenes of horror and cruelty as opposed to adhering to any of the aforementioned ideologies (Fig. 12.2). Examples of material viewed by this clientele can include violent images of Daesh and the Ku Klux Klan, Second World War footage, and violent pornography. The presence of this category of individuals attracted to violence, and the fact that case histories reveal that a number of our clients have shifted ideologies, suggests that for a significant number of potential lone actors, ideology may be an idiom of distress; the individual can channel feelings of rage and despair into a particular discourse, which both reflects their inner state and also serves to provoke, providing them with a sense of legitimacy and affiliation.

Client involvement in follow-up with the Polarization Team is voluntary, even in cases which are court-ordered and all clients are aware of the person or institution that referred them. The team's clientele has a wide variety of needs and requests, and these are vital to the alliance-building process. For example, clients may refuse an initial formal assessment but may want help

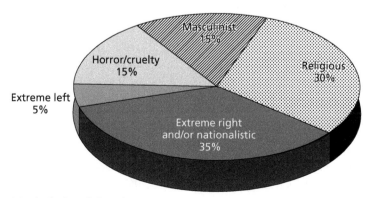

Fig. 12.2 Ideologies of clientele.

finding a job or accessing a gym. All clients who engage in follow-up present some form of psychological distress and most of them report some dysfunction in the intimate or social sphere. Among the few clients that were preliminarily assessed but declined any follow-up, lack of empathy, remorse, and insight, and a sense of pleasure in provoking fear in others suggested the possibility of psychopathic traits. Risk of violence is assessed through the National Consortium for the Study of Terrorism and Responses to Terrorism (START) [14], a clinical consensus instrument with an adult and an adolescent version. The START is designed for cross-sectional or longitudinal assessments of the levels of suicidal and homicidal risk in patients with a mental disorder. In order to monitor the patient's evolution, the START is repeated every 6 months. In terms of diagnosis, three main groups dominate: mood and stress-related disorders (with a high incidence of childhood adversity and trauma as reported in the literature) [15, 16]; autism spectrum disorders (ASD) [17, 18]; and psychosis (in particular delusional disorders). In the cases of autism and delusional disorder, while approximately half of the clientele was already diagnosed prior to being assessed by the team, the remainder was diagnosed by the team. In the team's clientele, two symptom clusters are often core to a complex differential diagnosis. Firstly, rigidity and obsessive thoughts may be central in autistic individuals, as well as in obsessive-compulsive disorder and delusional disorder. Secondly, impulsivity and grandiosity may signal a hypomanic phase, reflect a narcissistic personality disorder (or traits), or be a signal of episodic or regular drug abuse. ASD is diagnosed with the Autism Diagnostic Observation Schedule and Autism Diagnostic Interview, by a certified psychologist specialized in autism assessment. Other diagnoses are always established after repeated evaluations, by both the team psychologists and psychiatrist. In some cases a full forensic court assessment confirms the diagnosis.

The following vignettes illustrate some of the initial clinical presentations of patients seen by the team.

12.5.4 Case studies

Kevin is a 40-year-old man with three children, two girls aged eight and four years, and a boy aged six years. He has never held a regular job owing to academic failure, but since his youth he has obsessively gathered factual data on a variety of topics, which suggests at least a normal level of intelligence. The divorce of his parents was highly traumatic for the client owing to the sudden abandonment by his mother, with whom he lost contact. Initially, he became part of an extreme -left group; however, during a difficult transition period (separation from his wife), he switched to an extreme-right ideology and became a self-proclaimed Nazi, believing that feminism was a plague spread by the Jews, which ruined the family, and that his marriage would be saved if his wife submitted to his authority and wisdom. He was convinced that war was imminent and that he needed to protect his family and the endangered white population. He also condoned extreme right-wing terrorist attacks. The initial diagnosis was delusional disorder.

Sacha is a man in his early twenties, estranged from his family (who physically abused him), and who—at the time of referral—was living in poverty and in insalubrious housing conditions. He was referred to the Polarization Team by a security agency after having been charged with preparing an armed left-wing revolution. In the first meeting with Sacha, he was dressed extravagantly, had poor hygiene, and spoke at length and in detail about the early stages of socialism in Europe. His great-uncle, a very important identity and attachment figure for him, had died some years ago, and had been actively involved in the anti-fascist movement decades ago in Spain. Sacha was diagnosed by a team psychologist, with considerable experience in the field of autism, as having an ASD.

Liliane is a 25-year-old single mother of two boys. She converted to a radical form of Islam at the end of adolescence and departed for Syria during the war. She had grown up in a highly disturbed family environment and was the victim of a gang rape in mid-adolescence. In Syria, she experienced further physical and sexual abuse. She returned to Canada with her two-year-old son (born in Syria) and was reunited with her other son whom she had left in her mother's care during her absence. Security agencies were concerned because she had indicated that she was considering returning to Syria, in spite of the risks to herself and to her children. She has been diagnosed with complex post-traumatic stress disorder with dissociative features.

12.5.5 **Family members and significant others**

Families may self-refer or be referred to the clinical team for support and/or for indirect intervention and risk assessment when the radicalized person is unwilling to receive services. Parents, siblings, or spouses may also consult if they are worried for the safety or well-being of the individual at risk. Such cases require clinical interventions of great finesse, which take into account developmental factors, attachment issues, and short- and long-term risks for the child. Children of parents who have been imprisoned for terrorist offences may also be highly distressed. A systemic intervention is needed to help them overcome the loss and express their ambivalence toward the parental figure without forcing them into a loyalty conflict, which may push them toward idealization or demonization of the absent parent.

Intervening to protect children may also require forward planning with involved partners, as has been the case in preparing for the return of families from the war in Syria. Since 2018 a group composed of representatives of a federal security agency, youth protection services, and the Polarization Team has worked on an approach focused on the best interests of the returning children, to minimize attachment disruptions as much as possible and to prevent re-traumatization in the arrival and resettlement phases.

12.5.6 Addressing social and institutional polarization and radicalization

The clinical team receives a number of consultation requests, which illustrates the diverse consequences of the polarization climate on minority and majority groups. Firstly, some situations brought to the team's attention because of concerns about radicalization proved to reveal educational or health professionals' stereotypes and prejudices about minority groups [12]. Secondly, tensions and conflicts can affect not only individuals or families, but also groups, requiring on occasion, a neighbourhood or institutional intervention. For example, one team intervention involved addressing a conflict between tenants of a building where opposing factions supported extreme-left and extreme-right positions. The conflict had escalated verbally and there had been indirect threats of physical violence. In another instance, a regional team intervened in a heated conflict between refugees and Canadians in a low-cost housing area, which had led to racial abuse and hate crimes. Thirdly, the presence of radicalized individuals with mental health difficulties in educational institutions can provoke considerable anxiety, which may lead to burnout, work absenteeism, and workplace conflicts about the relative safety of students and staff. In such situations, the Polarization Team can reassure and provide guidelines and intervention tools.

12.6 Main treatment principles

The Quebec model of intervention is structured around five broad treatment principles: alleviating psychological distress; consolidating familial and social ties; addressing issues of identity, affiliation, and belonging; working to identify and develop a sense of purpose; and enhancing cognitive flexibility.

12.6.1 Alleviating psychological distress

Acute feelings of distress and despair dominate the clinical presentation of the majority of the Polarization Team's referrals. These feelings may manifest through symptoms of depression, anxiety, and anger, and are often compounded by suicidal and homicidal ideation. Dissociation and psychotic symptoms can also evoke confusion, fear, and distress. Addressing such psychic pain and any feelings of associated hopelessness is the initial objective in the therapeutic process. Any trauma issues also need to be explored in order to create an emotionally safe therapeutic environment. Unresolved trauma can lead to re-enactment and risk-taking behaviours, which are often associated with radicalization and an association with extremist groups, who may be representative of both saviour or aggressor to the client. The team's treatment approach is supportive and flexible, culturally sensitive, and often entails psychotherapies of different types (e.g. trauma-focused, cognitive behavioural or psychodynamic). It may also include medication and modalities such as artistic expression and physical activities. In situations of high impulsivity medication often serves a dual purpose of soothing pain and anxiety, while also partially buffering the risk of acting out. The clinicians' concern for the patient's well-being helps to establish a strong therapeutic alliance and opens up the possibility for other therapeutic propositions.

12.6.2 Consolidating a familial and social network

Most of our clients are either very isolated and/or live in dysfunctional relational environments. Even if ongoing feelings of rejection and exclusion can be addressed in therapy, therapy is not an appropriate option for all individuals and many of them benefit greatly from direct help to improve relationships with their families and entourage, as well as to foster social integration. Family and couple therapy is often proposed, but, in many cases, because of family violence and/or trauma, this may not initially be an appropriate means of restoring relational functioning. Intense work on daily relations in the patient's direct environment may involve support to restore a feeling of safety and comfort in the neighbourhood and an investment in everyday interactions with community organizations or street workers, among others.

12.6.3 Addressing issues of identity, affiliation, and belonging

Radicalized youth tend to value and be highly invested in maintaining a single identity, to the exclusion of other forms of identity. However, in-depth assessment can reveal a wide array of past affiliations that may still have value, although this may not initially be evident to them. Through respecting a young person's feelings of rebellion, and not pushing normative identities, which may be seen by them as oppressive, the intervention can build on diverse levels of identity to introduce some flexibility in their sense of belonging. For example, while parents may be dismissed as failures or as uncaring, a grandparent figure may become an identification model. This may also happen with a mentor, a teacher, or (somewhat surprisingly) with security agency staff such as law enforcement officers.

12.6.4 **Working on a sense of purpose and a vision of the future**

The quest for meaning is a driving force in the lives of radicalized youth [19]. For these individuals, envisioning an apocalyptic future and maintaining a dystopic view of the world is often a way to purge one's fears and regain a sense of control over one's destiny [20]. Relationships, work, and study, and also small daily accomplishments can help restore a feeling of being appreciated and useful, and help to grieve the loss of one's grandiose sense of self. Art, music, drama, and writing can all be effective means to fulfilling a sense of accomplishment for youth who may not have the skills required to participate in more formal and structured activities such as civic engagement [21].

12.6.5 **Enhancing cognitive complexity**

Confronting and challenging the client's ideology is usually to be avoided, not only because it may sever the alliance, but also because such interventions often feed the client's sense of grandiosity and may reactively reinforce their devotion to extremist beliefs. However, this does not mean that work on addressing erroneous cognition is not possible nor important. In this context, consolidating the client's mentalization skills [22] could be an objective of the treatment process. This type of approach may help the client make connections between the content of some of his ideas and some of his/her own mental states (emotions, reactions). It may also involve helping the client to understand that others have emotions/thoughts/reactions that might be different from what he or she thinks they are [22].

Having presented the broad treatment principles, the following is a summary of the clinical evolution of the respective cases of Kevin, Sacha, and Liliane.

As Kevin was reticent to travel to consultations, therapy was provided in the home by two of the team therapists. Medication was proposed, but this did not prove beneficial. The therapists listened to Kevin's ideologically-loaded discourse, avoiding addressing directly the radicalized content and emphasizing progressively the personal dimensions of Kevin's experience. Patiently, through the exploration of his marital problems, he began to voice his feelings of powerlessness and accept some help to connect to his family network and to envision involvement in some type of employment. Homicidal and suicidal risk remained high.

Following his ASD diagnosis, Sacha was referred to specialized support services. Intensive psychosocial intervention was required to help stabilize his living conditions. The risk for potential acting out was monitored through bi-weekly or monthly appointments, which he attended willingly. In order to re-direct his radicalized ideas away from violence, it was proposed that he record them in essay form. Sacha found it satisfying to write a long manuscript that paid tribute to his great-uncle and provided him with a real sense that he was contributing in his own way to social transformation.

Liliane's treatment involved psychotherapy to address trauma and relational issues, addressing, among other things, her dissociative symptoms. She grad-ually became more stable and more aware of her children's needs. Services were also provided to her children in order to address issues of attachment and trauma that were interfering with their school performance and social adjustment.

As some of our clinical partners have commented, in essence, the Quebec approach is simply based on sound clinical practice, with particular attention being paid to social and cultural factors. In terms of strengths, the combination of specialized approaches—sensitive to cultural and contextual factors—and local wrap-around services appears to enhance social integration and decrease des-pair and associated suicidal and homicidal urges. In terms of potential adverse effects, the provision of intensive services to very isolated individuals sometimes generates strong dependency links, and these should be handled with care in order to avoid repeating prior experiences of exclusion and rejection. While the model resembles certain approaches described in the literature, it clearly differs from others. Most of the available clinical literature on intervention (secondary and tertiary prevention) focuses on de-radicalization and disengagement pro-grammes. Deradicalization involves challenging the cognitive frames sup-porting the individual's radical ideology; however, there is little-to-no evidence attesting to the success of this type of approach [23, 24]. Disengagement ap-proaches, which promote reintegration of the individual into their social en-vironment, have been shown to be more successful [11]. However, for now, the lack of well-designed evaluations of the existing models, including the Quebec experience, requires prudence in recommending any particular service model.

12.7 **Conclusion**

Three years on from its inception, the preliminary evaluation of the Quebec clinical model by its partners and clinicians suggests that it could be considered a promising approach to addressing the specific challenges of individuals who present as potential lone actors at high risk of violent radicalization. However, the model does not appear to reach many members of extremist groups who do not present with individual vulnerabilities.

While initial signs are positive, a rigorous evaluation is warranted to establish the short-, medium-, and long-term efficiency of the model, and eventually to identify the key elements that may be transferable to other clinical settings. In 2020, a five-year evaluative research project will examine these questions.

However, it is important to consider that any intervention can be harmful or misfocused if due attention is not paid to structural discrimination and to violence stemming from the associated marginalization and exclusion [25–27]. The risk of medicalizing social suffering and pathologizing dissent is real, and constant awareness of the possibility to harm, despite the best of intentions, is needed. Clinical care can in no way replace social justice, equity, and human rights—all key pillars in primary prevention against violent radicalization. In the meantime, however, providing empathy and care in the face of despair and rage may prove most beneficial in decreasing the risk of violent acts.

References

1. **Misiak B, Samochowiec J, Bhui K, Schouler-Ocak M, Demunter H, Kuey L,** et al. A systematic review on the relationship between mental health, radicalization and mass violence. European Psychiatry 2019;**56**:51–9.
2. **Rousseau C, Hassan G.** Current challenges in addressing youth mental in the context of violent radicalization. Journal of the American Academy of Child & Adolescent Psychiatry 2019;**58**:747–50.
3. **Bhui K, Otis M, Silva MJ, Halvorsrud K, Freestone M, Jones E.** Extremism and common mental illness: cross-sectional community survey of White British and Pakistani men and women living in England. The British Journal of Psychiatry 2019, DOI: 10.1192/bjp.2019.14.
4. **Schmid AP.** Radicalisation, de-radicalisation, counter-radicalisation: a conceptual discussion and literature review. Available from: http://www.icct.nl/download/file/ICCT-Schmid-Radicalisation-De-Radicalisation-Counter-Radicalisation-March-2013.pdf [accessed 4 August 2020].
5. **Silver J, Simons A, Craun S.** A study of the pre-attack behaviors of active shooters in the United States between 2000 and 2013. Available from: https://www.fbi.gov/file-repository/pre-attack-behaviors-of-active-shooters-in-us-2000-2013.pdf/view [accessed 4 August 2020].
6. **Gill P, Silver J, Horgan J, Corner E.** Shooting alone: the pre-attack experiences and behaviors of US solo mass murderers. Journal of Forensic Sciences 2017;**62**:710–14.
7. **Ragazzi F.** Countering terrorism and radicalisation: securitising social policy? Critical Social Policy 2017;**37**:163–79.
8. **Kleinman A, Kleinman J.** Introduction. In: **Kleinman A, Das V, Lock MM,** eds. Social suffering. Berkeley, Los Angeles, and London: University of California Press; 1997, pp. ix–xxvii.

9. **Ben-Cheikh I, Rousseau C, Hassan G, Brami M, Hernandez S, Rivest M-H.** Intervention en contexte de radicalisation menant à la violence: une approche clinique multidisciplinaire. Revue Santé Mentale au Québec 2018;**43**:85–99.

10. **Kirmayer LJ, Guzder J, Rousseau C, editors.** Cultural consultation encountering the other in mental health care. New York: Springer; 2014.

11. **Anon.** Mentoring and deradicalisation. In: **Jayakumar S**, ed. Terrorism, radicalisation & countering violent extremism: practical considerations & concerns. Singapore: Palgrave Macmillan; 2019, pp. 19–28.

12. **Rousseau C, Ellis H, Lantos J.** The dilemma of predicting violent radicalization. Pediatrics 2017;**140**:e20170685.

13. **Bauman Z, Haugaard M.** Liquid modernity and power: a dialogue with Zygmunt Bauman 1. Journal of Power 2008;**1**:111–30.

14. Kronick R, Rousseau C. Rights, compassion and invisible children: a critical discourse analysis of the parliamentary debates on the mandatory detention of migrant children in Canada. Journal of Refugee Studies 2015. academic.oup.com

15. **START.** IVEO Knowledge Matrix. Available from: http://www.start.umd.edu/data-tools/iveo-knowledge-matrix [accessed 4 August 2020].

16. **Rousseau C, Hassan G, Oulhote Y, Lecompte V, Mekki-Berrada A, El Hage H.** From social adversity to sympathy for violent radicalization: the role of depression and religiosity. Archives of Public Health 2019;**77**:45.

17. **Faccini L, Allely CS.** Rare instances of individuals with autism supporting or engaging in terrorism. Journal of Intellectual Disabilities and Offending Behaviour 2017;**8**:70–82.

18. **Faccini L, Allely CS.** Rare instances of individuals with autism supporting or engaging in terrorism: a reply. Journal of Intellectual Disabilities and Offending Behaviour 2018;**9**:64–6.

19. **Webber D, Babush M, Schori-Eyal N, Vazeou-Nieuwenhuis A, Hettiarachchi M, Bélanger JJ**, et al. The road to extremism: field and experimental evidence that significance loss-induced need for closure fosters radicalization. Journal of Personality and Social Psychology 2018;**114**:270.

20. **Venkatesh V, Podoshen JS, Wallin J, Rabah J, Glass D.** Promoting extreme violence: visual and narrative analysis of select ultraviolent terror propaganda videos produced by the Islamic State of Iraq and Syria (ISIS) in 2015 and 2016. Terrorism and Political Violence, 2018:1–23.

21. **Ellis BH, Abdi SM, Horgan J, Miller AB, Saxe GN, Blood E.** Trauma and openness to legal and illegal activism among Somali refugees. Terrorism and Political Violence 2018, DOI: 10.1080/09546553.2018.1516209.

22. **Fonagy P.** Affect regulation, mentalization and the development of the self. New York: Routledge; 2018.

23. **Hassan G, Brouillette-Alarie S, Ousman S, Varela W, Lavoie L, Killinc D**, et al. A systematic review of what works in primary and secondary prevention programs that aim to counter violent radicalization. Public Safety Canada (Submitted).

24. **Stephens W, Sieckelinck S, Boutellier H.** Preventing violent extremism: a review of the literature. Studies in Conflict & Terrorism 2019, DOI: 10.1080/1057610X.2018.1543144.

25. **Kirmayer LJ, Kronick R, Rousseau C.** Advocacy as a key to structural competence in psychiatry. JAMA 2018;**75**:119–20.

26. **Eisenman DP, Flavahan L.** Canaries in the coal mine: interpersonal violence, gang violence, and violent extremism through a public health prevention lens. International Review of Psychiatry 2017;**29**:341–9.

27. **United Nations General Assembly.** Plan of Action to Prevent Violent Extremism. Available from: https://www.un.org/counterterrorism/plan-of-action-to-prevent-violent-extremism [accessed 4 August 2020].

Chapter 13

Deradicalization and rehabilitation: A case study of the Quilliam Foundation's decade-long approach in the UK, the United States, and worldwide

Muhammad Fraser-Rahim and
Mohammed Hassan Khalid

13.1 Introduction

Despite a great deal of research into the radicalization process of extremists, there has been significantly less study with respect to the deradicalization process of those who previously supported an extremist organization. When we study terrorism, extremism, and violent extremism at large, we often focus heavily on tactics and strategy. Yet we can learn a great deal if we look at the cognitive and emotional behaviour that underlies a particular set of beliefs.

As will be seen in this chapter, it is clear that a range of factors contribute towards radicalization and the actual ability for someone to mobilize into violent extremist behaviour and activities. Some of which induce feelings of shame, guilt, and vulnerability, and can often become the catalyst for radicalization.

These events often take place during times of transitions in life, including—but not limited to—divorce, adolescents, death, new friends, and, increasingly, an online space and world that provides an environment for new ideas and friendships—some of which are nefarious in nature. All these elements can amplify issues of identity crises within a person, which can affect both men and women, boys and girls, and enhance susceptibility to extremism. For Quilliam, the oldest counter-extremist organization in the world, hundreds of personnel accounts and stories have been at the centre of the work in understanding the reasons, motivations, and pathways to violent extremism. Its founders, Maajid Nawaz and Noman Benotman, both former extremists themselves, represent two distinct but similar experiences. Nawaz was involved in the ascendancy of

Muslim activism in Europe in the 1990s and Benotman's rise to fame in Islamist circles was based in his home country of Libya, where he came from a highly affluent Libyan family that contradicted the government and policy circle analytical line that equated poor, uneducated, and non-elite circles as the primary means for recruitment.

In the case of Mohammed Khalid, one of the people we worked to rehabilitate on his journey in and out of extremism, and whose case study is detailed in this chapter, the use of the Internet was a persistent and consistent medium for his journey to extremism, and one that was paramount to his transition from radicalization to mobilization in Islamist violence. Furthermore, Khalid's story of consuming propagandist content and disseminating extremist messages indicates that social media sites, in particular, are often exploited to reaffirm an extremist position discovered offline. Moreover, the absence of critical thinking and digital literacy skills seems to enhance susceptibility to extremism, as participants consume and regurgitate material without critically engaging with the underlying arguments. Simultaneously, conspiratorial websites and sensationalist reporting by some media organizations inflate the sense of threat, leading to negative perceptions toward 'the other'.

From this chapter the reader will gain first-hand insights into the struggle, the challenges, and the 'human' experience of someone who is journeying in and out of extremism. Quilliam continues to engage with individuals throughout the United States and worldwide, and works in finding good practices throughout the processes of deradicalization, demobilization, and rehabilitation.

13.2 **Deradicalization: the US and global context**

In the wake of terrorist attacks in France, Nigeria, the UK, the United States, and other places worldwide, it is evident that governments are struggling to find effective deradicalization programmes and efforts to stop the threat of violent extremism. The increase in the number of attacks by Islamic State and its metastasized affiliates, along with other transnational terrorist groups, shows sophistication and diversification of their techniques, tactics, and procedures, and have demonstrated these groups' adaptability, proving that local communities are more vulnerable to terrorist attacks than ever before.

The White House Countering Violent Extremism (CVE) summit in 2015, together with follow-up meetings and the January 2016 publication of the United Nation's Secretary General's Action Plan to Prevent Violent Extremism, served in many ways to rally the international community toward high-level support for a swift response involving private sector, civil society, religious, and government participants. In May 2017, the State Department and the Unites States

Agency for International Development released their first-ever Joint Strategy on Countering Violent Extremism to help communities identify the early signs of radicalization and intervene before violence begins. Countries all over the world, including Kenya, Nigeria, Pakistan, and the United States, are pulling together national CVE strategies in an effort to come up with tailored responses based on each country's specific demands and needs in order to steer citizens away from a path of radicalization.

As such, much focus has been dedicated to preventing individuals from joining or engaging in violent extremism—where they believe violence under-taken by non- state actors that is inspired or justified by, and/or associated with, an extreme political, religious, or social ideology. However, less attention has been given to the processes of disengagement and deradicalization, concepts key to effective rehabilitation and reintegration programming—components increasingly recognized as essential parts of any holistic counterterrorism/ countering violent extremism or terrorism prevention strategy. We provide the following definitions to help the reader distinguish how we define our key components: disengagement; deradicalization; rehabilitation; and reintegration.

- **Disengagement:** the process and physical removal of a person from a terrorist organization and going through the behavioural change away from violence.

- **Deradicalization:** a radical change away from previously held beliefs in the extremist mindset and ideology, and a mental/cognitive opening away and rejection of those views.

- **Rehabilitation:** a process borrowed from law enforcement/criminal justice field in which an individual willingly seeks to change their behaviour to find new ways of being to express themselves. As this has been utilized in the gang and drug prevention space, for those in the terrorism prevention field, this has been aligned closely with deradicalization.

- **Reintegration:** the process of an individual re-joining society in which they restore their family, personal, and community links in a process of self-restoration.

In no way are these terms to be seen as the end all or be all, but they begin to help the reader and practitioner think more deeply about how programmes and interventions are executed in finding solutions to assist individuals. For policy-makers, academics, practitioners, religious leaders, civil society, and laymen, different definitional uses and insights vary depending on their perspectives, and where they are in the process and chain of aiding individuals in and out of extremism. For victims, perpetrators, security professionals, or counsel-lors alike, we have all just begun to scratch the surface and time is the biggest indicator of how we can engage in iterative learning on this issue. All this becomes uniquely important and vital as we collectively think about creative and tailored strategies in healing individuals affected by transnational terrorism and violent extremism.

As a whole, the work to sway individuals away from extremist beliefs and behaviours is not an easy one. In fact, the work of both ad hoc and now organized programmes, like the efforts of Quilliam both in the United States and globally, can be slow, timely, and tedious. Many of these efforts do not interest people, but they are vitally necessary for communities. However, these efforts, with consistent engagement by experts who understand these issues from practitioner, policy, and academic perspectives, can see results and in time can create a radical transformation in the individual, resulting in them being a productive member of society.

The following subsection captures the personal and first-hand account of one such individual, Mohammed Khalid, with whom Quilliam has worked with on his journey in and out of extremism. This first-hand account and testimony provides further insights and perspectives from the youngest person in US history indicted on terrorism charges.

13.2.1 Mohammed Khalid: an autobiographical account

Born in Al-'Ain, United Arab Emirates (UAE), in 1993, I was the second of four siblings in a Pakistani family. Most of my distant relatives had migrated to Pakistan in the 1947 partition of British India. So I considered myself a confluence of different cultures: I was an Indian, a Pakistani, and an Emirati.

My father immigrated to the UAE with our growing family and worked hard to provide for us in this wealthy country. But our expenses kept piling up. The UAE was undergoing a developmental frenzy and our rental house, the house where I had grown up, was soon demolished to make way for a supermarket. Permanence for me was temporary, even then. I belonged somewhere only to have it replaced by somewhere—and later something else.

I was living in the country for about a decade when my grandmother's health worsened back in Pakistan. We returned to our ancestral home in Pakistan to care for her. Around this time, my father also decided to leave his mother and family behind, and leave for the United States. Pakistan could not provide us with a better future. He hoped to petition for his wife and children if his immigration case was successful.

The pain of separation was quite severe on all of us. After my grandmother's death, my extended family ran into a dispute over the house. For years, I lived with my mother and siblings in a single room upstairs. I soon became nostalgic for the UAE and searched for a semblance of a normal life. Eventually, I overcame my hesitations. I knew that we had come from a poor family, but restricted means did not have to restrain my dreams and ambitions.

All my parents ever wanted was to provide us with opportunities denied to them. Education, they insisted, was the surest way to self-sufficiency and success. Both of them had only graduated high school and worked in a variety of jobs to support their families. That was not the future they dreamt for us. Our future, they envisioned, would be far brighter and better. Our only job, they told us, was to focus on our studies.

To that end, my father spent all of his savings to put us through the best schools anywhere we relocated. I was privileged to enrol in schools generally attended by students from wealthy families, something that I only realized years later. It was a testament to my parents' prudence that I never felt the burdens of our straitened means. I was also enrolled in Arabic lessons to read and memorize the Qur'an, but I never read the translation of what I read and only half-heartedly listened to my Qaris' explanations.

Religion was important: I knew I was a Muslim and I was happy to be one. However, religion did not play a significant role in my life except as much as was culturally appropriate.

This changed after September 11, 2001.

I remember when I stood affixed before the television and watched the planes strike the twin towers of the World Trade Center. Even back then, I paid particular interest to news media and analysis, which provided me with a deeper exposure into the cultural climate and the political issues locally and globally. Having lived in one foreign country, I was eager to see how other countries were. That day, I acutely remember the sentiments of one news anchor contextualizing the attacks while speaking of the U.S. role in wars around the world. The anchor could be forgiven for thinking that way; anger perpetually simmered beneath the surface about a global superpower with a free rein to do as it wished. But wars were only a part of the equation. The economic power and moral standing of the United States was also consistently called into question by the general public.

Too preoccupied with grown-up affairs, my family and relatives gathered and talked about everything but politics. I cared just as less about the messy world of regional politics as the fanfare of local councils' never-ending elections. But in attending local mosques and listening to the often-fiery sermons, and in overhearing conversations among locals in shops and cafés, I encountered in the public sphere the same sentiments expressed by the news anchor that day. I began to hear about the West's 'indifference' to the loss of Muslim lives in multiple countries, especially Afghanistan. Many harboured grudges against the US foreign policy. Influential voices argued whether the United States 'deserved' it or not. But I did not talk about it, nor did I want to. It was the least of my concerns, if at all. I was too busy trying to do my best in what mattered to me the most: education. I did, however, latently absorb this hostility as reality.

My Qari Sahab in Pakistan never brought up any such matters and limited our infrequent discussions of religion to the fundamentals. He talked about the stories of Prophet Muhammad and his companions in Islamic literature, but he never spoke of any religious narrative or dogma. Maybe I was too young to notice the difference between the political atmosphere in Al-'Ain and Lahore, i.e. whether people cared more about important issues when they were assimilated (as in UAE) or when they coalesced under the banner of national identity (as in Pakistan). It is more likely, however, that I simply did not care about it. True to the wish of my parents, I wanted to attenuate myself completely to studies.

Around this time I was also exposed to computer technology. I learned about a thing called the Internet and was instantly fascinated by the ability to speak to my father thousands of miles away in a distant land simply through a dial-up modem. Orkut, a now-defunct social networking website, was the craze in school back then. I joined it. My main interests lied in academic groups and communities on the website. I also befriended an assortment of friends and felt more at ease messaging back and forth than talking in person. For the sake of wholesomeness, I also joined a few religious communities.

Along with the indirect exposure into religious extremism festering in parts of a society generally, if mutedly, antagonistic to the West, I found the direct signs of extremism on some community groups on the website. While the majority of these groups were dedicated to a hate-free discussion about religious affairs, several members openly advocated reprehensible views like hurting or even killing non-Muslims and their supporters. I maintained awareness of such people and realized that their views were not specific to one locale. Although these members resided in different countries around the world, the Internet brought them together for a shared purpose. But I chose not to interact with them. Life was too busy with studies anyway.

In school, I liked to be in my own zone. I forwent friendships and social interactions in favour of undivided attention in my subjects. Unlike my peers, I did not fool around or obsess over girls. I was just passionate about fulfilling my need for achievement as much as I could. The only extracurricular activities I participated in were those in which I was forced to participate. Preferring solitude instead of companionship, I was far from being a loner; in fact, I saw books and notebooks to be my best companions. Buried within the pages was everything I wanted to know, or thought I knew.

I always entertained great dreams and even greater ambitions. I wanted to become famous. I wanted to make my parents proud. In Pakistani culture, we refer to this as 'ma baap ka naam roshan karna'. Literally, it means 'brighten the names of parents'. Giving thanks to our parents is an inherently incomplete task: no matter how much we try, we can never fully pay back our parents. But I vowed to try to do so. On her part, my mother encouraged me to explore the world on my own, while also protecting me from unseemly influences as much as she could. Having our father abroad automatically made us suspect before others. There was always a lingering fear whether our family could be a target of certain criminal elements in Pakistani society.

I knew that my family lived in relative poverty, but of any pressing effects out of it, I was largely immune. So, I trained my eyes and mind to look beyond my family, while also being as close to them as possible. I was passionate about exploring the world, even if it had to be done in my head. Where I failed is when I could not imagine the world beyond the setting of a classroom, however much I wanted to; I knew not much about people besides what was portrayed in textbooks, cartoons, movies, and soap operas. To my eyes, all the drama was contained within these mediums. It was, I believed, all I needed to know.

Ignorance played as great of a role in my life as enlightenment in my studies. My parents encouraged me to know and serve others as much as I could, especially those I did not know. But the fact remained that I did not make any attempts to know others outside of school. I hardly played cricket with other neighbourhood children and spent my time mostly cloistered in a study room preparing for the next exam or test. Still, I did not consider myself a high achiever; I just tried my best in accomplishing whatever I set my mind to. That did not dissuade my classmates and teachers from advertising me as a nerd to the point that a whole school section knew who I was. I did not dispute this characterization, mostly because life in school was as enjoyable as it was happily challenging.

After years that felt more like decades, my father was granted lawful permanent residency status in the United States. He soon began the process of petitioning for our arrival in the country. When news came that the petitions were granted, I was the most elated of all. I did not harbour any resentment or animosity for the United States, which was to be our future—and permanent—home. Like most Pakistanis, I envied the United States, even as negativity persisted about its foreign policies. In fact, I aspired to make significant contributions in the United States if I was ever given a chance. Since I had little trouble integrating in the Emirati and the Pakistani society, I did not and could not foresee having any lingering doubts about my assimilation in the society of a distant land. To immigrate here and to be finally united with my father as one cohesive family unit was a dream coming true before I had a chance to explore the meaning of the American Dream. I was happy beyond measure.

I arrived in the United States with my mother and siblings in the fall of 2007. We encountered some hostility from the airport customs officers during the verification process, where (for some reason) questions were more barked than politely directed at us. I dismissed this as a one-time anomaly; we were inside the United States. That was all that mattered.

If only it was that easy. In Pakistan, the UAE, and now the US, I had gone through the same slow and steady process of making sense of my surroundings. I wanted to prepare myself for the unexpected challenges that would come in my way and I was confident I would overcome them. It had worked in the UAE and Pakistan. America was going to be an even more exciting place. And I was certain it wasn't wishful thinking, because I had heard, read, and seen everything about the United States—at least the good parts that I sincerely believed in—that I could have. So I never considered that, shortly upon my arrival, I would be so completely disillusioned that I would fail to make a distinction between reason and fanaticism.

My entrance into the path of extremist ideology had no clear beginnings. It certainly wasn't present when I was in Pakistan or the UAE. After I enrolled in school, I became an average high-school freshman who liked to focus more on studying than making friends. I was also very strictly purpose driven: for me, school was but a place to obtain one's education. In the UAE and Pakistan, this outlook was implicit if not widely encouraged and adopted. But in the United States, it almost instantly made me a target of ridicule by some of my fellow not-so-bright classmates. I was sneered at as a nerd as if I had inherited a non-communicable disease. I laughed and played along, taking the remarks as an unspoken sign of respect. That is what I had always done back in Pakistan. The difference was that this time, I felt not only like an outsider, but also an outlier.

The beginnings of my frustration and resentment came another way. I was deeply troubled by what was endearing to me was tattered into pieces without any sense of shame or decency: my religion. I was not a practising Muslim per se; I tried to pray five times a day, recited a few Arabic verses of the Qur'an daily, and tried to live a life of goodwill and obedience. As a Muslim, I held God in the highest esteem. Likewise, I held the prophet Muhammad—whose name I shared as my first name—as a model of the person I should aim to be in order to succeed in this life and the next.

After the events of 11 September, as I have mentioned, I had a growing awareness of the way others perceived the United States. Now in the country itself, curiosity and intrigue took over. I looked forward to seeing whether those suspicions were justified. Did Americans exhibit hostility or were they welcoming?

I clumped together the people with the government and considered them to be one and the same. After all, this is how I had seen Emiratis and Pakistanis. I was as eager to see the reality with my own eyes as I had been enthusiastic about the prospect of starting a new life in the United States. What followed was a barrage of disappointments, beginning with seemingly insignificant, crude insults.

In Pakistan, the tradition is to call people by their given names that are usually middle names. Mine is 'Hassan'. That is how my family and classmates knew me. But in the United States, I felt pleased with the change, even honoured. People now called me by my first name, Mohammed. The confusion came when my fellow high-school students ignorantly and almost immediately began to associate my name with terrorism. 'Mohammed' was apparently a nom de guerre of terrorists, of those who intended to blow Americans up. As I was the luckless holder of that name, I was automatically a terrorist. Several of my classmates did not hesitate to accuse me of personally being behind the 9/11 attacks.

This was something hard for my young mind to reconcile. I could take personal attacks. But facing unprovoked jabs at something as sacred to me as my name was quite jarring. At the same time, I was relatively unprepared for weathering this criticism. I did not know how to absorb this, nor could I formulate a worthy response. A young immigrant, I was unschooled in the ways to take things in stride and let them go. Challenges for me were dealt with in structured settings, i.e. in the form of lessons to promptly memorize or setbacks to heavily absorb. Nothing had prepared me for insults or *ad hominem* attacks.

Instead of having shouting matches as teenagers would, I began to internalize the growing resentment I felt. I never showed outward anger or frustration. In retrospect, it would have been better if I had, because the hostility I faced was soon transformed into musings of a practical reality: 'You want a terrorist? I will give you a terrorist'.

In my discussions with classmates willing to have a debate about religion and politics, I felt compelled to separate the two. I agreed that terrorists were responsible for many reprehensible acts, including suicide attacks and murders of innocent people from all walks of life. I desperately pointed out that people who justified violence in the name of any religion did not make that religion a diabolic enemy of humanity. I tried to maintain a barrier between the normative value of religion and the outlandish fevers of politics. But no combination of words worked. My words transformed into pleas that fell on deaf ears. I was still a terrorist, my classmates joked. I had come from a country that sponsored terrorism, they asserted. I laughed along, as always. But I also slowly bristled inside, not knowing how to manage the hurt I felt.

I wanted to keep my ethnic roots intact, but I also wanted to integrate. I sought to contribute in the only way I knew how: study. Within a year, I was on the Internet looking for the meaning of my Muslim identity and searching for something, anything, to extinguish the fire of a crisis I felt enveloping me. My search was broken down into three key themes: meaning, purpose, and a sense of belonging. The outward exploration I had envisioned had downgraded to an internal quest. I wanted to intelligently convince my classmates that they were sorely mistaken in adjudging Islam or Muslims under the classical stereotypes, and that no abstract sacred order of a religion was synonymous with terrorism. But I had several confusions of my own. I knew what Islam was. But what was this concept of terrorism? Which kind of people could enjoy striking fear in someone else's heart? Who were these terrorists, anyway?

At first, my Internet searches were mostly focused on general topics about Islam and Muslims. But the Internet was also on edge about the Middle East conflict, wars in predominantly Muslim countries and other dismal global affairs. Today, online companies are taking a more active role in policing the vast quantities of material created and shared on their networks, purging offensive content. But back then, good was mixed with the bad. A terrorist proclamation could be found next to an innocuous spiritual video.

In my online quest, I was directed to YouTube. The site provided the perfect avenue to further my inquiry; videos had held an innate appeal for me since my earliest days at Pakistan. I used to watch Hollywood movies with fascination. Enduring classics like *Harry Potter* and *The Chronicles of Narnia* had been my favourite movies; I even believed that the fantasy worlds reflected reality. Now that I was in the United States, I saw that the world of fairy tales had little to do with reality. It made me feel like I had been deceived, as if something had been taken away from me even before the dream had a chance to flourish. I had never felt this incomplete as I did now.

Something was missing. Something was, in fact, wrong.

I never really anticipated facing the kind of challenges I faced in this unfamiliar part of the world. I grew unhappy and missed my Pakistani friends more than ever. I felt isolated, lost, and alienated. Despite my best intentions I could not make high school friends, most of whom had taken to taunting me anyways. I shied away from social interactions. Outwardly, I was fine. But the confusion inside was too overwhelming. This happened in concert with my exposure to the alternative world of Internet. Living in this fantasy world to escape from reality had never been more appealing. It became my reality.

With the proliferation of extremist propaganda on YouTube, it was a matter of time that I began to ignore the walls I had tried to create in separating religion from politics. I browsed several websites that upheld Islam as more than a faith. I learned that Islam encompassed a system more than a regulating moral universe, that its precepts reigned over every aspect of our daily lives. This, by necessity, included as much a dominion over the political affairs as the social relationships between Muslims and others.

If Islam was a way of life, I deduced, I had to incorporate religion in all aspects of my life. This included the muddy grounds of politics. Soon, politically charged videos gave way to videos that incorporated ideological elements of religious extremism. I created a YouTube account and began to save these videos, imagining them to be an accurate portrayal of reality. After all, the grievances in them were informed by my own personal experiences.

Rating and commenting on YouTube videos led to my first online interactions with other YouTube users, mostly religious extremists. Soon, I was adding them to my 'Friends' list, subscribing to their channels, and messaging and commenting on their user channels. I was invited to join 'The Cause' and, considering them to be true representative of the faith, I readily agreed. The Cause began with postings of innocuous, religious videos but later encompassed the unquestionable embrace of extremist ideology.

Through the misguidance of the YouTube extremists, I began to repost videos that glorified violence in the name of protecting the Muslim nation, or Ummah. As such videos were taken down for violating YouTube Terms of Service, I began to create copies and repost them. My accounts were reported by other users and subsequently suspended by YouTube. I re-emerged under new accounts and persisted in reposting the videos. I was cursed and taunted by both neo-Nazi and pro-Israeli groups, the two disjointed opponents of extremists on YouTube. This time, I did not engage in a debate. I simply accepted their attacks as words of praise. I became immune to criticism.

Religious extremism is never an entirely self-propelled phenomenon. Aspiring extremists are actively goaded, lured, encouraged, and enticed to partake in either direct or indirect actions. Not all extremists are predisposed to committing acts of violence, especially when other overt means of support are readily available.

Internet forums and discussion boards usually fill this void. To be sure, I did not jumpstart from YouTube videos into full-fledged acceptance of the extremist cause. I had to start believing in it first. Several extremists on YouTube encouraged me to explore all facets of the ideology directly from the poisonous wellspring of jihadist forums. Once I was in the cult, extremist ideology could be pandered more effectively.

Jihadist forums are quite unlike other discussion portals on the Internet. The sole difference lies in the content purveyed to the Internet audience, as well as the active member base of extremist recruiters and sympathizers, which includes both curiously odd characters and calculating extremist propaganda disseminators. All of them are vehement supporters of extremist ideology with little-to-no tolerance for dissent. The forums are a way for extremists to plan and propagandize, to communicate and facilitate, and to inspire the naïve and the reckless into taking action. Much like militant groups vying for legitimacy by fashioning themselves as representatives of ordinary Muslims, extremist forums underline the pernicious effects of extremism by portraying extremists as virtual messengers of a faith under constant attack.

One of the most efficient means at the extremists' disposal was not in the everyday use of the Internet, but in shaping their message to bring it to a wider audience. The entire point of a jihadist forum was to provide an alternative to the mainstream narrative antagonistic to the whole idea of terrorists—who fancied themselves as resistance fighters—as evil criminals. In these forums, extremists' 'virtues' were extolled, and religious discussions were always tailored to justify any actions taken by established extremist groups. Portrayed as the voice for the voiceless, extremists were seen as defenders of the faith without whom the Muslim nation would collapse upon itself. Depending on the type of forum, certain extremist groups and their supporters could be banned for ideological or operational differences. Apparently, even extremists had discriminating standards. Being on the remotest margins of the society did not preclude them from adjudging themselves as *Ghurabaa*, or strangers. Their ways were strange but in their jaundiced eyes, that certainly did not make them outcasts. If anything, it only enhanced their eccentricity.

I watched countless video series, professionally made and aesthetically appealing, showing everything from on-the-field militant operations to periodic eulogies and Eid specials. I also took part in discussion threads, scouring the Internet for relevant media content that helped supported the Cause in any way. My indulging on the forum was shadowed by my age. I was open about the fact that I was just a teenager. While some extremists encouraged me to continue learning and participating on the forum, veteran members were not so forgiving in relinquishing their doubts about my identity.

I began to spend hours upon hours on the extremist forums talking to a handful of extremists about all of my grievances and difficulties in adjusting to the United States. I complained to them about my family and school problems. They lent me an ear where no one else had. As I opened up to them, I hid my online interactions from everyone, including my own family. I was instructed to hold dear to the rope of faith, the jihadist version of it, because this was the surest path to success. Online extremists became my best and only friends, and offered a viable alternative to the in-person interactions that I had never really cared for. I did not intend to commit any violent crimes, but I also began to make many sacrifices I did not need to make, including forsaking my own family to be a part of this new cult.

Extremist websites belong to the dark web. Operating under the testy assumptions of free speech and freedom of thought, the websites glorify violence against the 'enemy' and heavily promote their message through various mediums. Security of discussion forums is of paramount consideration. If a website is not secure, details and information about its members may be pilfered by any interested party, especially law enforcement. Password- or invitation-only access ensures that new members to the site are referred only by established forum members. Paranoia about spies and traitors runs wild. Every new member is a suspect and is vetted for any signs of dishonesty and deception.

Having a member who professed to be under 18 years of age was a risky proposition for any extremist forum administrator. Young people were courted even then but not nearly at today's levels. My membership represented an anomaly; I was automatically suspect and, to overcome the presumption that I was a spy, I had to prove my merit.

Never the one to be completely daunted by challenges, I was up for the task. My involvement became more intense as I scanned the forums for the overriding objectives: recruitment through inspiration. It was a cause near and dear to the hearts of the extremists. I had been recruited by other forum members to join the website. I was told that believing in this dogma was the surest way for success in this life and in the next. The right thing to do was to spread the word, to propagate.

Naturally, I picked up from where I had left off from YouTube. I had done some crude translations of both Urdu and English Islamic songs, subtitling videos whenever possible. Many YouTube viewers admired such videos and, at one point, I had several channels with hundreds of subscribers. But as my videos took on more morbid tunes and incorporated graphic, raw war footage from areas like Palestine and Iraq, my main accounts were reported by the users and suspended by YouTube. The videos I had worked hard to create and upload for days and weeks were gone in a matter of minutes.

I did not have to face such problems on extremist websites where video links were stored on file-sharing websites, mirrored, and even archived on an assortment of website servers to be perpetually preserved. Link were reported and uploaded anew in ever-sore battles between extremist veterans and reporting parties. I was happy to partake in such labours, in addition to subtitling and occasionally translating 'official' extremist media videos.

My efforts earned me the attention of interested parties. I was contacted by the forum administrators and offered 'unofficial' translation projects. I would submit my best translations and watch the same translations resurface under the brands of extremist media outlets, knowing that I had hit the jackpot. I was schooled in the methods of secure communications and utilization of specialized software for encrypted chats. I was also granted access to administrative-level accounts of two different extremist forums. In a matter of few months, I was not only able to bond with other forum members, but also work stealthily for official extremist media outlets. While I was informally called on as-needed basis, I had never felt more appreciated.

It was in this extremely vulnerable state that, despite never being a violent person my entire life, I subscribed to and fully succumbed under the political ideology of Islamism, including agreeing with its means and ends. I allowed myself to be manipulated and tacitly agreed to partake in a plot to target a European cartoonist who had drawn some offensive caricatures of the prophet Muhammad that many Muslims find offensive. Instead of seeing clearly and rationally as I normally would, I was lost beyond the point of no return. My involvement in this half-baked plot would soon be accompanied by severe and lasting consequences.

The deeper my involvement in the web of extremist ideology, the more secluded I became from everyone I knew. This included my own family. I stopped speaking with everyone and began to perceive my online 'brothers and sisters' to be the only, true Muslims. I had already been relatively estranged in high school. But now I saw almost everyone as the 'other'. My wish for discovery in this new country had taken a strange twist. Instead of learning about the humanity inherent in each and every one of us, I learned what made the other party worthy of contempt.

When I think about my past, I am unable to discern the fictitious line that was crossed between my immigration to the United States and involvement in religious extremism. If such a line was found, I imagine, it could provide substantive clues to how individuals—regardless of age, gender, race, and other classifications—are directed to the path of extremism. It would have the potential to solve the problem of extremism altogether. As my case shows, such a bright line cannot be constructed. Each story of religious extremism is unique. These solutions demand a no-less-novel approach.

My involvement in religious extremism stemmed from something as simple as a lack of knowledge. I was in my prime age, willing to learn about the world, but also a walking story of personal failure. Instead of upholding a mind of open inquiry, I narrowed my life to be a subservient subset of others' wishes. I became a servile follower instead of an objective, independent thinker. What I valued most in my life, i.e. my education, became nothing more than an abstraction. I did not honour the principles of self-discovery and exploration that could have saved me from the headaches of self-contained crises. Ideological, religious extremism became my life's governing principles instead.

In the end, it was ignorance that bred my defiance and hatred against the other. While I had never been the one to accept failure, my life spiralled directly into that path. I did not make any attempts to understand others and think for myself. I chose to reorient my life on the precepts of the society's worst fringes—those who are dedicated to destruction of everything a society should and can aim for. I did it knowingly but just as much unapologetically, believing that only I was headed on the right path. The difference that I had craved for since my early years had mutated into an unrecognizable force that insidiously and completely blinded my judgement.

I would not realize my errors until it was too late. Escorted in handcuffs from my family's apartment to an unmarked police sedan on the day of my arrest, I was told by an FBI [Federal Bureau of Investigation] agent that 'the time for talking is over'. I had difficulty understanding what he meant. But perhaps he was referring to my many meetings with federal agents over the past few years. Those meetings had served a purpose of their own, but they had also been conducted in an atmosphere in which I was more or less annoyed that I had to encounter the stern questioning and, as I saw it, the honeyed tones of those I saw as my opponents.

To be sure, I had largely scaled back my online activities at the conclusion of my high-school career. It was not so much due to my waning enthusiasm at the same monotony of disseminating extremist videos onto several platforms or undertaking official translation projects on behalf of jihadist media groups. I liked doing what I did for people I knew as my only friends—or even more than that as brothers and sisters. But even my veneration for extremist ideology could not supersede a more practical consideration: high school was over. College was to begin. I simply was short on time I could devote to my online endeavours.

I imagined myself a university student swamped with the rigor and intensity of academic life and having little time for online shenanigans. My achievements and accomplishments, as a practical matter, came not from the smug satisfaction of knowing that an extremist video I had helped translate had been posted online for the entire world to see. The virtual medium of Internet could only do so much.

Instead, I would only be as successful as I was studious. One had always led to another. I knew that if I worked hard, success would follow. So I always attempted to keep my studies and my thoughts separate, as one did not always complement the other. I did this not out of malice or hatred, but out of cowardice. I was too scared of admitting that viable alternatives to my perspectives may have existed. Once religious extremism became my life's overarching focus, I suffocated the ingenuity and critical thinking that a deeper self-study of my life could have elicited. I did not know if I could—or rather if I wanted to—deal with the real world when the virtual world provided so much satisfaction. It so happened in the form of an Islamist ideology that could relate to my personal circumstances.

If the time for talking was over, I did not see how I had talked in the first place. I shied away from engaging in any form of social interaction with the only people who fully knew of my activities: federal agents. I could not count my high-school acquaintances as friends. I kept my online life hidden from my own family. The few people I knew in my community could not be trusted with the knowledge of these activities either. I had never overtly broadcast my views to others, partly because I was conflicted myself. What confused me every single time was how I could harbour grudges against those people I did not even know.

Getting frustrated was the easy part: it was harder to know who I could direct my anger towards. Would the targets of my hate also include all of my respected teachers and fellow students? Were strangers, by the sole virtue of their American citizenship, entirely responsible for the calamities afflicting Muslims worldwide? Did the system of representative democracy in the United States, and the so-called War on Terror, directly or indirectly implicate each and every American?

These were just some of the conflicts I desperately wanted to resolve. But instead of engaging in a period of necessary self-inquiry, I adopted the Islamist ideology and allowed it to do its almost magical bidding. Because the answers were already there, I needed not search any further. I was satisfied with that. Anything that could help me avoid the potential pitfalls of my thinking was welcome.

It was those erected barriers that came crashing down on me, one after another, on that fateful 5th of July, 2011.

I was taken to a juvenile facility in Leesport, Pennsylvania, by three agents. On the way, the agents attempted to make small talk with me about the weather and food. One even offered to buy me something to eat. When I refused, the conversation turned to the difference between kosher and halal food. I responded only half-heartedly, looking intently beyond the windows and into the rushing landscape of a world I had never really understood.

After going through the first of many humiliating bouts of being strip-searched, I walked into the dayroom of the juvenile facility with a duffel bag containing my spare yellow jumpsuits, drawers, and some toiletries. Two juvenile correctional counsellors (JCCs) scanned me from top to bottom as they directed me to walk in a straight line from the door to my prison cell. They asked my name and where I was coming from. They asked if I was a student and what I studied. I told them I had just graduated high school and hoped to attend college soon. I was still in denial about all I had lost hardly a few hours ago.

One of the JCCs looked at me in disbelief as I stood before the prison cell. 'You were accepted to Johns Hopkins?', he asked.

I nodded, finding it hard to understand why he appeared to be so puzzled. 'What are you doing here?', he pressed.

'I ... I don't know', I stammered. 'They... they say I ran into some problems'. With that, I blushed as I stepped into my prison cell. I wanted to continue to refuse to accept reality, but I was not quite sure how much longer I could keep up the façade.

Over the course of the next few months, my prospects for release began to look dimmer. I encountered the most gruelling period of crisis in my life; I wanted to come to terms with my past thoughts and actions, but I was unwilling to accept that I was at fault. Prison had been a price I had instinctively, as any extremist should know, been willing to accept as part and parcel of my beliefs. I was fully geared for it. I just never thought it would actually materialize. Once it did, all the battle-hardened mental training I had received by reading about the virtues of being a prisoner for The Cause, slowly fizzed out. I began to realize that I could face decades in prison, and that it mattered less that I had never been a violent person or actively engaged in any overt terrorist activities.

I have maintained that I needed the hard reality of prison to come to terms with my past, to accept the present, and still come out in the future as a stronger and better person. My evolution came about as do most things in life: with patience, effort, and time. Understanding others, or the wish to learn and know, rescued me from the throes of ignorance that had brought me to prison in the first place. Initially, I was resistant to change because it is quite possibly the hardest thing for anyone to do. The world of religious extremism was the only world that I had ever known, and everything that life could offer was so compellingly if unreasonably resolved in my mind that I had been willing to gamble my real life sitting in jail—all for the promise of a hyperbolic afterlife—for however many years it took.

From the very beginning of my transformation, I wrestled with the question of whether the problem of extremism was isolated to its own realm or whether religion had something, if anything, to do with it. I had been, and still am, a born Muslim who used religion as an excuse for my actions. I was never taught to accept the use of violence for any purpose, religious or otherwise.

I had hardly ever read the Qur'an's English or Urdu translations—that is, unless I was translating media propaganda and cherry-picking the fiercest translations to merge with the overarching message. The verses most colourful and intense in their language appealed to me more than the 'boring' ones that dictated a true Muslim's way of life. I also perused the *hadith*, or the sayings and tradition of prophet Muhammad, to find those texts that resonated with themes of violence and extremism. I relegated the rest to be reflective of life's more mundane affairs.

My goal, as with all those who partake in the dissemination of extremist propaganda, was to invite as many people as possible into extremism. This could be done in many ways, the most effective of which was to broadcast graphic war footage, the likes of those that had been responsible for my own radicalization. It was also to counter the influence of mainstream media outlets that consistently attacked the ideological narrative of online extremists. Driven more by animosity and hatred than by any sense of moral superiority, I continued with my activities relatively unabated.

There is a dispute as to whether religion plays a role in religious extremism. To say that Islam is devoid of a pure, idealistic interpretation that was utilized by other online extremists in my indoctrination, is to deny the existence of the problem I had to internally and forcefully resolve for myself. Islam continues to remain my beloved religion, but instead of utilizing a Muslim-centric approach in dealing with societal issues, today I find greater comfort in focusing on the pluralistic elements of the religion. The individual identity that I sacrificed and merged with that of a cult-like group on the platform of 'sacred' values has been rebuilt. More than that, it has made me a wholesome, unique individual again.

I maintain trust in God and belief in His last messenger. But I am also more cautious, sceptical, and open to criticism and flexibility. The religion of Islam enhances my personal development and also informs my outlook on the world. It is now the means to an end (i.e. an objective or a challenge), not an end in itself. The black-and-white, with-us-or-against-us perspective has matured to include an implicit understanding that the world is as different only as much as I see it, and that there is a lot I have yet to know. Acceptance of my ignorance was the first step towards lasting change.

Prison provided me the necessary if inopportune venue to reflect on my past and realize that something had gone seriously wrong in my life. My interactions with others only confirmed it. In the juvenile facility itself, despite my pending case being under seal, JCCs became aware of my pending charges. Curious how a teenager could indulge in such serious allegations, many JCCs pulled me aside and demanded to know what happened. This was something new to me. I had never thought that people of a different faith or belief would be interested in knowing about my hidden fears and worst prejudices. Nevertheless, I had actively avoided interacting with people in general. Being in prison helped me and forced me to speak to others.

Every day for about four months, I met with JCCs and other correctional staff and spoke unreservedly about little and major aspects of my life. The more I spoke and discussed, the more I shed my shyness and indifference. I had made myself blind to the humanity of others, choosing instead to focus selectively only on those who shared my religion. Opening up to the JCCs allowed me to express my frustration, sadness, and anxiety about my past and the future. In return, the JCCs were even more open about their lives, goals, struggles, dreams, and hopes. It was an antidote to my pattern of thinking and permanently infused in me the values I had been utilizing for the wrong purposes. Empathy with others, especially those who were different than me, overrode all of my baser instincts. I no longer wanted to zone in on a group of people who happened to share the same faith with me. I wanted to understand those I had 'othered' and do so on my own terms.

My parents had brought me up to serve others. I had been of service, but only to the accomplishment of nefarious goals. I just did not realize what I was doing or where I was headed to. Though I was free to make my decisions and choices in life, I was young when I made those choices. Before I faced the full range of consequences and while I languished behind bars, I wanted to understand where the trajectory of my life had gone wrong. The pool of like-minded believers I had found in my online search for meaning and understanding had been severed from me, at least for the time being. There was going to be no guided navigation and I would have to find my own answers.

I had never intended to enlist in a terrorist movement or commit acts of violence from an early age. But I was mesmerized by extremist ideology because my personal life had undergone a radical shift itself. I had toggled between three different countries before I had turned 18 years old. I had begun to doubt the meaning of stability as I absorbed my surroundings. In the United States, the alienation I instantly felt upon arrival came about a full circle in my criminal activities.

What made my journey so dangerous was that, at the same time I was being radicalized, use of the Internet was evolving. I was shy and insecure, as most teenagers are. I eschewed face-to-face interactions because I possessed a form of social phobia and a permanent mental health condition. Finding like-minded believers online and enhancing my social connectivity had substantially narrowed my perception of the world, engendering a dismal outlook that had little to do with reality. I had trusted complete strangers over my own family and acquaintances because they fostered a sense of affiliation and identity. That is why I had come to accept the narrative.

Coming out of the shadows meant escaping the borderless world of the Internet and into the real world. Whether I liked it or not, I had to talk to prison officials and other prisoners. I was shocked by how well I was treated and accommodated. The staff at the juvenile facility went beyond what was ordinarily required in attending to my needs and, sometimes, wants. Similarly, I began to speak to other juvenile prisoners and learned about their lives and stories as well. The facility's regulations disfavoured social interactions with other juvenile prisoners except under staff supervision. I knew I was heavily monitored, but I took the risks and broke the rules to speak with those I wanted to know more about. I wasn't disappointed.

Contrary to my worst fears and prejudices, I encountered vulnerability. Perhaps more than I had been vulnerable to extremist influences, the juvenile prisoners represented the starkest examples of discrete life experiences. From frequent exposure to violence in unstable homes to suffering as victims of abuse themselves, these children were never afforded the kind of opportunities that I had been relatively privileged to receive in my life. I was never physically abused and grew up in a stable household. I was loved and cared for and enrolled in the best possible schools of three different countries.

I quietly absorbed the experiences of these juveniles—both girls and boys—and could not come to terms with how immature and impetuous I had unintentionally grown. In attempting to make sense of my own life, I had disregarded the conundrums that others faced in far more disadvantaged positions. Some struggled with their inability to ameliorate their behavioural issues, while others wrestled with the demons inside their heads. The specialized needs of these juveniles could hardly be met by consigning them to a penal institution where they were unable to receive treatment services or meaningful rehabilitation. And, in fact, many innately rebelled against any control or authority imposed upon them by the institution. To me, however, these juveniles represented an aspect of humanity that I had chosen to ignore.

My parents and siblings consoled me over the phone during this difficult time. I had shunned my family up to the day of my arrest, when an FBI agent actually prodded me to say goodbye to my crying parents. My incarceration changed the dynamic of our relationship and brought us closer than before. My parents drove every week from Maryland to Pennsylvania to see me for the allotted 30-minute visits and, in the remainder of the days, sent me letters almost daily. Upon my release, my brother told me that my family wrote letters, so I did not get bored or lose hope. But while I was greatly distraught and torn about my future, I was also embarking on a new journey in my life. I was now more concerned for my family's welfare despite seeing no light at the end of the tunnel in the abrupt resolution of my case.

My grievances had incubated while I was in Pakistan and morphed into full force after I watched YouTube videos depicting violence against Muslims around the world. These videos were supplanted by media production arms of terrorist groups that depicted a supposedly monolithic West against a monolithic Islam since the time of the Crusades. I had accepted and adopted the extremist narrative because I believed I had seen all there was to know about the West's animosity against Islam and Muslims. The confusion, distrust, and doubt I had engendered was only to be replaced by facing the practical consequences of my actions. For me, this came in the context of imprisonment.

After I turned 18 years of age, I was transferred to an adult institution under the custody of Bureau of Prisons (BOP). It seems safe to say that unless I had received my unplanned rehabilitation in juvenile custody, I would not have had the opportunity to change. I was immediately placed into the Special Housing Unit and segregated from the general population of the prison. For many months, I was left alone in a damp prison cell for 23 hours a day where I craved normal interactions. Stepping out into the caged enclosure of a recreation yard for an hour did not compensate for them.

When, after many warnings, I was finally transferred to general population, I gradually reoriented myself to the adult prison life. I hosted tutoring classes for other prisoners to obtain their GEDs [General Educational Development tests]. I also demanded of prison authorities to place me in a work assignment where I could be paid a few cents every day to take care of my prison needs from the commissary. Being able to work gave me a form of hope, the belief that I could look forward to an attainable future amidst the stinging uncertainty of how much time I would be doing behind bars. It also connected me to others. News of my case had been widely publicized at this point and shocked many staff and prisoners because they could not match the profile of a terrorist with my character. There were many exceptions, of course, as this was still a prison and certain prisoners and officials disliked me more than others. But by being open and empathetic towards others—and at times even a bit silly to escape the harshness of prison life—I was able to overcome my reticence. The distorted view I had held was gradually replaced with certain universal values that are held by most people everywhere, namely extending a willingness to understand and demonstrating responsibility towards others.

I was formally diagnosed with depression, anxiety, and later Asperger's syndrome in many psychological evaluations performed before my sentencing. I also actively searched for as many treatment and rehabilitative opportunities as I possibly could, only to be spurned by prison staff who thought I was being too demanding. Yet, in doing so, I met a handful of prison officials who became my mentors. With no counterextremism programme in place and my attorneys' meticulous attempts to obtain mental health treatment in suitable facilities either thwarted or ignored, I did what I could and searched for as many programmes I could take as possible. Only after sentencing, when I had served a majority of time in a pretrial facility with little-to-no programming, I was transferred to a low-security institution and able to enrol in several spiritual, victim-impact, educational, vocational, and programming courses and work details. The insight I gained further reinforced my rehabilitation and transformation.

Most importantly, my Asperger's syndrome diagnosis enabled me to reorient my responses and thinking in a way that brought out my complete potential. The prison environment can be quite imposing, and I was not always successful in trying to adapt to the constant changes. But just keeping in mind that I had characteristics of the syndrome and of related issues such as depression and anxiety allowed me to at least try to nurture the ability to see things from others' perspective. I was also more aware of my manner and tone of communication, and began to learn to cope with the challenges of the syndrome. I embraced my eccentricity and awkwardness instead of trying to adapt my personality to others' expectations. Self-awareness played a greater role than self-initiated endeavours to get accustomed to different social environments.

Prison quite possibly saved my life and made me a better person. Upon transfer to Immigration and Customs Enforcement (ICE) detention to undergo deportation proceedings for the civil violations I incurred due to my criminal conviction, I continued much of the same work I had done in the custody of BOP. Being in immigration detention, however, presented its own set of distinct challenges that were remarkably separate from and often harsher than those in criminal custody. Moreover, I was also forced to fight against deportation to a country where I could have faced near-certain death. Despite this, I resolved to pay it forward by extending to others the same level of care I had received during my most difficult times. In ICE detention, this took the form of assisting other detainees in their immigration cases in often last-bid attempts to stay in the United States.

Actions precede consequences. The consequences that I faced for my teenage actions came with their own distinct set of challenges. A jaundiced view of the world was followed by throes of tangible reality. My arrest and my incarceration brought my life into an even greater crisis than the one I had wrestled with. Resolution of this crisis entailed coming to terms with the magnitude of the problem itself. The harsh prison environment did not make it any easier.

At the onset, the problem that I encountered was never completely an ideological problem. Religious elements were merged with the ideological re-awakening I had in prison. From the time I was transferred to the custody of the Federal BOP and up to the time that I served an additional year and a half in ICE custody, I faced not only the inherent confusion of the transformation process, but I also attempted to reconcile the spectacle of religiosity in prisons. I was lucky to have been guided earlier through the process, but for the most part, I failed to see this guidance reflected in Muslim prisoners.

While my ongoing search for meaning and identity had taken a sharp turn in prison, there were some prisoners who continued to seek to understand themselves and their actions but went awry in doing so.

For such prisoners, radical beliefs were not adopted suddenly without any cause. It happened over the course of many months and years. Religion provided them with the means to foment inter-group loyalties. And besides the apparent illusion of religiosity, they had little to contribute to any debates about the meaning and significant of religious texts and traditions. It was doubtful whether fostering debates was even a goal; conformity came at the expense of suppressing dissent. A totalitarian prison environment hosted another totalitarian subculture. The fact that I came out of it relatively unscathed gave me the confidence that I was on the right path and that I had, finally, found my peace within.

Upon my release from prison, I was more than satisfied with who I had become. Although I felt that my detention was unnecessarily prolonged, I understood why it had to happen. I did not harbour any resentment or hatred for the government or the prison officials, even if most had good reasons to be sceptical of my transformation. I accepted that regaining trust would be harder than building it in the first place. The only control I had was over my own life and my own actions. In that respect, I pledged to live my life as transparently, as honestly, and as emphatically as I possibly could.

This was easier said than done. Although the prison administrators failed to provide me with opportunities available to others for mental health treatment and therapy, I was nonetheless able to maintain my sense of self and not allow disappointments to thwart my hopes for a better future. Reintegrating into a society I had formerly despised and getting reacquainted with the everyday blessings we take for granted daily was the perfect venue to test those disappointments.

Despite my unreserved sincerity, I faced obstacles and restrictions that almost entirely sapped my strength and demoralized me. This time, however, I did not keep it buried inside me. I actively searched for support to benefit from any resources I could find. Prison had given me the harshest training for dealing with life's worst disappointments. It was because of this that I was able to revitalize my commitment to apply the change I had nurtured behind bars. This even included maintaining touch with prison officials who had been instrumental in helping me foster that change. Having a supportive, caring family made up for my biggest losses and disappointments: it makes a world of difference knowing that when all doors are slammed in your face, one door will always remain open.

I am constantly transitioning in emerging from a fictionalized world I had imagined behind bars to the reality that I am privileged to see with my own eyes. Making an ethereal escape from the wretched reality of prisons was done by allowing dreams to carry one away. Being out, I learned that the dreams that provided me with solace served but to provide a transitory psychic sustenance. Reality was much harder and, admittedly, scary at times. Still, I felt confidently capable of dealing with it. At least I had the mental fortitude to do so. The key was persistence and patience at every step.

Just as the bulk of my change process had been self-propelled, I had to re-establish my foothold in society on my own. The uniqueness of my case presented unique challenges. At first, I was denied opportunities to volunteer in my very own community due to my charges. Restarting my college education presented its own host of problems. One local college denied me admission after a thorough review of my past conduct. My legal status precluded my receipt of any federal, state, or college-specific aid. I was prohibited from obtaining employment until a decision could be made to the contrary.

But uncertainty is as much part of the reintegration process as is the scepticism whether one's commitment to the extremist ideology has really been shattered. Although extremism in itself may not be indicative of a readiness to commit violence, it is still a potent force that thrives on a mixture of misery and confusion. It can be undermined, however, if it can be understood how anyone can be radicalized without regard to their age or background. With this understanding comes the need for open and honest engagement with the disaffected, not veiled hostility against an entire religious group or a religion.

Indoctrination can be undone as surely as reintegration back into the community can take place. At a time when extremist groups are suffering territorial losses and reverting to the same online frontiers that brought them new recruits, how can disengagement, deradicalization, and rehabilitation be integrated into an effective preventative approach? Will extremist ideologies continue to proliferate in concert with the combination of political, moral, religious, and social narratives propounded to radicalize and recruit others? What is the role of religion in countering extremism? Does secular liberalism provide a better alternative?

More than the simplistic narrative of perceived slights mutated into grievances—whether personal or political—extremism is also usually accompanied by a sense of loss, exclusion, alienation, confusion, and doubt. All of these factors underline the common reasons a person becomes vulnerable to the messages of extremists or the aura of extremism. By fostering a vision of a more inclusive world, the grip of extremism on insecure extremists (i.e. those who secretly harbour doubts but dare not voice their complaints) can be mitigated. Humanizing their stories does not provide extremists with means to harbour abhorrent views, but serves to dissuade them from adopting extremist views in the first place.

My deradicalization, like my radicalization, came out of the voluntary acceptance of an alternative narrative. From the point of my arrest, when I thought that it was all over, I was treated decently and humanely. My voluntary renunciation of extremism became a rewarding, not prohibitive, cost, because something as basic as fair treatment that I thought would have been denied to me was extended to me openly. The juvenile prison staff attended to my religious needs, such as praying and fasting, without any prejudgement. Ironically, some even encouraged me to study more about religion because they were religious themselves. The only difference between them and me was that I had used religion as a tool, while they embraced it as a guidepost. Still, religious talks did not serve a role in our frank discussions about suffering and empathy. One need not be religious to be more empathetic. All that was required was open-mindedness, a willingness to understand, and a means by which to be reassured.

The group dynamic that provided me with the identity I thought I had lost upon immigration to the United States was now being nurtured in belonging to a more tolerant and pluralistic group of people who engaged me and gave respect. What these prison staff had done was to expose me to an alternative perspective, an alternative way of looking at the world. By them doing so, I did not need any ideology to help me focus on our similarities and appreciate our differences. All that was asked for was to be as susceptible to understanding as I had been susceptible to extremism.

The greatest challenge I faced in overcoming my extremism was the absence of formal efforts to rationalize my thinking. What the prison staff did through their engagement was not part of any structured programme that could help me rationalize my thinking and expose the pitfalls of the path I was headed to. Overcoming extremism became a problem I had to deal with and that I had to resolve. At least I was up for the task and willing to overcome my ignorance. I do not doubt that someone else in my position could have opted differently depending on lack of support or resistance to change. Alternative pathways cannot be seen in blindness even if most of the work of change and transformation is necessarily self-propelled.

In my particular case, there were more than typical challenges. My personal characteristics, including my mental state, made me more vulnerable to the extremists' message. As mentioned earlier, I was formally diagnosed with depression, anxiety, and later Asperger's syndrome in many psychological evaluations performed before my sentencing. There was nothing 'wrong' with me, I learned, but possessing traits of these conditions at a young age helped me understand my behaviour and the role of my emotions. Awareness of my conditions enabled me to emerge from the traps of extremism with the hurtful knowledge of how I was manipulated and misused, and what made me more impressionable than others. I finally understood how and why my vulnerability was exploited to serve others' agendas.

Sadly, mental health treatment was lacking in almost all of the facilities that I was transferred to. I was expected to seek help when I was not even cognizant of how I could do so and whether anyone could understand the type of journey I had made. Stigmatization associated with having an illness partly kept me from confiding in others. Mental health professionals who were aware of my past had seen nothing like what happened to me. While their guidance was very much appreciated, they could not assist me with a complete evaluation of facets of extremism. That guidance came from within. While I was forthcoming about my past, the same cannot be said of others in need of counselling who suffer from mental health disorders and, consequently, are more susceptible to the influence of extremist ideology. Such individuals need more than a pathway to disengage from extremism; they require active support in the form of individualized care and treatment.

Being highly motivated in studies and versed in intellectual endeavours did not necessarily translate into possessing critical thinking skills. I was at an age where I was busy piecing together the fragments of my worldview with little-to-no measure of rationalization. I did not verify what I was told once I read, heard, or watched it. If extremists advertised a utopia where no man ever suffered, I gullibly believed it. I did not even begin to think in my trance that chaos in the world—including in the world I had created in my own imaginations—would throw into complete doubt all that I was being taught. Considering the world from this point of view is necessary to understand why someone in their youth—such as myself—was able to partake in offensive behaviours and adopt an antagonistic posture against anyone not part of my newfound beliefs.

We live in a world too frequently marred by acts of extremist violence, so it is with good reason that we begin to think of jihadists as murderous automatons dedicated to wholesale violence. But understanding extremist mindset and worldview necessitates more than a normative condemnation of jihadism. The extremist ideology is typically prohibitive in the scope of human activities allowed beyond the rigid interpretation of texts and traditions of the seventh century unless, that is, the same ideology is represented as the only 'authentic' expression of Muslim identity in a world where true Islamic principles are in regression. In trying to resurrect a past divorced from the reality of modern world, online extremists allow themselves a wide latitude in benefiting from the tools of modernity (i.e. the Internet, imagery, and literature) insomuch as those tools are used to further the cause.

Jihadi poetry, songs, hymns, films, essays, and magazines may initially seem superfluous to the strategic purpose of extremists. But new recruits to the cause are less likely to spend their time studying the finer nuances of extremist ideology than participating in the romanticized jihadist culture as a gateway to the doctrine's acceptance. Instead of having the extremist narrative boringly drilled in one's mind, it is presented in a more attractive, more sentimental, and more grandiose form on extremist venues and forums. When YouTube videos became my first-hand exposure into this unknown world, I became blind to the human suffering of the ideology's victims and slowly became prone to romanticize my own suffering and problems, which I superficially paralleled to the adversity of the occupied and the oppressed. Effectively, I adopted a form of twisted empathy and dismissed the pain and suffering of the 'other' as a deception.

Jihadist extremists are further moved by a desire to right the wrongs, but only if such wrongs can be ascribed to anyone else but their own actions. They are empathetic to the suffering and violence inflicted on the vulnerable, but only if they are at the receiving end of it. Terrorism and extremism is perpetuated by the aggressors, so extremists do not accept the proposition that the responsibility for pains and casualties lies with them. Victimhood is a concept imputable to their particular group and followers and an alien concept if their targets are brutalized or killed in acts of militant violence.

With the intensity of belief overpowering any rational conception of their actions, potential extremists settle into this powerful flow without realizing what they are getting into. Short-term emotional rewards become more valuable than long-term thinking about the consequences of their actions. But our capacity to feel empathy is not as immutable as it may seem at the first glance. Exposure to varied perspectives can be fostered by immersive counternarratives to extremist ideology, narratives that highlight the real human costs of militant violence. Kindness and understanding has to be an inherent part of the process of reorienting one's perspective, and despite the religious nature of extremism, this needs not to be accomplished in a purely religious environment.

Staff at the juvenile facility who helped me see the world in a different light were not attempting to educate me in a religious context. They were correctional counsellors who engaged me as they would have engaged any other juvenile: with love, care, and understanding. Similar to the supportive role of my parents after my incarceration, the counsellors listened with an open mind and did not impel me to agree with their perspectives and opinions. They simply stated their dreams, hope, and wishes—and talked about all the little things in everyday life that makes one happy or sad. They spoke to me about facing challenges and difficulties in their personal lives and about attempting to escape a prison of their own making. Ignorance had led me to isolate them from their personhood. Once I was forced to see reality, it was matter of time that I was able to scale the walls of my own creation. I finally was able to rediscover empathy not as a selective emotion, but as the kindling that fires compassion in our hearts and impels us to help others in distress. What I had found was grace and it is something I have since pledged to pay forward.

Having a moral code can be a strong deterrent to knowingly participating in immoral acts, especially if such acts inherently promote violence. Unless, of course, subscribing to extremist ideology is considered to be a moral act in itself. Living in a Western country and being lost in the radical discourse meant that I was left torn between two worlds. After the process of dehumanizing others, I still could not resolve how violence could be justified against innocent civilians, especially those who cared more about living their everyday lives than harming Muslims. I was brought up in a traditional, loving household and taught laudable family values. In accepting extremist ideology, I had serious doubts whether anyone unwilling to subscribe to my newfound set of beliefs was automatically a target. The ideology itself somehow became a suspect in this way. I shied away from such a blanket indictment and tried my best to keep the online and the physical worlds separate. I was slowly attenuating myself to the extremist ideology, but I was also doubtful whether I could resolve this deficiency.

In preventing extremism of those in a similar position as I was, it is even more critical to emphasize the common, unbreakable bond between the opponents of the ideology and those subscribing to it, i.e. the underlying humanity. Targeting innocent people, no matter which side of the equation they are on, is inherently wrong. Most extremist recruits may be driven by a strong sense of justice and may not be ready to participate in blatant acts of violence at the onset. If the remnants of their morality can be recovered before it is too late, their extremism can be mitigated as well. For my part, the realization that targeting the other side could be wrong, especially if they did not have anything to do with direct violence perpetrated against Muslims was enough to stop me in my tracks for at least as long as to take a second look at my beliefs.

Still another major turning point in my transformation was when I saw that non-Muslims spoke out and even defended Muslims against aggression or violent acts levelled against them. Many people I interacted with, including correctional officers, immigrant advocates, court-ordered psychologists, and religious leaders, condemned hateful speech against Muslims in the strongest terms. Some were even vocal about the excesses of the US foreign policy and military manoeuvres in other countries. Knowing that there were those in sympathy, if not in solidarity, with the affairs of Muslims around the world was something that shocked and surprised me. For example, several people protested against the indiscriminate killings of victims of drone attacks. The extremist hype of Islam being under attack by enemies of Muslims began to look more outlandish in this context. Bringing further exposure to credible supportive voices within—and outside—the Muslim community is an important precursor in diminishing the attractiveness of extremist narrative and ideology.

Because of online radicalization and religious extremism, I not only lost six years of arguably the most experimental years of my life, but also suffered a barrage of setbacks and disappointments that will accompany me for a very long time. After the years I lost, I was lucky enough to receive a second chance to re-join my community and have the opportunity to reorient the essence of my dreams and ambitions. My career goals remain much the same as they were when I was a child, except that I can now share my past experiences to help others avoid the distortions and pitfalls of my past actions. I realize that it will take me twice the amount of work as others to reach a stage where I want to go. I also understand that my intentions and endeavours will be questioned and perhaps even distrusted. However, being at peace with who I am today is as meaningful as the work I do daily to learn about others and build empathy. Radicalization and extremism—especially on the online frontiers—are bound to affect and entrap more vulnerable youth. But if against all odds we can still invoke the best within us and guide those youth before it is too late, perhaps we can also uplift their prosperous future and save the very fabric of our humanity.

13.3 Analysing programmes: what works and what doesn't work?

For practitioners, academics, policymakers, and analysts alike globally, the vast spectrum of the violent extremism rubric makes the responsibility in measuring its impact particularly difficult as there is not a standard method to evaluate efforts both within government and among civil society and academic communities. In the case of Quilliam—and even in the experience of Mohammed Khalid—numerous questions arise on how, if ever, one person is truly rehabilitated. Is there a magic pill that works, or is there some sort of full-proof ability to determine if someone is truly healed? Equally important, the case of Usman Khan, the British-born extremist who appeared to have been rehabilitated from his actions in 2012, when he was jailed for his part in an al-Qaeda-inspired terror plot against the London Stock exchange, and then went on a killing spree in 2019, in which he attacked innocent recent college graduates at a rehabilitation conference, further shows the thin line between violent extremism and the journey out of it. In the example of Khalid and the hundreds of other individuals worldwide that Quilliam has worked with, there is never a 100% guarantee that our efforts will work every time. But, what Quilliam and similar organizations like us will argue is that there is a constant and iterative process in which our work and engagement recognizes this effort from the beginning and willingness to seek solutions in the long, arduous and slow process to heal, reform, and aide individuals.

All over the world, countries have been experimenting with such efforts, as has Quilliam. Denmark, the UK, Saudi Arabia, and Singapore have all been highlighted for their various approaches to helping individuals in their transition from extremism. These myriad strategies and approaches range from utilizing cognitive development, community reintegration, ideological reform, and mental health counselling, to name a few.

Despite conventional wisdom to the contrary, findings by the FBI and social science research now substantiate the view that domestic terrorists—specifically acts of violence carried out by white males—are a greater threat than actions carried out by Islamist extremists like al-Qaeda or the Islamic State of Iraq and Syria (ISIS). The horrific white nationalist terror attack in New Zealand, which left 49 Muslim worshippers dead in 2019, is the most recent example of the threat and how to respond adequately. Domestically, in the United States, the most salient example of this can be found in the case of the Coast Guard Lieutenant, Christopher Hasson, who stockpiled weapons, hoping to use them to establish a 'white homeland', and created a digital spreadsheet identifying House Speaker Nancy Pelosi, as well as other high-ranking Democrats, as targets. All of this raises the question of how we should respond to the threat posed by terrorists both at home and abroad. What are the common threats that these groups pose and how does the United States, as a nation, come up with appropriate measures for prevention, rehabilitation, and reintegration? The historical record shows that the United States has relied on strategies to prevent radicalization but has rarely taken stock of, let alone utilized, the unique skills of individuals who are or have been involved in extremist activity to deradicalize others, opting to prosecute such individuals instead. Furthermore, partisan politics represents a formidable obstacle to the formation of organized off-ramping programmes, such as those seen as being model examples ranging from the UK and Denmark, to name a few.

As highlighted earlier, the range of activities in the CVE rubric makes measuring their impact even that much more challenging. Because of this, a limited number of publicly available evaluations exist. A range of government practitioners and university-based entities have sought to provide some level of rigour to understand what works and what doesn't using a mixed-methods approach, measures, and designs some of which show new thinking, innovation, and creativity. As a whole, there are a number of similar themes and roadblocks that further complicate providing an evidence-based approach to monitor and evaluate CVE programmes and policies. Three overall themes have been highlighted by evaluators of CVE efforts and many have lobbied to have better monitoring and evaluation of programmes.

1. **Causation:** like in other fields and disciplines, the CVE methodology of evaluation has challenges in proving that a certain action was prevented because of a specific intervention. Various factors and variables certainly impact outcomes, and CVE interventions in many evaluators' perspectives are no exception.

2. **Data and metrics:** depending on where individuals who evaluate programmes are viewing the problem set (academics, policymakers, and practitioners) also determines how to respond adequately. In various instances, there is an overdependency on qualitative and quantitive data, while dismissing anecdotal stories and hands-on experiences. Because there are various levels of understanding of extremism in all its forms, there is no clear and streamlined effort in how to respond and look at the necessary tools required to engage in this issue.

3. **Changing information and bias perspective:** various security factors worldwide can radically impact on how research is perceived and impacted by these circumstances. Using a diverse range of approaches to understand this problem set using a mixed-methods evaluation strategy, along with technologically savvy tools, can prove to be quite helpful, but constant learning must be explored.

Needless to say, forward leaning, and collaborative and innovative new techniques are underway. As Quilliam has been experimenting and engaging in innovation for close to 20 years, our work and efforts are iterative, like other efforts worldwide. As the global community seeks to find solutions for the future on what works and what doesn't, sharing, comparing, and learning from good practices that are ever evolving will aide us all in understanding this phenomenon of radicalization and extremism, and the appropriate responses to solve these issues.

13.4 **Policy recommendations**

Based on Quilliam's experience in working with Mohammed Khalid and others around the world, the following are suggested recommendations.

13.4.1 Leverage former extremists and establish a former extremist's network globally

Through Quilliam's experience in the United States and worldwide, the support network of individuals who have previously belonged to extremist movements and their exit out of that mindset are extremely important. By having the necessary support network, individuals will have less of a chance of recidivism, and can be a helpful tool for families, mental health counsellors, and experts who work on this issue.

13.4.2 Prison rehabilitation services

While they are in prison, incarcerated on terrorism-related charges, prisoners should be assisted, mentored, and advised on various forms of rehabilitation (i.e. ideological and mental health) so as to help them slowly on their journey in and out of extremism. Working with organizations who have experience in this domain will be vital for long-term success.

13.4.3 Mental health facilities and services

In the case of Mohammed Khalid, he was diagnosed with Asperger's syndrome and was not able to find the appropriate mental health services until much later. As in the cases of other individuals Quilliam has worked with, training and working with mental health services, ensuring they are equipped with understanding the signs and indicators of transnational extremism, and working with subject matter experts as partners are vitally important for the short- and long-term assistance for patients.

13.4.4 Engage organizations with crossover experience with all forms of extremism

There are organizations who have dealt with other forms of violent extremism, including gang and drug addiction, that have good practices that can be applied to the rise of Islamist rehabilitation. By working with organizations who have experience in other fields, along with organizations with expertise in dealing with the Islamist extremist threat, the continuity of learning from good and best practices can take place.

13.4.5 Establish and create a coordinated domestic rehabilitation programme

Worldwide, including countries such as Denmark, Singapore, and the UK, to name a few, there are country-specific rehabilitation efforts that bring together all of society's approaches to prevent extremism in a coordinated fashion. In the

United States, we have not engaged in such an effort that brings together expertise from former government officials, former extremists, and so on. As such, without a robust agenda and coordinated effort that is not ad hoc, the United States is faced with new and emerging threats, and current threats that require rehabilitation strategies and policies that have to be responded to in the immediate term.

13.4.6 Support more local, private, and government-funded initiatives on rehabilitation

More resources, money, and time must be dedicated to the growing number of individuals who are returning home after serving al-Qaeda-related convictions and others who are being incarcerated for ISIS-related terrorism offenses. Public–private partnerships are needed more than ever, and individuals also need the necessary support while they are in prison and throughout their process to reintegrate back into society.

Further reading/resources

1. **Atran S.** Talking to the enemy: an alternative approach to ending intractable conflicts. Solutions 2012;**3:51–51.**

2. **Bakker E, de Leede S.** European female jihadists in Syria: exploring an under-researched topic. Available from: https://www.icct.nl/download/file/ICCT-Bakker-de-Leede-European-Female-Jihadists-In-Syria-Exploring-An-Under-Researched-Topic-April2015(1).pdf [accessed 5 August 2020].

3. **Barrelle K.** Disengagement from Violent Extremism. Available from: https://www.academia.edu/1370945/Disengagement_from_violent_extremism [accessed 5 August 2020].

4. **Cohen J, Ballou B.** SAVE Supporting Document: Becoming a Former. Available from: https://www.cfr.org/report/save-supporting-document-becoming-former [accessed 5 August 2020].

5. **Dalgaard-Nielsen A.** Promoting exit from violent extremism: themes and approaches. Studies in Conflict & Terrorism 2013;32:99–115.

6. **De Guttry A, Capone F, Paulssen C,** eds. Foreign fighters under international law and beyond. The Hague: Asser Press; 2016.

7. **Demant F, Slootman M, Buijs F, Tillie J.** Decline and disengagement: an analysis of processes of de-radicalisation. Available from: https://dare.uva.nl/search?identifier=4f819bfb-4ea9-4196-a7fd-3c107594205f [accessed 5 August 2020].

8. **Ebaugh H.** Becoming an ex: the process of role exit. Chicago, IL: University of Chicago Press; 1988.

9. **Fraser-Rahim M.** America's other muslims: Imam WD Mohammed, Islamic reform and the making of American Islam. London: Rowman and Littlefield; 2020.

10. **Horgan J.** Deradicalization or disengagement? A process in need of clarity and a counterterrorism initiative in need of evaluation. International Journal of Social Psychology 2009;24:291–8.

11. **Horgan J.** Individual disengagement: a psychological analysis. In: **Bjørgo T, Horgan J**, eds. *Leaving* terrorism behind: individual and collective disengagement. Abingdon: Routledge; 2008, pp. 17–29.

12. **Horgan J, Taylor M.** Disengagement, de-radicalization and the arc of terrorism: future directions for research. In: **Coolsaet R**, ed. Jihadi terrorism and the radicalization challenge. Farnham: Ashgate; 2011, pp. 173–86.

13. **Koehler D.** Family counselling as prevention and intervention tool against 'foreign fighters'. the German 'Hayat' program. Available from: https://journals.sfu.ca/jed/index.php/jex/article/view/49/83 [accessed 5 August 2020].

14. **Koehler D.** Understanding deradicalization. Methods, tools and programs for countering violent extremism. Abingdon and New York: Routledge; 2016.

15. **Koehler D, Kruglanski A, Webber D.** The radical's journey: how German neo-Nazis voyaged to the edge and back. Oxford: Oxford University Press; 2019.

16. **Mironova V.** From freedom fighters to jihadists: human resources of non-state armed groups. Oxford: Oxford University Press; 2019.

17. **Nadhif A.** New study explores Tunisia's jihadi movement in numbers. Available from: https://www.al-monitor.com/pulse/originals/2016/11/tunisia-center-study-terrorism-distribution.html [accessed 5 August 2020].

18. **Neumann P.** Victims, perpetrators, assets: the narratives of Islamic State defectors. Available from: https://icsr.info/wp-content/uploads/2015/10/ICSR-Report-Victims-Perpetrators-Assets-The-Narratives-of-Islamic-State-Defectors.pdf [accessed 5 August 2020].

19. **Porges M, Stern J.** Getting deradicalization right. Available from: https://www.foreignaffairs.com/articles/persian-gulf/2010-05-01/getting-deradicalization-right [accessed 5 August 2020].

20. **Rafiq H, Malik N.** Caliphettes: women and the appeal of Islamic State. Available from: https://www.quilliaminternational.com/shop/e-publications/caliphettes-women-and-the-appeal-of-islamic-state/ [accessed 5 August 2020].

21. **Rosenblatt N.** All Jihad is local: what ISIS' files tell us about its fighters. Available from: https://www.newamerica.org/international-security/policy-papers/all-jihad-is-local/ [accessed 5 August 2020].

22. **Roy O.** France's Oedipal Islamist complex. Available from: https://foreignpolicy.com/2016/01/07/frances-oedipal-islamist-complex-charlie-hebdo-islamic-state-isis/ [accessed 5 August 2020].

23. **Sageman M.** Leaderless Jihad: terror networks in the twenty-first century. Philadelphia, PA: University of Pennsylvania Press; 2008.

24. **The Soufan Group.** Foreign fighters: an updated assessment of the flow of foreign fighters into Syria and Iraq. Available from: https://wb-iisg.com/wp-content/uploads/bp-attachments/4826/TSG_ForeignFightersUpflow.pdf [accessed 5 August 2020].

25. **ZDK Gesellschaft Demokratische Kultur GmbH.** EXIT-Germany: we provide the way out. Available from: https://www.exit-deutschland.de/Datei-Download/29/Broschuere-EXIT-Engl_PDFDS_11.4.pdf [accessed 5 August 2020].

Chapter 14

Counter-radicalization, public health, and racism: A case analysis of Prevent

Tarek Younis

14.1 Introduction

In December 2019, the British public elected Boris Johnson and the Conservative Party as the majority government of the UK. The success and proliferation of nationalist parties across the Global North[1] is significant for any public venture to counterextremism or radicalization. According to a recent survey prior to the 2019 election, 62% of Conservative voters agreed with the statement 'Islam threatens the British way of life', corroborating previous surveys made in this regard [1, 2].

Insofar as radicalization is increasingly framed as a public health issue, mental health is increasingly viewed as a dominant pre-emptive position to prevent prospective political violence [3]. The UK's 'Prevent' policy is significant in this regard, in that (1) it already performs the role of a public health policy in all but name and (2) it significantly centres on mental health as the locus of intervention [4]. Indeed, as Freedom of Information requests have recently uncovered, several mental health trusts across the UK now screen for radicalization among all their patients [5]. This chapter will explore what a public health approach to radicalization entails in the UK, a country in the throes of mounting nationalism. It will argue that any public policy addressing radicalization and extremism, without addressing how these concepts permeate public consciousness, is exemplary of how prejudice is given institutional legitimacy in contemporary times—institutional racism.

----

[1] The Global North replaces the 'West' or 'Western world' throughout this text to remain consistent with literature underlining this region's geopolitical dominance across the globe. 'The West' connotes civilizational supremacy.

14.2 **Islamophobia, nationalism, and the War on Terror**

Despite the rising antagonism towards Muslims and Islam on political platforms across the Global North, Islamophobia is often reduced to overt displays of discrimination or so-called 'hate crimes'—physical and verbal abuse. While important, the exclusive focus on the physicality of discrimination serves to dismiss the political context that gives Islamophobia its legitimacy. Thus, a necessary understanding of Islamophobia recognizes it within a system of meaning that is culturally and politically reproduced by State structures, and particularly nationalist projects [6]. The challenge remains how to understand Islamophobia as a form of racism within a system of meaning as it might relate to countering violent extremism. Herein lies the significance of racialization. The political project of nationalism seeks to separate those who belong to those who do not—the Other—in the production of its cultural and political boundaries [7]. Although the designation of Others vary across the historical trajectories of nation states, one element remains consistent across the Global North: a racialized ethnonationalism serves a central, performative pivot that delineates 'us' from the 'them' [7, 8]. Moreover, one can trace the racialization of fanaticism within a historical Eurocentric trajectory dating back at least to the Enlightenment; European philosophers have long viewed Islam as a fanatical religion par excellence [9].

Individuals and groups are thus *racialized* according to the dominant social conflicts in modern nation states. In the War on Drugs, for example, criminality is racialized to black people, whereas in the War on Terror threat and cultural backwardness is racialized to Muslims and Islam. Such an understanding of Islamophobia sees then the contemporary management of Muslims—as the *de facto* Other—historically congruent with the treatment of 'Others' across nationalist projects (e.g. such as Germany's 'the Jewish question' prior to the Second World War). The devastating outcome of nationalist projects was best summarized by Hannah Arendt, who observed that, in Germany, 'the Nation killed the State'.

None of these social conflicts is fixed, however. We see how the War on Terror, for example, securitizes long-standing assimilation discourses, thereby subsuming the question of integration within the prism of national security. This explains why the Prevent policy wedged 'fundamental British values' as a mandatory framework within British education. Thus, while integrated Muslims deserve their status of belonging, the onus is on them to perform their Britishness continuously. The War on Terror, insofar as it seeks to catch those who turn away from nationalism, reproduces a system that reifies the political salience of the 'Muslim Question'. This was most acutely demonstrated in a report outlining how governmental counterextremism strategies *enable* the far-right's Islamophobic counter-jihadi movements across Europe [10]. In this way, both Islamophobia and the threat of extremism take their proper historical and political context. The question then is how the Prevent policy—which emphasizes mental health in its current iteration—fares in such a context.

14.3 Prevent: institutional racism in practice

In the fall of 2018, a Muslim woman admitted to me in confidence she consulted a mental health professional in the National Health Service (NHS). During the consultation, the therapist suggested that one of the signs of 'successful treatment' would be her ability to remove her headscarf. As egregious as this might be, what followed was just as significant: the woman was then afraid of sharing her concerns any further, for fear of a Prevent referral. I have since documented four other cases of Muslims who refuse to see a mental health professional for fear of an erroneous radicalization referral, more broadly associated with the current political climate. To presume these are simply aberrations, or that a more 'evidence-based' mental health approach to countering violent extremism (CVE) will mitigate the fear of false referrals, is missing the woods for the trees. There is a particular logic to why the woman feared a counter-radicalization referral, even if no mention of Prevent was made on therapist's part. As I will outline from my fieldwork, the very introduction of extremism/radicalization judgements and assessments into mental health institutions played a significant role.

How is Prevent training understood and practised by (largely mental health) NHS staff? This was the guiding question of our fieldwork, based on ethnography, carried out in London between May 2017 and January 2019. The research draws upon government policy and training documents, and attendance at Prevent training, as well interviews and focus groups conducted with NHS staff and the British Muslim community (for more on the methodology, see [4, 11]). We found that Prevent training in the NHS employed a combination of psychological and ideological frames to convey the importance and then meanings of radicalization to healthcare staff, consistent with the literature on (de)radicalization [12]. The following subsection will provide a synthesis of this work, which will present the themes in a stepwise manner to illustrate the logic of institutional racism.

14.3.1 **The moral valence of counterterrorism**

Firstly, one cannot begin a discussion of Prevent or CVE without emphasizing its political impetus, which is reflected in the burgeoning military–academic–industrial complex devoted to terrorism—a low-probability event. The salience of terrorism can be further observed when viewed in contrast within the complete list of statutory and mandatory training prescribed to NHS staff (see Box 14.1).

We see that that the moral salience of terrorism, situated here between 'Moving and Handling' and 'Resuscitation', is given primacy to the exclusion

---

Box 14.1 The full list of online statutory and mandatory training options for a clinical psychologist registered at Camden and Islington NHS Trust, taken from e-lfh.org.uk [accessed December 2019]

Conflict Resolution—Level 1
Data Security Awareness—Level 1
Data Security Awareness Survey
Equality and Diversity and Human Rights—Level 1
Fire Safety—Level 1
Infection Prevention and Control—Level 1
Infection Prevention and Control—Level 2
Health, Safety and Welfare—Level 1
Moving and Handling—Level 1
Moving and Handling eAssessment—Level 2
Preventing Radicalisation—Basic Prevent Awareness
Preventing Radicalisation—Awareness of Prevent (Level 3)
Preventing Radicalisation (Mental Health)—Level 3
Resuscitation—Level 1
Resuscitation Adults—Level 2
Resuscitation Paediatric—Level 2
Resuscitation Newborn—Level 2
Safeguarding Adults—Level 1
Safeguarding Adults—Level 2
Safeguarding Children—Level 1
Safeguarding Children—Level 2
Health Education England Learning Path

of a plethora of other social ills. For example, there were more than 400 domestic homicides in the UK between 2013 and 2016, with only 13 recorded terrorist deaths in that time span [13]. Yet the number of domestic homicides has not resulted in a nationwide training programme to help staff identify and report preabusers, who appear to be largely white males [14]. Such an analogy is only indicative of counterterrorism's moral and political salience, a field of study that, since its inception, has sought to manage the fine line between insiders and outsiders [15]. Given the widespread budget cuts in mental health provisions through austerity policies, the political impetus financing counter-radicalization incentivizes mental health professionals to make Prevent referrals in order for patients to receive the support they would otherwise not receive [5].

To substantiate the moral dimension of counterterrorism in health care even further, an unexpected but consistent finding was the self-censorship that critical NHS staff experienced during Prevent training [11]. This is largely owing to the political and moral subscript underlying counterterrorism, whereby the 'good' position is to accept the Prevent duty, and the 'bad' position is to reject it. A racialized white woman, for example, shared the following experience. During Prevent training, she raised her hand and questioned why staff were being trained in counterterrorism. To this, one of her colleagues turned to her and affirmed, 'We're just trying to save lives!' As such, the moral salience of counterterrorism raises significant concerns of ethical distress among healthcare staff and their liberty to question how their professional practice is being dictated by political rhetoric. This is not a novel observation and is, in fact, well documented in the field of terrorism more broadly [15]. The moralizing dimension of counterterrorism, however, impedes all forms of resistance, dismissing the need for accountability and privileging a system of coercion (to be discussed later).

Although the moral dimension of counterterrrorism affects all, it was more acutely experienced by critical British Muslim healthcare staff who shared a unique, embodied fear of speaking out against the Prevent duty. This was often stated in explicit terms, such as admitting their apprehension of speaking out for fear of being vilified by their colleagues, or more covert behaviours, such as engaging in critical discussions about Prevent in secure WhatsApp groups. In fact, in one instance, a Prevent trainer claimed that counter-radicalization training was about 'Muslim terrorism'. Although Muslim NHS staff voiced their objections, as far as my participant was concerned, both the trainer and the discriminatory repercussions of this incident remain overlooked. It is important to affirm that it is unnecessary for there to be *any explicit statements about Muslims* to evoke discomfort. In one instance, a Muslim psychiatrist admitted he felt awkward when the trainer insisted exclusively on 'white' terrorists, as if they were beating around the bush. Again, this is the result of the hegemonic association between Muslims and security threats, which is further elaborated upon later.

14.3.2 **The primacy of (racialized) intuition**

Secondly, the pedagogical utility of Prevent training must be questioned, given that there is no validated criminological or mental health profile of radicalization. On the contrary, this deficiency in evidence has not stopped the government from relying extensively on the Extremism Risk Guidance (ERG 22+, a highly criticized and non-validated measure, which a report to US Homeland Security admitted would lead to a large catchment of innocents (see [16]). Indeed, the ERG22+ is now embedded within the comprehensive risk assessments of British mental health trust [5]. Now all patients are screened for a number of elusive factors such as anger, us-and-them thinking, and grievances. Given this ambiguity, it becomes clear that Prevent largely hinges upon training staff to *trust their intuition* when they experience a 'concern' [4]. Reliance on intuition is not exclusive to Prevent; it can be gleamed from wider risk-averse strategies, for example the instruction to 'see it, say it, sorted' on London public transport.

In one case example, the Prevent trainer—in a train-the-trainers session, which involved the participants returning to and training their respective institutions—remarked that a vulnerability towards radicalization may be an adolescent who *gains or loses confidence*. Given the preposterous implications of this statement, I asked if the trainer can elaborate any further, to which they admitted it was confusing but that one must 'trust one's gut' and, in another instance, 'refer every minuscule concern'. In another Prevent training session, a group exercise entailed unearthing the possible risk factors associated with radicalization from case examples. A participant in my group observed that, in one case, the mother was single. When I asked for her to elaborate, she simply affirmed (a popular belief) that single mothers are prone to parenting issues. The participant then raised this vulnerability towards radicalization with the Prevent trainer, who nodded and reminded participants that anything can be a risk factor in its proper context. The bottom line of Prevent training then is that it is better to be safe than sorry in the case of uncertainty; the primacy of one's 'gut feelings' is framed as a natural extension of healthcare staff's clinical acumen, giving an opening to prejudicial attitudes to be legitimized rather than regulated, negated, and cautioned. In other words, insofar as clinical judgements *always* rely on often hazy and uncertain criteria, so too should the threat of radicalization enter this diagnostic evaluation. The reliance on intuition is foundational in explaining how racial prejudice enters the picture.

14.3.3 **Performative colour blindness in counter-radicalization**

The third and most significant observation deals with the normative association between threat and Muslims/Islam in public consciousness. Insofar as 'intuition' is raised as integral in counter-radicalization, the government appears to recognize its discriminatory potential. This is especially evident in Prevent training, which engages in what I call *performative colour blindness*: the *active* recognition and erasure of a common sense that associates racialized Muslims with the threat of terrorism [4]. This performative colour blindness takes shape in two ways during Prevent training.

The first is the endless posturing that *anyone* can be vulnerable to radicalization, irrespective of belief or race. Colour blindness, as Michelle Alexander [17] outlines in great detail, is integral to the very perpetuation of racist structures in twenty-first century policies. The drive towards colour blindness in Prevent—especially in light of its historic accusation of discrimination towards Muslims—is vitalized by psychologization. Psychologization denotes a process that essentializes complex social/political issues within individuals and is particularly favoured by neo-liberal forms of governance. In the process of psychologization, all individuals are reduced to a universal set of risk and protective factors according to our shared human vulnerability [4]. As such, the positivism within 'psychology talk' provides the ultimate colour blind platform.

Secondly, counter-radicalization training involved an explicit rehearsal of training staff *not* to focus on Muslims—herein lies the *performative* dimension of colour blindness. This attempt to control for prejudice took place both formally and informally. Formally, Prevent training slides might present 'attending the local mosque' beneath a list of potential vulnerabilities to radicalization. If a participant were to choose this option, they would be informed their choice is incorrect and returned to the list to choose the correct options (I discuss the implications of this 'correction' later). Informally, Prevent trainers are incessant in reminding participants not to mistake religiosity for vulnerabilities of radicalization. They might say, for example, that a headscarf is not meaningful to counter-radicalization in and of -itself. It is in this informal space that the perpetual raising and erasing of radicalization's hegemonic association with Muslims reveals itself more fully. The trend to shift towards the 'far-right' will be discussed in its own section.

This, then, begs then the following question: Can unconscious bias—the hegemonic association of threat, foreignness and regressiveness—towards Muslims be trained away? Beyond performances of colour blindness, this question remains vital for policy interventions seeking to tackle extremism/radicalization more broadly (i.e. without specifying any particular group affiliations).

In an interaction with a Prevent senior official, for example, I was told that better training will be able to control for racial prejudice in radicalization referrals [18]. However, as we know from training that privileges intuition—as is the case in police stop and search training in the War on Drugs—the result will always reflect hegemonic and racialized prejudices [17]. Indeed, even individuals who do not think they are racist still act upon racial, unconscious bias in controlled settings [19]. As such, given the racialization of threat, it is questionable if population-wide counter-radicalization policies can develop effective antiracist postures in training.

14.3.4 Counter-radicalization referrals: prejudice in practice

All of what has been discussed naturally culminates in a system-wide institutionalization and legitimization of prejudice, irrespective if the Prevent duty inevitably catches potential criminals in its scattershot. In my fieldwork, I relate to a number of stories, including but not limited to:

1. A nurse referring a disabled Muslim adolescent because he was watching a video in Arabic.
2. A mental health team who suddenly prioritized radicalization in their clinical formulation when a white, female convert donned the hijab.
3. A non-Muslim male refugee from the Middle East who was referred because he hailed from a conflict zone [4].

In consultation with a non-governmental organization that collates and provides legal counsel for individuals distressed by their Prevent referrals, I have also been informed of a particular detail: there appears to be a larger incidence of NHS staff *referring their colleagues*, compared to other public bodies such as education. This corroborates the fear that Muslim staff shared in our interviews with them [11]. This is best captured by the story of a Muslim chaplain: he was contacted by a staff member, who feared for a patient's potential radicalization. The staff member had noticed that the Muslim patient suddenly began wearing a *kufi* (a small head garment worn in many Muslim-majority countries), to which the chaplain responded, 'I have one, too'.

14.4 Islamophobia in counter-radicalization: a systemic issue

The growing popular support of nationalist politics is fundamental to any discussion on counter-radicalization strategies. I have catalogued a number of Muslims who spoke of going on *hajj*, but these only represent the tip of the iceberg in the growing body of literature documenting the impact of CVE on civil society. Kundnani and Hayes [20] recently reviewed CVE policies across the Global North and found they are vaguely defined; empirically incoherent and operating largely on common-sensical but erroneous logics; eroding (Muslim) civil society by employing 'soft power' to develop pro-Western Muslim identities; used to justify the expansion of surveillance systems; limiting digital rights and freedom of expressions; being applied to legitimate political activities such as protests, demonstrations, and direct actions such as those related to Palestinian activism [21]; and, finally, lacking formal accountability, beyond the state's own bureaucratic framework (the State reviews itself), given that CVE policies are largely implemented as executive decisions. Accordingly, the focus of this section will further elucidate major hurdles in counter-radicalization policies, especially as it shifts towards mental health.

14.4.1 Issues of expanding CVE towards the far-right

Here I will explicitly address the growing trend of 'shifting' CVE towards the far right, and highlight several major concerns with the recent Prevent referral statistics. As I have argued, insofar as a counter-extremism strategy is employed nationwide, whiteness was always privileged for 'their bodies alone were insufficient to conjure the threat of radicalisation' [4]. Thus, my research raised concerns over the question of thresholds, as it relates to distinguishing between acceptable and extremist behaviours in the public imaginary. This distinction, as one might imagine, is highly racialized. In one example I elaborated upon, a racialized Muslim's rather banal mention of wanting to homeschool his children raised the thought of radicalization in a general practitioner's mind. This is not an arbitrary; it belongs squarely within the now-securitized logic of integration, whereby Muslims who appear to distance themselves from society are viewed with suspicion.

But there is a far more significant error in this trend to 'capture' the far right within the auspices of general CVE policies: its reification of racism and xenophobia unto the margins of society. Nationalism and Islamophobia are hardly 'extreme' political positions in our current sociopolitical climate, irrespective of group affiliation. In her seminal book, Liz Fekete [22] demonstrates how the 'far right' has, indeed, entered every level of governance across Europe. Furthermore, research across European nations has shown that harsher immigration rhetoric is largely not partisan—as in not exclusive to the political right [23]. In other words, a whole range of actors technically fall within the auspices of xenophobia—but we see that counter-extremism has no claim over them. Prevent and CVE policies more broadly are instead more focused on particular groups such as the English Defence League than nationalist ideologies, thereby not only defeating the purpose of a broad counter-extremism strategy (given the focus on particular group affiliations), but also privileging the rising tide of nationalist rhetoric associated with racist violence towards Muslims and immigrants. The threshold differential of *who* and *what* constitutes extremism also has severe legal ramifications for individuals. One of the confounding changes to the Terrorism Act 2019 has been the legalistic addition of 'reckless' in the support of terrorism (as in, unintentionally supporting a terrorist group). In other words, as Clive Walker [24] explained in written evidence to the UK parliament, this addition results in the criminalization of associating oneself with extremist views—for example, supporting the broad notion of jihad—and allow the subsequent charge of terrorism for *recklessly* supporting the ideology of the Islamic State of Iraq and Syria (ISIS). Here we must ask the question: Is there an extremist equivalent of a *reckless* nationalist claim?

14.4.2 Issues of coercion and accountability

Coercion is a weighty theme in counterterrorism. How does coercion figure in a mental health strategy under the auspices of counter-radicalization? Simon Cole, who was previously the national police lead for Prevent, admitted that counterterrorism police might inspect anyone refusing to cooperate with a counter-radicalization intervention (i.e. such as mental health). Even without such admissions, we know very little about how Prevent referees experience the point of referral and the intervention proposed, except for those publicized by the government. Taking again from the War on Drugs, we know that black people significantly comply with discriminatory stop and searches, even when police disclose that the procedure is voluntary [17]. Thus, coercion can never be discounted when resistance to counterterrorism measures reflects poorly on the individual and their families. Indeed, a NHS safeguarding guide explicitly states that 'perceptions that UK government policy is discriminatory (e.g. counter-terrorist legislation) [. . .] may play an important part in the early indoctrination of vulnerable individuals' [25]. It remains significant then not to essentialize 'mental health interventions' as an unconditional good. The dismissal or infringement of individual agency—especially through coercive structures managed by and in the interest of the State—potentially exacerbates the very experience of depoliticization, which has been associated with political violence [26, 27].

The possibility of coercion must be followed by a discussion on accountability. Nowhere is this more pertinent than Prevent training itself. In online Prevent training, a slide poses the question, 'What factors might make a child vulnerable to radicalisation?', to which the respondent must choose three of the following options: deprivation; bullying; attending the local mosque; and adolescence [4]. If someone happened to be prejudiced towards Muslims and checked 'attending the local mosque', what happens next? During training, they are simply returned to select the 'correct' answers before moving on to receive their certificate of completion—that is all. Such a scenario is not difficult to conjure: a recent large-scale survey found that one-third of Britons preferred not having a mosque nearby [2]. Thus, prejudice towards Muslims and the need for accountability is erased in Prevent training—the issuing of a certificate effectively proving one has been 'cleared' of bias. Furthermore, as I also noted among Muslim NHS staff, there is no one to speak with if one experienced Islamophobia, let alone if they perceived Prevent training to be discriminatory. This experience was not limited to racialized Muslims either: a black psychologist distinctly felt uncomfortable with Prevent training as well. She admitted then that she self-censored because she felt experiences of racism were not handled seriously. What is important in all these cases is the difficulties of discussing race and racialization as a structural concern in the NHS.

14.5 **Conclusion: if not this, then what**

The racialization of threat in our current political climate is significant. I have argued that even if a public, colour blind counter-radicalization strategy were to exclude explicit references to any one group, *it would still be about Muslims*. This is the significance of nationalism in both the *raison d'etre*, as well as function of counterextremism. This is not to disparage the potential of efforts to prevent violence and co-opting a public health approach. For example, if anxiety was observed to be associated with incidence of violence, then perhaps a public health approach to address anxiety *without* reference to elusive racialized constructs such as extremism might benefit. But such a strategy must reject the political impetus fuelling the push towards counterterrorism, eschew the false equivalence drawn between Islamists and the far-right ideologies (given the privileging of nationalism), and recognize the depoliticizing repercussions of interventions that legitimize racial prejudice.

The causes of political violence in these politically and economically turbulent times are manifold. The damage done by policies executed by politicians—who seek political clout by tackling the spectre of terrorism—necessitates a systemic rethinking of counter-terrorism and its institutions. The explicit objective should be to go beyond the War on Terror, not ameliorate it. Alternatives do exist: the Transnational Institute recently provided an inspiring, progressive alternative to the UK's counter-terrorism apparatus [26]. As it has been said repeatedly, a central thrust to disrupt the threat of political violence is a trustworthy social contract between those most vulnerable in society and the State.

Herein lies a vision for the future, one which takes both public health *and* racism seriously.

References

1. **ICM Omnibus.** Avaaz Islamophobia & anti-Semitism poll. Available from: https://www.icmunlimited.com/our-work/avaaz-islamophobia-anti-semitism-poll/ [accessed 29 December 2019].
2. **Perraudin F.** Third of Britons believe Islam threatens British way of life, says report. Available from: https://www.theguardian.com/world/2019/feb/17/third-of-britons-believe-islam-threatens-british-way-of-life-says-report [accessed 13 September 2019].
3. **Bellis MA, Hardcastle K.** Preventing violent extremism in the UK: public health solutions. Available from: https://www.fph.org.uk/media/2475/preventing-violent-extremism-in-the-uk_public-health-solutions-web.pdf [accessed 6 August 2020].
4. **Younis T, Jadhav S.** Islamophobia in the National Health Service: an ethnography of institutional racism in PREVENT's counter-radicalisation policy. Sociology of Health & Illness 2020;**42**:610–26.
5. **Heath-Kelly C, Strausz E.** Counter-terrorism in the NHS: evaluating Prevent safeguarding duty in the NHS. Available from: https://warwick.ac.uk/fac/soc/pais/research/researchcentres/irs/counterterrorisminthenhs/project_report_60pp.pdf [accessed 6 August 2020].
6. **Kundnani A.** Islamophobia as ideology of US Empire. In: **Massoumi N, Mills T, Miller D**, eds. What is Islamophobia? London: Pluto Press; 2017, pp. 35–48.
7. **Valluvan S.** The clamour of nationalism: race and nation in twenty-first-century Britain. Manchester: Manchester University Press; 2019.
8. **Meer N.** Racialization and religion: race, culture and difference in the study of antisemitism and Islamophobia. Ethnic and Racial Studies 2013;**36**:385–98.
9. **Toscano A.** Fanaticism: on the uses of an idea. London: Verso; 2017.
10. **Aked H, Jones M, Miller D.** Islamophobia in Europe: how governments are enabling the far-right 'counter-jihad' movement. Available from: https://research-information.bris.ac.uk/ws/portalfiles/portal/192414854/Aked_Jones_Miller_Counterjihad_report_2019.pdf [accessed 6 August 2020].
11. **Younis T, Jadhav S.** Keeping our mouths shut: the fear and racialized self-censorship of British healthcare professionals in PREVENT training. Culture, Medicine, and Psychiatry 2019;**43**:404–24.
12. **Silva DMD.** 'Radicalisation: the journey of a concept', revisited. Race & Class 2018;**59**:34–53.
13. **Home Office.** Domestic homicide reviews: key findings from analysis of domestic homicide reviews. Available from: https://assets.publishing.service.gov.uk/government/uploads/system/uploads/attachment_data/file/575232/HO-Domestic-Homicide-Review-Analysis-161206.pdf [accessed 6 November 2018].
14. **Violence Policy Center.** More than 1,800 women murdered by men in one year, new study finds. Available from: http://vpc.org/press/more-than-1800-women-murdered-by-men-in-one-year-new-study-finds/ [accessed 8 January 2019].

15. **Stampnitzky L.** Disciplining terror: how experts invented 'terrorism'. Cambridge: Cambridge University Press; 2013.

16. **RTI International.** Countering violent extremism: the application of risk assessment tools in the criminal justice and rehabilitation process. Available from: https://www.dhs.gov/sites/default/files/publications/OPSR_TP_CVE-Application-Risk-Assessment-Tools-Criminal-Rehab-Process_2018Feb-508.pdf [accessed 6 November 2018].

17. **Alexander M.** The new Jim Crow: mass incarceration in the age of colorblindness. New York: New Press; 2012.

18. **Younis T.** The UK's PREVENT policy would not prevent white supremacist attacks like Christchurch—it's part of the problem. Available from: https://mediadiversified.org/2019/04/01/the-uks-prevent-policy-would-not-prevent-white-supremacist-attacks-like-christchurch-its-part-of-the-problem/ [accessed 2 April 2019].

19. **Penner LA, Dovidio JF.** Racial color blindness and Black-White health care disparities. In: **Neville HA, Gallardo ME, Sue DW**, eds. The myth of racial color-blindness. Washington, DC: American Psychological Association; 2016, p. 330.

20. **Kundnani A, Hayes B.** The globalisation of Countering Violent Extremism policies. Amsterdam: Transnational Institute; 2018.

21. **Malak A.** Prevent: silencing Palestine on campus. Feminist Dissent 2019;4:8.

22. **Fekete E.** Europe's fault lines: racism and the rise of the right. London and New York: Verso; 2018.

23. **de Haas H, Natter K.** The determinants of migration policies. International Migration Institute 2015;117:32.

24. **Walker C.** Written evidence from Professor Emeritus Clive Walker (CBS0001). Available from: http://data.parliament.uk/WrittenEvidence/CommitteeEvidence.svc/EvidenceDocument/Human%20Rights%20Joint%20Committee/Legislative%20Scrutiny%20CounterTerrorism%20and%20Border%20Security%20Bill/written/85566.html [accessed 29 December 2019].

25. **NHS England.** Safeguarding adults: a guide for health care staff. Available from: https://www.england.nhs.uk/wp-content/uploads/2017/02/adult-pocket-guide.pdf [accessed 4 October 2019].

26. **Blakeley R, Hayes B, Kapoor N, Kundnani A, Miller D, Mills T,** et al. Leaving the War on Terror: a progressive alternative to counter-terrorism policy. Amsterdam: Transnational Institute; 2019.

27. **Davies J.** Back to balance: labour therapeutics and the depoliticisation of workplace distress. Palgrave Communications 2016;2:16027.

Chapter 15

A discourse for the prevention of radicalization in the Netherlands: Curbing the radical inflow

Carl H.D. Steinmetz

15.1 Introduction

Although terrorism is not a new phenomenon, with globalization and the consequent increased movement of people, and the escalating use of social media and the Internet, its impact on communities is evident and worrying. Different countries have chosen different pathways into combating terror attacks and dealing with the post-attack situations. In this chapter my focus is on the Dutch government's response and contrast it with those of other countries.

15.2 The Dutch scene

According to the National Coordinator for Security and Counter-terrorism (Dutch abbreviation: NCTV), terrorism is defined as 'threatening with violence, intimidation, forcing the state (not) to do something, and the recruitment of members' [1]. The Minister of Security and Justice of the Netherlands entrusted the NCTV with the control of national security and crisis management, counterterrorism, and cybersecurity. An amount of €266,427 million was made available for this in the State Budget Ministry of Justice and Security [2, p. 3]. This money was largely meant for bodies such as the police, the Dutch Public Prosecution Office and the Royal Netherlands Marechaussee, which are responsible for the actual implementation of these tasks. These funds are used to arrest individuals in a timely fashion and deal with radicalizing persons via a repressive, individually targeted approach. The recent attacks in Europe, the United States, Africa, and Asia, and the consequent polarization between ethnic groups not only encourages repressive measures, but also promotes strategies to curb the perceived influx of 'radicals'. However, counterterrorism can only succeed with a more forceful commitment to a preventive community-based approach with more resources from the central government.

During a broadcast of the Dutch daily talk show *De Wereld Draait Door*, which discussed terrorism, Beatrice de Graaf [1] reflected on the recent attacks by arguing that we are blinded. 'Contemporary terrorism (post-9/11) is regarded as new', which is obviously not true. To provide evidence to the contrary, she claims that Saddam Hussein's colonels were trained by the East German Stasi to set up terrorist movements. These colonels, she says, now work with Islamic State (IS). According to de Graaf, terrorism has known four major global wave-like patterns since the nineteenth century. These increase and decrease, and every new wave uses the insights gained from previous movements; for example, the strategy of the propaganda[1] of the deed, the 'Gideon's gang', the national right to self-determination, extreme provocations, negotiation, metropolitan guerrilla warfare, social media, and 'youth culture'. The aim of terrorist movements is intimidation of larger communities and provocation to extreme responses that endorse their position and mobilise their followers.

In short, the public is challenged to review its assumptions about terrorism as perhaps a reasonable and proportionate response to repressive counter-terrorism measures.

A better understanding of the causes and consequences of terrorism may well lead to less fear, fewer reactions, and adjustments of behaviour. We need to learn about the impact of counterterrorist actions on those who carry out terrorist activities and those who deal with the consequences, as well as those who are directly and indirectly affected by terrorism.

Possible interventions to address radicalization will be elaborated further later in this chapter. We will consider these interventions from the perspective of the individualism–collectivism dimension. The plea for investing more manpower and money in the prevention of radicalization will subsequently be elaborated in order to prevent the recruitment of more 'radicals'.

15.3 **Individualism–collectivism dimension**

The levels of individualism and collectivism in populations and terrorist movements means that interventions to tackle radicalization must reflect these [3].

---

[1] 'Propaganda is a set of the messages intended to influence opinions of the masses, not giving the opponents any opportunity to rebut the idea. Instead of telling people the truth, propaganda often aims at manipulation of ideas to influence the behaviour of a large number of people. So, it presents ideas selectively. Propaganda is related to advertising, where it is about promoting a product. It is also used to influence religious beliefs of society' (https://marketingwit.com/types-of-propaganda-techniques).

15.3.1 **Case history (a constructed narrative)**

Kacey (courageous, 'hawk-like eyes'; not her real name) considers going to Syria. She is 21 years old. She feels vulnerable and is emotionally isolated. Her older sister has died, her father beats her mother and is involved in drug trafficking. At school, she was assaulted by a classmate. On the tram, bus, and metro, she has the feeling that everybody stares at her. At primary school, the advice given to her was to follow a preparatory secondary vocational education (a non-theory-oriented type of secondary school education in the Netherlands), which was way below her ability. At the time she thought: 'Of course, I am not one of them, since I am fully veiled'. She has the feeling she is on her own. She reflects on her identity and seeks it in faith. She is in need of affection and chats with a young man in Syria by telephone and falls in love. He tells her about the Muslim community that is attacked worldwide, with conflict and a war of 'unbelievers' against Islam and Muslims on many fronts. This reinforces her feeling of being treated unfairly. She feels understood by him and would rather leave for Syria tomorrow. But this is not simple. Her grandmother is fiercely opposed to this.

15.3.1.1 The individualist approach

Kacey's teacher in secondary school reports her radicalizing behaviour to the 'higher' authorities, who immediately take action. Kacey's Internet use is investigated. The conclusion is that she is radicalizing. The police raid her house in the middle of the night. She is taken alone, interrogated at the police station, and confronted about her behaviour. Her passport is seized. She cannot go to Syria. Kacey is even lonelier than before. A year later she manages to escape from the Netherlands.

15.3.1.2 The collectivist approach

Kacey's grandmother gathers all the women from the extended family. There are lots of them. They give Kacey the opportunity to explain what is on her mind. Several women start crying. Nobody knew that Kacey was in such a bad state. Mother and grandmother take Kacey in their arms. They talk, cry, eat, and drink tea. Together, the women decide that Kacey will go and live with a single aunt. This aunt is assigned the task of talking to Kacey and taking Kacey to a different family member every week. The extended family seeks the solution in promoting mutual connectedness. A year later, Kacey completes the course 'Care and Well-being' at the level of secondary vocational education.

This history illustrates the differences between individualist and collectivist approaches and it is worth noting that immigrants will belong to different types of communities, some of which may well be more traditional than others.

15.4 **Individualists and collectivists: responsibility and interventions**

According to theory, individualists and collectivists have a different view of responsibility and causes of criminal behaviour, and therefore also of violent protest, committing attacks, travelling to war zones in order to go into battle there or supporting warriors in war zones. We expect these differences in sense of responsibility and causation to have consequences for interventions depending on whether developed and implemented by the state, the municipality, the neighbourhood, society, the extended family, and educators.

15.4.1 **Individualists: responsibility and interventions**

Individualism mainly occurs in mostly Western societies and stands for independence and autonomy. Individualists remind people of their own responsibility. Individualist words belonging to their approach to radicalization include warn, infiltrate, detect, arrest, and imprison.

Individualists use 'tit-for-tat' interventions, such as detainment, harassment, and pushing away, in combination with a community that facilitates this. Step 1 is carrying out risk assessments, the timely detection and discouragement of criminal behaviour with risk prediction, and following people from having beliefs to committing acts. Step 2 is arrest, seizure of passport, preventing a return to war zones, prevention of fighters, their wives, and their children from returning to Western states, and imprisonment in high-security cells, in particular for those on the security watch lists. Criminal law objectives are normative here. These objectives include prevention (deterring others from committing the same), protection of society (during detention the same crime can no longer be committed by the same person), re-education (the convict has to better their life), and retaliation (victims and society may take revenge via criminal law).

Risk assessments, detection, and subsequent approaches [4] focus on (A) hotspot locations/high-risk times; (B) high-risk victims (repeated victimization); and (C) high-risk perpetrators (habitual offenders). This integral approach is secured in various effective theoretical frameworks, namely: opportunity theory and routine activity [5, 6],[2] a personalized and TOP-X (a Dutch focus on known neighbourhood criminals/radicals; the 'X' stands for the number of criminals or radicals) approach. The focus extends beyond just

---

[2] These theories are simple in essence: the extent of crime is determined by three factors: numbers of potential offenders, numbers of attractive targets (attraction factor), and the level of monitoring and control over and the protection of these targets.

the police and criminal law. The neighbourhood, the family, the school, friends, work, housing, and so on, are included in a personalized approach. This 'trawl' of which the scope is broader than that of criminal law might also be referred to as the Communities That Care approach. The 'trawl' includes cousins, brothers, and sisters. With individualists, the emphasis is mainly on action against the perpetrators and less on prevention, as described in the earlier case history.

It seems as though individualists lack something in their approach to radicalization. Opportunity theorists would say the attraction factor (see footnote 2) is lacking in the approach of individualists, such as 'the higher good' in radicalization. Furthermore, individualists seem to demonstrate a panic reaction. They recruit 'informers' in all kinds of institutions who pass on signals to the 'higher authorities'. These 'informers' are to detect whether students radicalize (a type of Stasi practice).

15.4.2 Collectivists: responsibility and interventions

Collectivism mainly occurs in more traditional societies and in the non-Western world, although as a result of globalization and urbanization many cultures are in transition, and these are changing. In the Netherlands, collectivism is apparent in some groups of immigrants, refugees, and expats. Individuals from collectivist cultures are seen to be more empathic and community oriented, with mutual dependence and connectedness. Collectivist cultures believe in 'we-ness' and may feel that they have or have not addressed the problems of poverty and exclusion outside the family or in their upbringing. They may look for causes and consequences, such as predictors of sympathy for radicalization. They put the responsibility for what goes wrong with the system, the family, the educators, the neighbourhood, and society with the extended family, clan, or tribe. Using this as a starting point, they attempt to find tools for such an approach. This interesting approach will not work for everyone and we will briefly focus on several lesser-known collectivist risk factors in the Netherlands.

Bouchra Ftitache [7] examined the learning achievements of immigrant primary school pupils. These children often have poorer Cito test results (this is a selection test to check if a child is at the right level of education; it is comparable to the Eleven-plus exam in England and Northern Ireland) and lower school attainment levels, compared to Dutch children. This study shows that (A) children of non-Western immigrants have more psychological and social problems (including oppositional–rebellious behaviour, antisocial behaviour, aggression, and relational problems with peers) than Dutch children; (B) immigrant children are more often bullied at school than Dutch children; and (C) the aforementioned disadvantages that already existed in group 1 (year 1 in England) of primary school have not disappeared in group 8 (year 6 in England).

In his book *Marokkaan in Europa, crimineel in Nederland* (*Moroccan in Europe, criminal in the Netherlands*), Frank Bovenkerk [8] compares their presence in Spain, Italy, Germany, France, Belgium, and the Netherlands. The core of his explanatory argument is that 'parents have lost grip on their sons' and that the transition from an agricultural to an urbanized community, initially as pathfinders and immigrant workers, and subsequently through reunion with relatives and family, has been accompanied by poverty and exclusion. Bovenkerk [8] seeks the explanation for 'Criminal in the Netherlands and not in Europe' with the crumbling authority of patriarchal fathers. This starts with the enforced absence of fathers in the young years of boys (i.e. attachment phase), the judging of fathers for a corrective slap (this clearly will be child abuse in the Netherlands), seeing that fathers are discarded after their work is finished (sons see their father falling from a pedestal), and not becoming familiar with customs such as the negotiating culture and a policy of tolerance, and with the language of the fatherland because these fathers often had to work hard (often in heavy industry) in order to secure a scarce income.

Esmah Lahlah [9] compares adolescent Dutch boys with Moroccan boys in order to find out the reason why the latter group commits more violent crimes. She discovers familiar and less familiar factors that explain this difference. Well-known factors include low socio-economic status, traditional masculinity norms, and a less close relationship with the parents. Lahlah [9] says: 'that Moroccan youngsters experience the emotional relationship with their parents as being less warm than Dutch youngsters, and that they experience more violence in the family than Dutch youngsters'. The latter is a lesser-known fact. Lahlah says:

> 'over 60% of Moroccan youth have been exposed to physical violence by a parent. With Dutch boys this is 21%. 17% of these adolescent Moroccan boys have been subjected to sexual abuse by a family member compared with 5% of Dutch boys; 45% of Moroccan boys have been subjected to physical violence between parents compared with 17% of Dutch boys.'

Lahlah establishes a solid link between two potential risk factors for the emergence of radicalization, namely committing serious crime and repeatedly falling victim to serious crimes.

Elisabeth van der Ven [10] researches the nature, scope, and consequences of psychotic complaints (symptoms that persist for longer than one week) and autism spectrum disorders of second- and third-generation immigrants and Dutch people. She notes,

> that the risk of immigrants with a dark skin colour suffering from psychotic complaints is five times higher than Dutch people, while immigrants with a white skin colour run a risk that is twice as high. The risk of North-African males and especially Moroccan males suffering from psychotic complaints is five times as high as that of North-African females.

Her conclusion is 'that immigration itself is not a key explanatory factor, but being a member of a (minority) ethnic group'. These results are explained on the basis of bullying (non-clinical psychotic symptoms emerge because of bullying at school) and the 'social defeat' hypothesis (growing up in an urban environment, low IQ, traumatic experiences, drug use, and a pre-history of immigration). van der Ven [10] argues:

> all in all, a growing group of young people are emerging who feel displaced. They do not feel at home in Dutch society. Some of them even retreat in their own (religious) community, others withdraw and threaten to become lonely, develop serious psychological complaints or become susceptible to the seductions of radicalism or criminality.

Entirely different studies exist that map out risk factors and causes in terms of the emergence of radicalization. Relevant to this argument are studies that hold the prison system and the Internet responsible for the dissemination of radical ideas (both work like a pressure cooker). An example is the research into 'jihadi cool' and the combating of it [11].

These risk studies are in line with assumptions of collectivist individuals. The contexts of educators, extended family, neighbourhood, and society are responsible for the emergence of these risk factors. According to collectivists, the conclusion to be drawn from this is that the prevention of radicalization should 'dovetail' all these contexts for the emergence and tackling of risks.

15.5 A forceful, preventive approach for tackling radicalization

In short, a forceful, preventive approach is required to remove these causes. Prevention should be interpreted in a broad sense here, being geared towards the prevention of crimes in the house, family and public environment, the prevention of health complaints, and the prevention of poverty and exclusion. A landslide will be required for such an immense effort. Collectivists struggle to place their plea for such a forceful, preventive effort in a framework to which policymakers can say 'yes'. Kamaldeep Bhui [12] has the following cynical comment about this: 'a preventive approach to radicalisation is not part of the current in the UK counter-terrorism policy, which focusses on those likely to commit terrorist acts'.

15.6 Ingredients for a forceful, preventive approach for tackling radicalization

The themes for a forceful, preventive approach for tackling radicalization are elaborated further. Theme 1 is the scope of an intervention. Theme 2 is the introduction of prevention of radicalization in businesses and institutions. Theme 3 is the development of interventions via process phases and cost–benefit models.

15.6.1 **Theme 1**

We believe the potential scope or impact of an intervention should be determined beforehand. I wish to coin the term 'telescope model' here for the scope/impact of an intervention. The telescope shows that poverty and exclusion are visible and therefore easier to tackle than radicalization. Seventeen per cent of the Dutch population lived in 2017 in poverty [13, p. 60; 14, 15], and experience (social) exclusion. Bhui [16] shows that in two cities in the UK, including London, up to 2.4% of the Muslim population sympathize with radicalization. Translated to the Dutch population, this number is significant. The situation looks different for people who radicalize. According to the NCTV [17], there are several hundreds of supporters and several thousands of sympathizers in the Netherlands. In the case of 2000 sympathizers, we still talk about less than one ten-thousandth of the Dutch population. Sympathizers cannot be easily traced. It is only possible to trace them with an enormous effort on the part of the police, the judicial authorities, and 'informers'.

An important interim question related to the scope is the following one: Suppose we manage to reduce exclusion and poverty by 10% every year, what would be the impact of this on supporters and sympathizers of radicalization? Regretfully, we do not have the answer to this question. And there are views that poverty is important as a driver of radicalization, as well as it being unimportant, yet we know poverty and inequality are related to exclusion, and protest and violence can be a consequence; thus, considering similar processes in radicalization is not unreasonable, and, I argue, essential.

15.6.2 **Theme 2**

Persons who radicalize may also be employees or self-employed professionals with institutions or businesses such as education, care, municipalities, the police, the army and airports, e.g. Schiphol. Up to now, the approach for tackling radicalization in the Netherlands has been lacking a business organization approach. An approach geared towards businesses and organizations consists of the following elements: (A) the reformulation of the mission and vision of an institution/business in such a way that students, customers, and patients recognize themselves in terms of profile and presence in the organization Our Kind of People (Dutch abbreviation: OSM); (B) working with a reporting code for radicalization (from detection to tackling and forwarding to the 'triangle', i.e. the police, the public prosecution service, and the local government); (C) working with a top team in charge of de-radicalization (using people, knowledge, and resources in an economical way); (D) the development of an organizational guideline for tackling persons who radicalize or who are on the path of radicalization; and (E) the organization of information meetings. Australia, for example, has focused on potential radical attacks on businesses and institutions since 2005 [18].

15.6.3 **Theme 3**

Prevention programmes should have the following intervention strategy: (A) ensure that (young) people do not get on the path of radicalization; (B) ensure that (young) people who are on the path to radicalization are encouraged and supported in being removed from this path; and (C) ensure that individuals, educators, the extended family, the neighbourhood, and society are integrated and dovetailed in any prevention programme.

This intervention mission is crucial for the design of primary, secondary, and tertiary prevention. The primary factor is to prevent an attack from being committed, to prevent people from joining the fight in war zones, and to prevent the emergence of sympathy for radical ideas. At a secondary level, it is important to reduce the impact and suffering as a result of attacks, going to war zones, dying there, or returning. Secondary prevention is curbing the effects of venturing on the path of radical ideas. Prevention will only work if there is early intervention, in which case the impact of intervention will be substantial. An original approach is the 'Broken Windows' approach [19], which tackles exclusion and discrimination 'head and tail' in risk areas. Tertiary prevention is offering assistance to radicalized people and their extended family in order to minimize the adverse effects of radicalization and its precursors. Tertiary prevention may produce primary and secondary effects because sisters, brothers, and cousins are not dragged into radical ideas.

Furthermore, process phases of (Islamic) radicalization Bhui are guidelines in the development of preventive interventions [16, 20]. These process phases include pre-radicalization (developing sympathies for extreme or terrorist movements without being personally involved in them), self-identification (seeking a new identity, 'they–we'), indoctrination (indoctrination is the influencing towards a new direction in life, the higher 'good', which transcends the personal 'good'), and jihadism (participating in the jihad as mujahideen or holy warrior; planning and preparation of an attack).

Crucial in the development of preventive interventions is the conclusion that during the process of radicalization [21], an individual changes from being passive to being revolutionary, militant, or extreme. Salafi-jihadi (Islamic), extreme left or right-wing ideologies might be considered as the 'context' within which such change may occur.

With radicalization, a close affiliation emerges with people, including information technology, as well as breeding places of terrorism. A second starting point in the development of preventive interventions is the knowledge that, during the radicalization transformation process, vulnerable people are taken advantage of, in particular. Very vulnerable people are those who have experienced traumatic events or those with factors that speed up developments (e.g. living in a neighbourhood with a relatively high number of recruiters and criminal gangs). In all phases of radicalization, we notice a correlation with individual vulnerability as a result of depression, poverty, low socio-economic status, committing petty and serious crime (including drug trafficking), discrimination, and exclusion.

For the development of preventive interventions, we can furthermore use the cost–benefit model that builds on the pull-and-push framework [22]. This can be combined with the process phases model. Push-and-pull factors are about interventions that remove persons from the path of radicalization. Examples of push factors that may be used include expectations that are not fulfilled, frustrations due to strategy and actions of terrorist, and not being able to cope with violence that occurs with radicalization. Examples of pull factors that may be used include demands imposed by the extended family, and/or opportunities to get out via education, work, and financial incentives.

The cost–benefit model is used in psychology, sociology, and criminology [22]. The key element of this model is that the decision to turn away from society and venture on the path of radical ideologies is informed by the excessively high costs involved in remaining part of the same society. There will be room for preventive interventions once the conclusion is drawn that seeing and committing gruesome murders is too high a price to pay to remain involved in a radical ideology. The development of intervention will also have to focus on the emotional process involved in turning one's back on radicalization in Ebaugh's role exit theory [22]. Exiting is seldom the result of a single decision. Exiting is preceded by a long process of doubt. It is possible to respond to this with preventive interventions.

15.7 **Conclusion**

Every year, the Netherlands spends €266 million on tackling terrorism and radicalization. The largest portion is spent on repressive techniques. Little money is left over for prevention. This article presents two novelties for the prevention of radicalization and terrorism. The first is learning to work with the social and cultural heritage of immigrants and refugees, which is bundled in the extended family. After all, the collective can be held accountable for their responsibility for the derailing individual. The second approach is to hold institutions and companies accountable for their responsibility for social security. In the Netherlands this is simple because the Netherlands has laws that regulate aggression, violence, and sexual harassment in the workplace. With some ingenuity, these laws can also be applied to radicalization and terrorism. Experience with this has been gained in Australia. Relevant institutions include community centres, places of worship, schools, and care institutions, including mental health institutions.

References

1. **de Graaf B.** Terugkijken: college terrorisme door Beatrice de Graaf. Available from: https://www.bnnvara.nl/dewerelddraaitdoor/videos/104 [accessed 6 August 2020].
2. **Ministerie van Justitie en Veiligheid. Rijksbegroting** 2020. VI Justitie en Veiligheid. Tweede Kamer der Staten Generaal 2. The Hague: Ministerie van Justitie en Veiligheid; 2019–20.
3. **Noor S.** Vrouwelijk IS-gangers: waarom gaan ze? Available from: https://www.kis. nl/sites/default/files/bestanden/Publicaties/vrouwelijke-isis-gangers.pdf [accessed 6 August 2020].
4. Sherman LW, Gottfredson DC, MacKenzie DL, Eck J, Reuter P, Bushway SD. Preventing Crime: What Works, What doesn't, What's Promising. National Institute of Justice, Research in Brief, July 1998.
5. **Felson M, Clarke R V.** Opportunity makes the thief: practical theory for crime prevention. Available from: https://popcenter.asu.edu/sites/default/files/opportunity_makes_the_thief.pdf [accessed 6 August 2020].
6. **Steinmetz CHD.** Een aanzet' tot een victimologische risicoanalyse; een denkmodel bij het voorkomen van kleine criminaliteit. Justitiële Verkenningen. **Number 2.** The Hague: Wetenschappelijk Onderzoek- en Documentatie Centrum, Ministerie van Justitie; 1980.
7. **Ftitache B.** Psychosocial and educational adjustment of ethnic minority elementary school children in the Netherlands. Amsterdam: Academisch proefschrift VU Amsterdam; 2015.
8. **Bovenkerk F.** Marokkaan in Europa, crimineel in Nederland: een vergelijkende studie. Amsterdam: Boom Lemma Uitgevers; 2014.
9. **Lahlah E.** Invisible victims. Ethnic differences in the risk of juvenile violent delinquency of Dutch and Moroccan-Dutch adolescent boys. Tilburg: Universiteit Tilburg; 2013 [dissertation].
10. **van der Ven E.M.A.** Ethnic minority position as risk indicator for autism-spectrum and psychotic disorders. Maastricht: Academisch Proefschrift Maastricht; 2016.
11. **Huey L.** This is not your mother's terrorism: social media, online radicalization and the practice of political jamming. Journal of Terrorism Research 2015, DOI: 10.15664/jtr.1159.

12. **Bhui K, Warfa N, Jones E.** Might depression, psychosocial adversity, and limited social assets explain vulnerability to and resistance against violent radicalisation? *PLoS One* 2014;9:e105918.

13. **Dutch Central Bureau of Statistics.** The Netherlands on a European Scale. Available from: https://www.cbs.nl/en-gb/publication/2019/20/the-netherlands-on-the-european-scale-2019 [accessed 6 August 2020].

14. **Factsheet WRR:** Economic Inequality in the Netherlands in 8 figures. Available from: https://english.wrr.nl/publications/press-releases/2014/09/03/factsheet-economic-inequality-in-the-netherlands-in-8-figures [accessed 6 August 2020].

15. **European Commission.** Poverty and social exclusion. Available from: http://ec.europa.eu/social/main.jsp?catId=751 [accessed 6 August 2020].

16. **Bhui K, Warfa N, Jones E.** Is violent radicalisation associated with poverty, migration, poor self-reported health and common mental disorders. *PLoS One* 2014;9:e90718.

17. **Ministerie van Binnenlandse Zaken en Koninkrijksrelaties. Jihadistische beweginin in Nederland.** Available from: https://www.aivd.nl/onderwerpen/terrorisme/dreiging/jihadistische-beweging-in-nederland [accessed 6 August 2020].

18. **Bowie V, Fisher BS, Cooper CL.** Workplace violence: issues, trends, strategies. Milton: Willan Publishing; 2005.

19. **Harcourt BE, Ludwig J.** Broken windows: new evidence from New York City and a five-city social experiment. University of Chicago Law Review 2006;**73**:271.

20. **Bhui K.** Mental health and violent radicalization. Mental Health Today 2013;24:6.

21. **MCGilloway A, Priyo G, Bhui K.** A systematic review of pathways to and processes associated with radicalisation and extremism amongst Muslims in Western Societies. International Review of Psychiatry 2015;**27**:39–50.

22. **Altier MB, Thoroughgood CN, Horgan JG.** Turning away from terrorism: Lessons from psychology, sociology, and criminology. Journal of Peace Research 2014;51:647–61.

Chapter 16

Tackling radicalization and terrorism in Dutch mental health institutions: Outcomes of a Dutch population survey

Carl H.D. Steinmetz

16.1 Introduction

In 2015 the municipality of Amsterdam (Department of Public Order and Safety) gave 'Expats & Immigrants' (a business specializing in creating tolerance and justice in the Netherlands) the assignment of discussing the approach to dealing with radicalization and terrorism in mental health institutions in the greater Amsterdam area [1]. The municipality of Amsterdam wanted to cooperate with mental health institutions in the greater Amsterdam area on radicalization and terrorism. In 2015, there was no working relationship to tackle radicalization and terrorism between the municipality of Amsterdam, the Amsterdam police, and the Amsterdam office of public prosecutors and mental health institutions. Arkin—the largest mental health institution in the greater Amsterdam area with 3000 patients annually—responded positively. Therefore, the municipality of Amsterdam organized an expert meeting (1 July 2015) of mental health professionals of Amsterdam and the surrounding environment. This expert meeting was attended by psychiatrists, psychologists, and social workers with treatment experience in radicalization and terrorism. Participants were from five institutions in the greater Amsterdam area and totalled 30 people. For the expert meeting a discussion paper was written based on evidence at the time [2–5].

In this expert meeting the following definitions were used. Terrorism was defined according to the General Intelligence and Security Service (AIVD):[1]

---

[1] General Intelligence and Security Service (*Algemene Inlichtingen en Veiligheidsdienst*).

The (active) pursuit and/or support of fundamental changes in society that would endanger (the continued existence of) democratic legal order (purpose), possibly by undemocratic methods (means) which may be detrimental to the functioning of the democratic legal order (effect).

The process of radicalisation was seen as the (increasing) willingness to pursue and/or support such changes (possibly by undemocratic methods), or encourage others to do this. [6, p. 75]

For terrorism the NCTV (Dutch abbreviation for National Coordinator for Security and Counter-terrorism) definition was used:

Terrorism is the ideologically motivated threat, preparation or act of serious violence aimed at people, or acts, aimed at causing property damage that disrupts society, with the aim of bringing about social change, creating serious fear among the population or influencing the political decision-making process. [6, p. 23]

16.2 Mental health, radicalization, and terrorism

The key question of the expert meeting was [1]: How should mental health institutions in the greater Amsterdam area work together if they want to address radicalization and terrorism among their patients? The focus of the municipality of Amsterdam at that time was on suspects and offenders of radicalization and terrorism. Mental health patients, who were victims and witnesses, were not included at all.

In the past, racialization and terrorism were not an issue for Dutch mental health institutions. The arguments within the meeting were many and included the following; radicalization and terrorism are not a Diagnostic and Statistical Manual of Mental Disorders (DSM) disorder, there is an absence of a clear privacy code (a code that regulates the transfer of data from a mental health institution to, for instance, the office of the mayor), and a lack of treatment knowledge. The first argument is in accordance with the conclusion of Kiran Sarma [7, p. 2]:

More than 50 years of research has failed to produce a body of research that has causally linked involvement in terrorism with mental disorders. Rather, the best research has concluded that individuals who become involved in terrorism do so due to psychosocial processes—where they increasingly accept the moral legitimacy of terrorism due to their social experiences.

An apparent contradiction is the historical case-based research in The Hague, the Netherlands, which showed that 60% of the radicals known in police files had a mental health history [8]. These data suggest that mental health institutions could be an important partner in tackling radicalization and terrorism. These data are more or less in accordance with the data of Anton Weenink [9], who studied known radicals in police files:

Preliminary results indicate that individuals with histories of behavioural problems and disorders are overrepresented. The results are at odds with the consensus view on terrorists [sic] alleged 'normality'. A focus on individual psychology could complement existing social–psychological approaches to radicalization. It may also assist in broadening awareness among policy makers and law enforcement officials that disengagement efforts need to be tailored to the individual, and that mental health specialists might have to play a role here.

Despite these concerns, at the expert meeting it was agreed that the mental health institutions in the greater Amsterdam area should commit themselves to an approach of dealing with radicalization and terrorism. According to the participants, the following factors were drivers of further partnership work: improvements in knowledge of radicalization and terrorism, in general, and improvements in treatment methods, in particular. Furthermore, the privacy of patients had to be protected, and confidentiality and ethical handling of data was to be addressed. The municipality of Amsterdam tried to establish a close alliance with mental health institutions, and produced a juridical privacy code that now regulates the transfer of relevant mental health patient data to the police, the public prosecutor, and the mayor. This perhaps contrasts with many other countries where such data are not transferred directly, but communicated through partnership meetings, and only if there is a high index of suspicion are data released. This desire on the part of the city of Amsterdam to put together all the pieces of the puzzle about the suspect with, for example, an intention to commit a terrorist attack—according to information from the police, the public prosecutor's office, and psychiatry—is at odds with the privacy regulations of mental health care. Thought is being given to consultation between 'officials' of these three institutions, as is currently applied in Security Houses in various Dutch cities. In short, not a whole file is exchanged, but only pieces that are relevant to arrive at a thorough approach to the person or persons suspected of the intention to commit an attack, for example. Knowledge about that intention usually comes from the AIVD.

The Ministry of Health, Welfare and Sport, and the Ministry of Justice and Safety (National Coordinator of Terrorism and Safety) followed the meeting with an assignment for Arkin to carry out a project that develops and tests mentioned instruments for addressing radicalization and terrorism in mental health institutions in the Netherlands, like guidelines, risk assessments, treatment protocols and organization, and a dedicated privacy protocol. The ultimate goal is dissemination of instruments, procedures, and guidelines. Here we report the outcomes of a survey conducted in order to find out how many of the 65 mental health institutions in the Netherlands up to 2016 were spending on radicalization and terrorism (including the availability of dedicated materials/

instruments). Before setting out our responses, I wish to place the work in a historical and organizational context.

16.3 Dutch history since 2002 on radicalization and terrorism and psychiatry

In 2002 the populist right-wing Dutch politician Pim Fortuyn was assassinated by Volkert van der Graaf. Fortuyn said: 'I don't hate Islam, I think it is a backward culture'.[2] On 11 November 2004 the first jihadist terrorist attack by Muhammed Bouyeri on Theo van Gogh took place in the streets of Amsterdam. Just before this incident a critical film of Islam had been produced by van Gogh and Ayaan Hirsi Ali. In court, Bouyeri said:[3]

> I cannot suspect van Gogh of any hypocrisy because he was not hypocritical. He was not and I know he said things because of his convictions. So the whole story that I would be offended because I am called Moroccan or that he called me a 'goat fucker' that's not true at all. I acted out of faith and I even said before that if it was my father or brother, I would have done exactly the same.

Many attacks on holy Koran, houses, and Islamic schools in all over the Netherlands took place after the murder of Theo van Gogh, such as the attack on the Islamic Bedir school in Uden [6]. According to researcher Ineke van der Valk,[4] based on the database of the Dutch researcher Martijn de Koning, mosques in the Netherlands during the period 2005–10 have been 117 times the target of violence that resulted from fear of Islam. Mosques were besmirched (43 times) or there was destruction of Islamic religious houses (37 times). In a Canadian review, a similar trend was shown in the West [10, p. 16]. A recent statement by the Dutch national Coordinator of Terrorism and Safety [11][5] indicates that attacks on Islamic institutions in the Netherlands have increased.

Since the jihadist attack in 2002 on Theo van Gogh no similar attack in the Netherlands occurred. The only other Dutch attack took place in 2009. This was an attack on the family of the then Dutch Queen, Beatrix. Karst Tates, who committed this attack, did it with the intention of hurting the queen's family. Tates was mentally disoriented.

---

[2] As reported in *Volkskrant*, 9 February 2002 (not archived).

[3] https://nl.wikipedia.org/wiki/Moord_op_Theo_van_Gogh

[4] See http://www.republiekallochtonie.nl/update-lijst-met-incidenten-rond-moskeeen

[5] There is an increase in the number of incidents in mosques and, at a local level, additional preventive measures such as camera surveillance are taken, said National Coordinator for Terrorism and Security, Dick Schoof, after consultation with six Muslim domes.

During this period, Dutch psychiatry discussed whether it had a task concerning radicalization and terrorism. The following quote clearly explains the position of Dutch psychiatry concerning radicalization and terrorism:

> We can conclude from the information in this review that individuals with mental illness, when appropriately treated, do not pose any increased risk of violence over the general population [12, p. 46]. However, this 'truth' does not significantly affect the imaging. From our field of expertise, it remains an important task to keep public opinion, together with patients, on the basis of hard data. [13, p. 136]

A more nuanced statement was subsequently released by the International Centre for Counter-Terrorism [14]:

> Existing research—and the discussions thereof during the expert meeting—point to the need for further research on for example the relationship between societal/situational factors and personality traits; the role of the social defeat hypothesis on the radicalisation process; the relation between profiles and discrimination as the lead-up to radicalisation; the correlation between individual psychological processes on the one hand and social and political processes affecting the (mental) life of individuals on the other; and the different typologies susceptible to different trigger factors.

16.4 **Organizational approach and instruments**

The Parnassia Group, the largest Dutch mental health institution with a total of about 153,000 patients in 2015, started some years ago to develop tools for dealing with radicalization and terrorism [8].

Carl Steinmetz [15] suggested linking tackling radicalization and terrorism in mental health institutions with a known body of work, namely that of an organizational approach to workplace violence that has already been performed by Bowie et al. [16]. The rationale behind this is that, in the Netherlands, there is a 25-year experience with workplace violence [17, 18]. If we use the content, procedures, guidelines, and legislation regarding workplace violence, it would relieve us of the obligation to develop from scratch the methodology for the approach of tackling radicalization and terrorism in and around the workplace. Furthermore, Steinmetz [19] experimented with the organizational approach (implementing tools and procedures with the school board, students, and teachers) to dealing with radicalization at a vocational education institute with 5000 students. A large simulation was performed with the school as a whole. The final result has been that the tool and procedures were accepted after a redesign by all school parties.

The organizational approach of radicalization and terrorism consists of two elements: (A) cultural awareness and sensitive treatment of patients [20];[6] and

---

[6] Integrating cultural awareness and sensitivity into your work means (definition by Bhui, [5]): 'To work towards a conscious and sensitive attitude towards the cultures of the

(B) all-inclusive multiculturalism [21],[7] which also means the reformulation of the mission and vision of a mental health institution in such a way that health workers (psychiatrists, general practitioners, psychologists, nurses, and social workers) and patients recognize themselves as being included.

Instruments of the organizational approach of radicalization and terrorism are:

1. Working with a reporting code for radicalization (covering all stages from detection up to and including forwarding to the 'triangle', i.e. the police, public prosecution service, and the local government).

2. Working with a small team of mental health care practitioners in charge of signalling, handling, treatment, and, finally, de-radicalization (and thereby using people, knowledge, and resources in a focused way).

3. Developing an organizational guideline for tackling people who radicalize or who are on the path of radicalization, as well as people who want to exit the path of radicalization.

4. The development of a Structural Professional Judgement (SPJ)[8] for monitoring treatment results [8, p. 284].

5. A juridical privacy code. This is a code that, in addition to the usual privacy protection, also regulates the transfer of parts of the medical file with third parties.

6. The organization of information meetings for both patients and care professionals.

Sarma (personal communication) suggested that the use of these instruments might depend on the kind of vision for the treatment of radicalized patients and (potential) terrorists. For instance, a dominant vision in treating patients is the systems approach, which could implicate extended family and community in the treatment. If, for instance, this vision is accepted, then the implication for

---

various groups of immigrants and refugees within mental health care. Culture refers to shared viewpoints, practices and ideas of a group of people (including Dutch people, immigrants or refugees). In the real world of service there are, however, many subcultures with various layers of refinement.'

[7] By all-inclusive multiculturalism we mean (definition by Stevens et al. [20]): 'All-inclusive multiculturalism helps organisations to tackle the restrictions of colour blindness and to deal with multicultural ideology by encouraging feelings of inclusion among staff via positive organisational change.'

[8] The philosophy of SPJ is that 'risk identification is *informed* by risk indicators while the evaluator develops a risk narrative and engages in careful case formulation for the individual being assessed in making the overall risk prediction'.

a SPJ is that we have to investigate the existence of role models—both positive and negative—in the extended family, neighbourhood, and ethnic community.

16.5 **Method and expectations**

The concepts of the organizational approach and instruments were translated into a questionnaire. The questionnaire[9] was created in Survey Monkey by the DSP Group (a commercial Dutch research business in Amsterdam). The DSP Group collected the data during the period December 2016–March 2017. Three reminders and one round of phone calls were implemented in order to increase the response.

With this questionnaire we were trying to achieve the following goals: (A) a positive response (60%) from mental health institutions completing this questionnaire (non-responses will be studied via public information, like city and area); (B) an estimation of the number of patients of concern regarding radicalization; (C) examine how many mental health institutions have experience with the organizational approach and instruments; and (D) examine how many mental health institutions actually have semi-finished products of the organizational approach and instruments.

16.6 **Results**

The key outcomes of the survey of the 65 Dutch mental health institutions are listed in Table 16.1. Themes such as (non)response, tackling radicalization and terrorism, percentage of patients who radicalize, interventions like training, psychoeducation, and working with instruments and policy documents are given in the table.

The data in Table 16.1 show that radicalization and terrorism in mental health institutions in the Netherlands receive a higher priority in the Randstad municipalities (7.1 million inhabitants) than in provinces outside the Randstad, such as the provinces of Groningen and Zeeland. Quite a large group of the mental health institutions in the Randstad render that this priority is based on their estimation that in 0% and 10% of their patients raise concerns about being radicalized. Even with conservative assumptions, the results indicate that, potentially, the Netherlands has thousands of patients who are of concern and need some sort of judgement. Surprisingly, only two-fifths of Dutch mental health institutions are tackling radicalization and/or terrorism in reality. Popular

---

[9] A copy of the questionnaire translated into English can be obtained from the chapter author.

Table 16.1 Schematic rendering of commitment of mental health institutions in the Netherlands to addressing radicalization and terrorism

Themes	Results
Response and non-response	
Response	Total number of institutions = 65 Response = 37 (57%) mainly with headquarters in the four largest cities of the Netherlands (Amsterdam, The Hague, Rotterdam, and Utrecht); 21/37 (57%) in four big cities
Motives for non-response	12 institutions: (A) it does not fit my corporate philosophy; (B) I have no time for this; (C) I am not busy with this subject; and (D) no headquarters in the four big cities No information for 16
Tackling radicalization/terrorism and % of patients who radicalize	
Tackling radicalization and/or terrorism	15/37 (41%)
% of patients who radicalize >0–10%[a]	20/37 (54%)
Intervention	**Results**
Training personnel	16/37 (43%)
Psychoeducation about radicalization and terrorism	3/37 (8%)
Cultural consciousness and sensitive working	23/37 (62%)
All-inclusive multiculturalism	9/37 (25%)
Developing instruments	9/37 (24%)
Policy documents	Results
Radicalization	3/37 (8%)
Terrorism	3/37 (8%)
All-inclusive multiculturalism	3/37 (8%)
Cultural conscious and sensitive working	3/37 (8%)

[a] Quite a number of mental health institutions gave a blank answer to this question. By studying the response answering patterns in the questionnaire we concluded that this means that these institutions had no patients who radicalize.

interventions are training personnel, cultural consciousness, and sensitive working. Virtually no mental health institution documented their efforts in policy documents. The explanation for these slight efforts used by commenters in the survey is: (A) we just started; and (B) why is the approach of tackling radicalization and terrorism not an element of workplace violence?

16.7 **Conclusion**

It is clear that there is a gap between the practice (radicalization and terrorist incidents and attacks) and reality of Dutch mental health institutions concerning radicalization and terrorism. The survey of Dutch mental health institutions (including the largest institutions) shows that the approach to radicalization and terrorism takes place mainly in areas around the four major cities (Amsterdam, The Hague, Rotterdam, and Utrecht, constituting 7.1 million out of a total of 17 million Dutch inhabitants in 2016) taking response and non-response into account. More than half of the 37 mental health institutions that responded claimed they have patients who radicalize. Only a minority of the mental health institutions documented the way they approach radicalization and terrorism in policy documents and/ or instruments.

In other words, most Dutch mental health institutions can be compared with a baby who puts takes her first steps in the field of radicalization and terrorism. Only 8% of the mental health institutions have policy documents and instruments such as a SPJs, reporting codes, and organizational guidelines. The decision to implement a concrete policy is, of course, hampered by the debate. Are radicalization and terrorism related to a DSM disorder? Viewed from the perspective of workplace violence, this question is hardly relevant as the public wants mental health institutions to provide relevant and evidenced services than stating that radicalization is not a psychiatric disorder, as was suggested by Geert Dom [13].

Radicalization, terrorism, polarization, and extremism should be adopted in the institutional and business programme as preventing 'violence in the workplace'. Adoption means using existing instruments, procedures, guidelines, and organizational approaches. With adoption, the only adjustment necessary is to implement a policy instrument concerning (A) cultural sensitivity and consciousness, and (B) all-inclusive multiculturalism, as most Western cities are super-diverse. In the Netherlands, and also in many Western countries, adopting this approach would be in accordance with other objectives. This would provide a general solution for all institutions and businesses, and will be more efficient and financially sensible.

References

1. **Steinmetz, Carl H.D.** (2015). Psychiatrie en radicaliseren. Working Paper, 2015. DOI: 10.13140/RG.2.1.1627.9921.

2. **Bhui K.** Mental Health and violent radicalization. Mental Health Today 2013;24:6.

3. **Bhui K, Warfa N, Jones E.** Is violent radicalisation associated with poverty, migration, poor self-reported health and common mental disorders. *PLoS ONE* 2014;9:e90718.

4. **Bhui K, Warfa N, Jones E.** Might depression, psychosocial adversity, and limited social assets explain vulnerability to and resistance against violent radicalisation? *PLoS ONE* 2014;9:e105918.

5. **Bhui KS, Owiti JA, Palinski A, Ascoli M, De Jongh B, Archer J,** et al. A cultural consultation service in East London: experiences and outcomes from implementation of an innovative service. International Review of Psychiatry 2015;**27**:11–22.

6. **Bakker E, de Roy van Zuijdewijn J.** *Terrorism.* Amsterdam: Amsterdam University Press B.V.; 2016.

7. **Sarma KM.** Chapter 9: Understanding terrorism: research of relevance to health and social care professionals. Presentation at the World Psychiatric Associations Taskforce on Social Divisions & Extremist Violence: gangs, cults, terrorists, and violent offending. 25–26 October 2016, Queen Mary University of London, UK.

8. **Sarma KM.** Risk assessment and the prevention of radicalization from nonviolence into terrorism. American Psychologist 2017;**72**:278–88.

9. **Weenink AW.** Behavioural problems and disorders among radicals in police files. Available from: http://www.terrorismanalysts.com/pt/index.php/pot/article/view/416/826 [accessed 7 August 2020].

10. **Cauchy D.** Preventing radicalisation. A systematic review. International For The Prevention of Crime, 2015. DOI: 10.13140/RG.2.1.4862.1682.

11. **Schoof D.** NCTV Schoof: de werkelijkheid is soms bizarder dan Homeland. Available from: https://nos.nl/artikel/2166880-nctv-schoof-de-werkelijkheid-is-soms-bizarder-dan-homeland.html [accessed 7 August 2020].

12. **Rueve ME., Welton RS.** Violence and mental health illness. Psychiatry (Edgmont) 2008;**5**:34–48.

13. **Dom G.** Radicalisering, terrorisme en psychiatrie: een alternatieve waarheid? Available from: http://www.tijdschriftvoorpsychiatrie.nl/issues/511/articles/11261 [accessed 7 August 2020].

14. **Paulussen C, Nijman J, Lismont K.** Mental health and the foreign fighter phenomenon: a case study from the Netherlands. ICCT report. Available from: https://icct.nl/wp-content/uploads/2017/03/ICCT-Paulussen-Nijman-Lismont-Mental-Health-and-the-Foreign-Fighter-Phenomenon-March-2017.pdf [accessed 7 August 2020].

16. **Steinmetz CHD.** Radicaliseren voorkomen: Nu of Nooit. Maatwerk vakblad voor professionals in sociaal werk; 2016;**17**:14–17.

16. **Bowie V, Fisher BS, Cooper CL.** Workplace violence: issues, trends and strategies. Milton: Willan Publishing; 2005.

17. **Steinmetz CHD, Regeer L, Hollander LB.** Veiligheidsbeleid in de instelling vanuit verpleegkundig perspectief. Houten/Zaventum: Bohn Stafleu Van Loghum; 1993.

18. **Steinmetz CHD, Savornin-Lohman PM.** (1995, pp. 37–56). 5 Agressie en geweld: de feiten; 6 Agressie en geweld: de aanpak en 7 Agressie en geweld: de opvang. Zaventum: Arbo & Milieu: praktijkreeks Seksuele intimidatie, agressie en geweld; 1995.

19. **Steinmetz CHD (2016). Radicaliseren Voorkomen. Nu of Nooit. Nummer 1 – Februari 2016 Vakblad voor Professionals in Sociaal Werk. Maatwerk.** Bohn Stafleu van Lochum.

20. **McGilloway A, Priyo G, Kamaldeep B.** A systematic review of pathways to and processes associated with radicalisation and extremism amongst Muslims in Western Societies. International Review of Psychiatry 2015;**27**:39–50.

21. **Stevens FG., Plaut VC, Sanchez-Burks J.** Unlocking the benefits of diversity: all-inclusive multiculturalism and positive organizational change. The Journal of Applied Behavioural Science 2008;**44**116–133.

Chapter 17

Leadership, conflict, and cooperation

Lord John Alderdice

17.1 Introduction

Leadership generally describes the effect of certain individuals who, by the power of their personality, substantially influence others and impact on processes and events. Such influence has been a source of fascination for writers from time immemorial, and the psychology of political leaders is a matter of regular discussion, from bar-room chat to substantial research and writing [1, 2]. I have thought a good deal about leadership in the context of violent conflict, and the cooperation necessary to address political disagreements through peaceful, democratic means. As a young person growing up in Northern Ireland as it broke down into the violence known euphemistically as 'The Troubles', I wanted to deepen my understanding of the causes of the conflict and develop more effective interventions. Indeed, a major element in my motivation for going into psychoanalytical psychiatry, was to understand why my community was consistently behaving in ways that were not in their own best interests. The cycle of destruction in my community advantaged no one and I wondered how to make sense of it. As psychiatrists worked with people who behaved in self-destructive ways, I thought, perhaps, there were lessons to be learnt that could be applied to a whole community.

My questions were simple. What had gone wrong that people had turned to violence? What motivated those who were leading the terrorist campaigns? Why did the violence become intractable? Why did 'normal' politics and the rule of law not bring about a resolution of the conflict? Was it possible to change the behaviour into something more lawful, constructive, and democratic? I spent much of my adolescence reading and debating these issues, and wondering how I might contribute to a better outcome. After qualifying in medicine, I undertook a psychoanalytic training analysis that helped me find a route to channel my passion for the issue. Becoming a journalist, commentator or political scientist, undertaking some responsibility in the security sector, and engagement in voluntary community dialogue and development were possible options. I decided on direct political involvement and wrote to all the parties across the democratic political spectrum in Northern Ireland. They replied, and one party seemed to fit my requirements. The Alliance Party attracted significant numbers of people from both sides of the communal divide and was specifically focused on addressing the violent conflict. It was promoting a liberal democratic political agenda with whose style and substance I could enthusiastically identify, and it seemed a suitable platform for therapeutic engagement. I joined and started to learn how a political party functions in the development of policy and the promotion of its aims. I also started to learn some things about political leadership and what James MacGregor Burns called 'followership' [2]. I was training in psychoanalytic psychiatry, as well as in family therapy, cognitive behavioural therapy, group analysis, and the various psychiatric subspecialities necessary for the full training of a consultant psychiatrist. This meant that I had a different perspective than those who were entering politics with legal training, business experience, a teaching career, or community involvement [3].

17.1.1 **Lessons in leadership**

The first lesson was that you are only a leader if you have followers. It is not simply a matter of accession to a title or position. Over the first few years I watched the leadership of my own party face extreme pressures as increasing violence pushed political opinion towards the extremes. It was not only the bombings and shootings, and the fact that many of them faced personal threats, but there was also increasing polarization as a result of terrorist violence and political initiatives. The first election in which I stood was in 1981, and the poll was held just two weeks after the Irish Republican Army (IRA) leader in Maze prison, Bobby Sands MP, starved himself to death. During that hunger strike in 1981, 10 republican prisoners died, the nationalist community was radicalized, and many of our supporters moved away from the centre to support a more nationalist position.

The British and Irish Governments then focused on creating a political dynamic that would win nationalists away from supporting the IRA and in 1982 a new Northern Ireland Assembly was established with the offer of power-sharing; however, the nationalists and republicans boycotted it. When, in 1985, the two governments tried further to address nationalist alienation by signing the Anglo-Irish Agreement, for the first time giving the Irish Government a say in the affairs of Northern Ireland, the whole Protestant Unionist community reacted with fury, and the support that we had lost from Catholic nationalists because of the hunger strike was now mirrored by an exodus of people in the Protestant Unionist community because of the Anglo-Irish Agreement.

Shortly after that the Northern Ireland Assembly was closed. All the leadership of Alliance who had been Members of that Legislative Assembly lost their jobs, and most of them had to leave active politics in Northern Ireland. I was now confronted with being a member of a party that had lost most of its senior leaders and many of its voters. This was the first of many lessons in the challenges of leadership. Being in a leadership position does not guarantee that you have followers, and without them you cannot survive as a leader. However, if you are simply following the crowds without standing for fundamental principles you are part of the problem, and from my point of view, there would be no purpose in being involved. I threw my hat in the ring for the vacant leadership position and, to the surprise of many leading people in the party, every political pundit, and indeed myself, I was elected with a handsome majority. Leadership lesson number two—in situations of existential crisis, experience and long service count for little. At such a time, people want someone who they believe brings a new prospectus that brings hope.

Having been elected Leader of the Alliance Party, I now had to address lesson number one myself. Being the leader of a party did not guarantee that anyone in the public domain would pay any attention. As a party of the centre, the previous leaders had always been careful to train their fire on the political leaderships of both sides—unionism and nationalism—with a wish to appear balanced, and a fear of appearing to favour one side or the other. Unfortunately, this meant that their statements were entirely predictable and not very interesting to the media or to the public. Almost every press statement had the same format. 'On the one hand', they would criticize one side, and 'on the other hand' they would also criticize the other side—the verse might differ, but the chorus was always the same. I decided to try to identify the site of the current resistance (as we would say in therapy) and address whichever side represented the key problem at the time. This meant that I would often focus my criticism on one side, causing anxiety to my colleagues who feared that I would be regarded as partisan. I knew that it would not be long before the other side provided a similar opportunity, but by being specific in my critique I created interest from the press and public. Which side would I identify as being the problem of the moment? Lesson three—leadership requires that observers pay attention to what you say. Sometimes it is called thought leadership, and it can be positive or negative, but it is not leadership if it is easily ignored.

17.1.2 The personality of the leader and the type of leadership

I often heard complaints that if there were different leaders things would be better, but I came to recognize that the personality of a leader is a representation of key elements of the 'way-of-being' of the group she/he leads, as well as reflecting particular qualities and providing an inspiring role model [4]. When the group's perspective and requirements change, it will find another more representative leader. In frozen conflicts the same leaders may be in place for a long time, because external factors remain constant. A transformational leader will take the community out of its current position and pass the leadership on to the next generation with the community in better shape.

One such transformational leader was Provisional IRA (PIRA) leader, Martin McGuiness. Subsequent to the 1998 Good Friday/Belfast Agreement that brought the violence in Ireland to an end, we were working together in Baghdad with a few other Northern Ireland and South African colleagues, trying to persuade the political leaders of the parties in Iraq to see negotiation as a better alternative than continued violence. In a very persuasive speech, Martin insisted that leadership was one of the key requirements for bringing communal violence to an end. 'Peace was not something that just happened'. he said. 'Peace, progress, and an end to violence only came through strong, persistent, persuasive, and courageous leadership'. He told the Iraqis how the IRA had concluded that while the British security services could not defeat them, neither could they defeat the British. Once they realized they were in a stalemate they concluded that it was wrong to send their young Republican colleagues out to be injured, imprisoned, and killed for no real purpose. They had to find another way to implement their vision of a United Ireland and sought a route into the political process. There were other pressures too, but whatever contributed to their considerations, once they decided to move towards negotiation, leadership was of critical importance on that long, complex, and often dangerous road. I know from conversations with them they had not thought it would take so long. Mistakes were made along the way, but determined and sustained leadership was crucial.

17.1.3 Challenges and requirements of leadership

One of the challenges for the psychologically informed leader is the appreciation that one may be mistaken. However, practical political leadership requires great confidence in one's abilities and perspectives. If I am not unduly confident, why should anyone suspend their own judgements in favour of mine? Leaders often feel that a preparedness to question oneself in a crisis, and ask whether 'my people' are in the right, may be the beginning of the end of one's leadership. One may wish that people gave more reflection space to leaders to have doubts, but most leaders feel that is not something in which practical politicians can indulge. Even if they hold to their community's traditional political beliefs, a leader may need to explore alternative forms of delivery. A commitment to working-class interests may be best served by being *in* the European Union (EU) at one point, but at another time they may believe that the same purpose would be better served by being *out* of the EU. Transformational leaders often need to reframe the narrative to enable their community to move forward. Given my background and personal agenda, I would sometimes find my thinking more influenced by my psychotherapeutic 'self' and at other times by my political one. The process of transformation of a group's way of thinking is a most difficult leadership challenge and I was trying to function both as a 'therapist' and as political leader as the latter role gave me the opportunity for therapeutic interventions in the political process.

What, then, are the key elements of political leadership in such situations of conflict? While the historical, political, social, and economic backgrounds of a community all contribute to the context in which violence breaks out, removing the 'root causes' does not of itself bring the conflict to an end. To use a medical analogy, while it is necessary to remove a patient from the toxic environment that has caused their illness, this intervention may not cure them of a disorder that has taken hold. Groups also form powerful attachments in situations of high emotion, and people become fused with their group and its aims, so any threat to the group or change in approach will meet with resistance. Leadership is a key requirement for getting groups to the negotiating table, but it only gets more challenging as one tries to reach an agreement and then attempts to implement it. There is a real threat of damaging and even fatal splits between those who want change and those who want to fight on. Courage is a key requirement of leadership in such circumstances; physical courage to put one's life at risk, intellectual courage to think the unthinkable, and emotional courage to hold two or more conflicting ideas in one's mind at the same time.

For leadership to be successful, the context must also be conducive. People do not become leaders of communities just because they are the most ambitious or talented candidate. An angry community will choose a truculent leader, a smaller community with an ambivalent attachment to the metropolis may elect a dependent personality, and a passive-aggressive leader may be chosen because the community feels resentful and unhappy. Studying the psychology of leaders can shed an interesting light on the community that follows them [5–7].

I have also noticed that a key requirement of successful leaders is an element of good fortune. Academics are hesitant to acknowledge such a thing, but however strategically shrewd and tactically adept a leader may be, she/he needs a context with some chance for movement. Even the extraordinarily charismatic leadership of Nelson Mandela did not stop apartheid in South Africa until the Cold War ended. Leaders can take active steps to resolve situations, but they need the good fortune to be leading at a time when the key stakeholders are prepared to build a new context. Context and timing are vital for successful leadership. A shrewd leader may, with persistence and perspicacity, contribute to good timing and a positive context, but being born at the right time helps.

In her analysis of how terrorist campaigns end, Professor Audrey Kurth Cronin identifies six outcomes: decapitation, negotiation, success, failure, repression, and reorientation [8]. These outcomes are not mutually exclusive, but leadership plays a role in all of them, as a requirement for success, or as a cause of failure. Decapitation involves the removal of the leadership by assassination or imprisonment. Failure is a failure of the strategy of the leaders. Negotiation is a role of the leadership, and reorientation requires the leader to reframe the group narrative and lead in a new direction. I found her analysis helpful, but our task as social scientists is not only to understand current theories, but also to search out and follow the evidence where it takes us and be prepared to amend and sometimes radically overhaul our ideas as the situation changes. As in religion, the progressive speculations of one generation can become the conservatism of the next, so we must continually challenge our theories. During the Irish Peace Process, my own appreciation of the emergence and ending of violent political conflict underwent substantial changes. Later I found that my new understandings were relevant in other conflicted parts of the world with different histories and cultures [9, 10]. Since the publication of Professor Cronin's book, the world and how it works has changed further and there has been widespread destabilisation of states from Afghanistan and right across South Asia and the Middle East to North Africa. In the late nineteenth and early twentieth centuries, anarchist terrorism was the tactic developed by weaker groups against a powerful state apparatus. World War II ended with the realization that a nuclear conflict could be catastrophic and terrorist groups became a modality though which superpower rivalries could be channelled without endangering world peace. The end of the Cold War brought this phase to a close and with it some long-standing terrorist campaigns were no longer sustainable. There were relatively peaceful, negotiated results in South Africa, Northern Ireland, and Nepal. Others were 'decapitated', as in Peru, and a number brutally put down, as in Sri Lanka, but now a new set of problems has emerged. If, in the past, the tactic of terrorism was the strategy of the weak against powerful states, the chaotic violence now resulted from the failure of weak states to sustain themselves against powerful terrorist networks. We do not fully understand the role of leadership in these networks, how they function in a world of complex communications, and whether this is a result of regional instability or a fundamental crisis of liberal democracy. It was assumed that free and fair elections would result in liberal democracies. This turned out not to be the case with the election of illiberal governments in South Asia, intolerant chiefs in sub-Saharan Africa, and fundamentalist Islamists in Gaza and Egypt. Free and fair elections can result in intolerant regimes that are a nightmare for minorities. Interestingly, Sheikh Ghannouchi, the intellectual leader of the Muslim Ennahda Party in Tunisia, pointed out that liberal democracy requires a complex culture of democracy, not just elections and institutions [11]. In complex adaptive systems, such as conditions in which terrorism and fundamentalism emerge, identifying a single key leader may not be the solution. As with a 'murmuration' of starlings that swoop, dive, and wheel, the science of complexity may be more relevant than the traditional understanding of leadership in the spread of large group phenomena [12, 13].

On the 'official' political side more traditional leadership studies remain relevant and the Irish Peace Process gives examples. Then British Prime Minister, John Major, agreed to address the issue, not because he was certain how the benefits measured against the risks, but because of his relationship with the Irish Taoiseach, Albert Reynolds, whom he had known when both were Finance Ministers for their respective EU member governments. The Peace Process was no small undertaking given the instability of Major's own government, and it is a testament to the leadership of both men that they took the necessary risks. It also speaks well for their successors that though they came from different political parties, they carried the process forward as a national rather than a merely governmental commitment. This is a requirement I have often urged to leaders in other places. Where conflict resolution is seen as a party initiative, it falls prey to electoral politics. It must become a 'national' commitment that stands above partisan politics and carried forward even when there is a change of government—a matter of national leadership, not party political leadership.

In the Irish conflict, which is often misrepresented as religious in nature (although religious identity does play a key role), the four main church leaders generally presented moderate attitudes and Pope John Paul II during his visit to Ireland in 1979, addressed the IRA in these very moving words:

> On my knees I beg of you to turn away from the paths of violence and to return to the ways of peace ... Those who resort to violence always claim that only violence brings about change. You must know there is a political, peaceful way to justice.

Sadly, this had no impact, and the PIRA formally rejected his appeal. While these churchmen were clearly in *positions* of leadership, they were unable to exercise effective community leadership away from violence, although there was effective behind-the-scenes work by some church figures.

17.1.4 **Communicating the message and convincing the followers**

When a leader has decided that for the good of his/her people, things must change, and is courageous enough to move forward, a key element in their role as a leader is re-framing the narrative of his/her community. This narrative identifies key elements in the group culture and Vamik Volkan [14] has identified how *chosen traumas* and *chosen victories* play a powerful role in determining this culture. While many events are not remembered, others have a seminal role in shaping how a group of people identify with each other and respond to friends and enemies. In emphasizing or underplaying different elements of historical narrative, the language a leader uses about the nature of the problem is crucial. Let me give some examples.

In Ireland/Northern Ireland the territorial 'zero sum game' seemed not amenable to resolution as 'shared space' connoted a loss of control by one side or the other (or both). The Northern Nationalist leader, John Hume, realized this, and began to develop a new political language based on relationships. 'It is not the island that is divided', he frequently observed, for it was still one physical territory. There is a political border, but that is because 'the people are divided about how they should share the island'. The message was that the political task was neither to maintain control of territory nor wrest it from the others, but to resolve the question of how to share the territory—to address the problem of disturbed historic relationships between the different groups on the island. When he engaged with the IRA leadership, he asked whether the method (terrorism) was more sacred than the cause (Irish unity). They replied that the cause was more important and he enquired whether violence could be abandoned if there was a better alternative. When republicans replied in the affirmative, Hume's challenge to the British and Irish governments was to develop an opportunity for Irish republicans to abandon the argument of physical force and espouse the force of democratic argument. This development of a 'peace process language' was crucial. Republicans did not speak of abandoning a failed violent struggle but characterized their efforts as 'courageously taking risks for peace'. The Ulster Unionist Leader, David Trimble, did not describe his approach as defeating, or even accepting, Sinn Fein (which later would have seemed a concession), but told his people that 'just because someone has a past does not mean they cannot have a different future', putting the onus on Sinn Fein to prove itself and making it axiomatic that such a change should receive a positive response from unionists.

Communication through action is at least as important as that of words, and much of the process of peace (and war) involves political choreography. Volkan [15] describes how in 1989 Slobodan Milosevic raised the ghosts of the past by having the remains of Prince Lazar exhumed, 600 years after defeat in the Battle of Kosovo in 1389, and paraded the coffin around villages and towns, collapsing the sense of time and making the feelings of confrontation and struggle from the past feel acute for his people in the present. He excited dangerous feelings that overwhelmed current reality, including the humanity of their neighbours, and led to catastrophic violence.

In the Irish Peace Process, the opposite outcome was achieved. The past was recognized as tragic and a new agenda was created to make possible a shared, non-violent, and respectful future for all the people of the island. Leaders began to share programmes in broadcasting studios, have meetings, and shake hands in public, but all was carefully calibrated to move an exquisitely delicate process along. The language and the drama were also able to convey subtly different messages depending on which community was receiving them. I experienced this as Speaker of the new Northern Ireland Assembly. Those who had formerly advocated physical force to solve the historic problems of British–Irish relations worked, albeit with difficulty, with those who wanted to maintain the British state. For Irish nationalists, the emphasis was on changes that they had achieved. This could be symbolic. When I allowed them to use the Irish language in the Chamber and welcomed the Irish President on an official visit, they felt they were no longer second-class citizens because their culture was being recognized at the highest level. For unionists, the symbolism of the Union Flag still flying over Parliament Buildings on designated days and the visits of Her Majesty, The Queen, to Stormont demonstrated the maintenance of the union with Britain.

The communication of new narratives through creative symbolism and language are examples of 'cultural leadership' and are necessary (although rarely sufficient) solutions. If the community has been torn apart and lives destroyed by guns and bombs, real change must be seen if it is to be believed, so it is vital that the weapons of war and the organisational structures that directed their use be transformed or decommissioned. In passing, I should point out that the term 'decommissioning' is an example of linguistic creativity. The word removed the connotation of victory/defeat and became the accepted description of the process by which paramilitaries acknowledged that the weapons were no longer appropriate, and they must dispose of them to the satisfaction of the wider community. The British and Irish Governments jointly established an Independent International Commission for Decommissioning and later an Independent Monitoring Commission (IMC) to exert pressure on the paramilitaries to decommission their weapons and stand down their organizations. At the same time, the British Army and the Police Service of Northern Ireland embarked on a programme of security normalization that was also monitored by the IMC and publicized in 26 reports over a seven-year period, all published in full by the British and Irish Governments. The purpose was to monitor activity and address two leadership issues so that the community could believe that things really were changing. The first issue was the relationship between the leadership of paramilitary groups and that of political parties, and the second was the holding to account of the leaders of paramilitary groups for any continuing violence or other criminal activity. It was recognized that leadership was a key element in bringing this long and bloody campaign of terrorism and counter-terrorism to a close and the leaders needed to demonstrate delivery on their undertakings through a process of external monitoring.

17.1.5 Feeling is part of how we think in conflict

In addition to all the qualities I have described so far—various types of courage, context and timing, commitment, creativity in developing new narratives and communicating them persuasively, and external monitors holding leaders to account for the agreements they have made—there is at least one other critical element.

People from stable societies expect individuals and groups to be rational actors operating in their own best social, economic, and power interests. However, in societies under existential threat people become devoted actors who think in a different way and will defend 'sacred values' at the cost of their lives and those of their loved ones. Sacred values are not necessarily religious values. The life of my child, the flag of my country, and the language and culture of my people are all examples of sacred values that not amenable to socio-economic metrics, and cannot traded for economic benefit, or subjected to simple cost–benefit negotiations [16]. However far along the process away from the use of physical force and violent conflict we find ourselves, there are elements of functioning as individuals and communities that are not driven by solely rational principles. Those leaders who are moving societies from conflict to cooperation, need to understand the challenges they face, and possess courage and commitment to do it, but they are also well advised to remain humble about what we do not know and be vigilant for signals of how their people think and feel. David Owen, in his book on hubris in political leadership [17], describes the disaster in store for any leader, however experienced, who fails to recognize this. Leaders are no longer leaders when they lose their followers. If hubris takes over and they lose empathy with the feelings of their people, they will not stay leaders for long. Maintaining a sense of how people feel is a vital component in leadership, in conflict, out of conflict, and in developing cooperation between communities with different histories, values, and identities. Learning about leadership is not something that is ever finally achieved. It is an ever-evolving process of engagement and change.

References

1. **Paxman J.** The political animal. London: Penguin Books; 2002.
2. **MacGregor Burns J.** Leadership. New York: Harper & Row Publishers; 1978.
3. **Little G.** Political therapy: an encounter with Dr John Alderdice, psychotherapist, political leader and peer of the realm. International Journal of Applied Psychoanalytic Studies 2009;6:129–145.
4. **Benson J.** The Northern Ireland Conflict and Peace Process: the role of mutual regulatory symbiosis between leaders and groups. In: Klein RH, Rice CA, Schermer VL. Leadership in a changing world. Lanham, MD: Lexington Books; 2009, pp. 203–22.
5. **Falk A.** Fratricide in the Holy Land. Madison, WI: University of Wisconsin Press; 2004.
6. **Robinson A.** Bin Laden—behind the mask of the terrorist, Edinburgh: Mainstream Publishing; 2001.
7. **Volkan VD, Itzkowitz N.** The immortal ataturk: a psychobiography. Chicago, IL: University of Chicago Press; 1984.
8. **Cronin AK.** How terrorism ends. Princeton, NJ: Princeton University Press; 2009.
9. **Atran S.** Talking to the enemy: faith, brotherhood and the (un)making of terrorists. New York: HarperCollins; 2010.
10. **Perry M.** Talking to terrorists. New York: Basic Books; 2010.
11. **Tamimi AS.** Rachid Ghannouchi: a democrat within Islamism. Oxford: Oxford University Press; 2001.
12. **Alderdice J.** Fundamentalism, radicalization and terrorism, part 1: terrorism as dissolution in a complex system. Psychoanalytic Psychotherapy 2017;31:285–300.
13. **Alderdice J.** Fundamentalism, radicalization and terrorism, part 2: fundamentalism, regression and repair. Psychoanalytic Psychotherapy 2017;31:303–13.
14. **Volkan V.** Enemies on the couch. Durham, NC: Pitchstone Publishing; 2013.
15. **Volkan V.** Blind trust. Charlottesville, VA: Pitchstone Press; 2004.
16. **Alderdice JT.** Sacred values: psychological and anthropological perspectives on fairness, fundamentalism, and terrorism. Annals of the New York Academy of Sciences 2009;1167:158–73.
17. **Owen D.** The hubris syndrome. York: Methuen & Co.; 2012.

Chapter 18

Extremism, violence, and mind: Apprehending the super-complex

Kamaldeep Bhui and Dinesh Bhugra

18.1 Conceptual constructions of terrorism

Definitions of who is and is not a terrorist are subject to critical debate, and political constructions, as well as a need for artificial ones in legislation that outlaws or incriminates such acts. Protecting citizens against terrorism through the mechanism of law necessarily requires broad legal definitions, offering flexible practice by criminal justice, law enforcement, health and social care, and educational agencies to accommodate diverse judgements that are appropriate for a wide range of individual situations and risk scenarios. The type of offence, the degree of lethality and precontemplation, the number killed or injured, and the stage a person is at in the pathway models of how terrorists are made, are all important influences in assessing risk, and such features might not be easily compared or applied for people with markedly differing biographies, narratives, and contexts of how they engage with terrorism. A variety of factors can be more influential in one or another person who is likely to commit terrorist acts, without necessarily raising similar risks in all people.

As is evident from earlier chapters, terrorists may or may not be non-state actors, criminals, minorities or migrants, or people with compromised capacity or mental functions. They may act alone, or in informal or highly organized groups, operating locally, nationally, or globally. Local histories, narratives of latent identities and conflict, *chosen conflict, or identities*, as Lord John Alderdice suggests (see pages 9, 83, 248), trigger reactions when group interests are negotiated; historical latent identities are reactivated at times of distress and threat to an in-group. Furthermore, terrorist activities do not exist in isolation from criminal activity or networks, most obviously in prison settings, and also where violence is already part of an individual's make-up. People at the margins of society also encounter a range of life-course hazards that heighten their risk of criminalization, including poor education and unemployment, histories of victimization and discrimination, extreme poverty and hurtful, harmful, or absent experiences of receiving parental care, and an absence of sufficient protections in schools and neighbourhoods.

In recent decades, terrorism studies have concentrated almost exclusively on Islamic fundamentalism and religious ideologies as the drivers of violent radicalization and terrorist actions, inventing appropriate vocabularies and hypotheses about causation. Several authors unpack this (see Chapters 2 and 14). The grounds for this are invariably anecdotal, biographical, case study-based, and prosecution-focused, seeking to be consistent with national policies and laws, so as to not contradict or undermine state responses, wherever possible. Yet where state actions are believed to be undermining citizenship rights, or democratic processes, subsections of the population have protested and sought a revision of the approach [1]. There are also international differences in terms of how the terrorist is constructed; religious ideologies seem to be central to the US and UK positions. In Canada, a different set of tensions exist between indigenous peoples and descendants of migrants, and then there are regional disputes about independence and autonomy.

Attention to other forms of violence and non-Islamic extremism lags behind the interest in Islamic terrorism, although the National Academies of Science now propose that countering violent extremism can best be tackled by a public health and population-based approach to combating violence in general [2]. This means we must understand multiple pathways to terrorism, including violent protest and violent offending, but also social, cultural, place-based and behavioural and attitudinal antecedents or facilitators, when involvement of the public and societal effort is part of the solution [3]. In any behavioural phenomenon, and one involving violence, the role of emotions, grievances, and propensity to violence through nature or nurture are critical to consider. The public health approach has been applied to violence in general, drug use, suicide, gun crime, and knife crime, as well as to health problems like obesity, diabetes, and heart disease. The prerequisite is that we understand the range of risk factors and how they interact to lead to a chain of causation and the adverse outcome. Small reductions in the levels of risk factors in the population then translate into significant effects, by the so-called 'shift of the curve of risk factor and outcome to the left' [3].

Therein lies the challenge for any approach. Understanding what is a stable risk factor, how it operates in an individual, or a group, and more generally, and then how it interacts with other risk factors is not easy to discern; and how these combinations of risk respond to changes of context, different political histories, and historical traumas waiting to be re-enacted. Such a consideration still suggests that understanding is possible, and a general approach might be captured. That a detailed mechanism, for example, how social support can be protective or social isolation harmful, operates in the same way in young Muslim heritage men in London, or Arabs in Palestine, or a US-born descendent of Nigerian parents. In each of these scenarios, representing real offenders, the relevance of social support or isolation may be remarkably important or truly trivial. Furthermore, the types of terrorist offending and the understandings presented in this book may not easily sit side by side. This does not mean they are wrong, or that we have failed, but that we are dealing with a special type of problem that does not lend itself to conventional approaches to science or crime prevention and one size does not fit all.

18.2 **From simple, complicated, and complexity to super-complexity**

Most systems problems and solutions are tackled by simple or complicated explanations and solutions rather than complex solutions that address system dynamics [4, 5]. There will be compromises in developing systems for multiple purposes; for example, in health systems population-level screening and intervention will not easily marry with personalized individual care, leading to a need to separate the two functions but still see them as part of a whole [6]. Thus, solving complex problems may not best be done from a description of causation, which may be inadequate or flawed, but to what a solution can look like and adopt a design-thinking approach, including the structure of relationships and feedback loops to better approximate to a solution that works for now [7]. A knowledge-to-action framework is proposed to deal with complex problems, including five elements [8], which we interpret here to include:

- nurture and sustain trusting relationships;
- co-produce and co-curate knowledge;
- introduce feedback loops;
- frame as systemic interventions not finite projects with predictable or linear consequences;
- consider variations by time and place.

We argue that complexity approaches may fail, when dealing with terrorism studies, as the subject of study changes over time and by place, and the ecological niche in which thinking occurs. Thus, definitions of terrorism change, and types of act and the means to coordinate and the sources of such actions will and do change over time. Furthermore, the analysis of a problem is constructed by national political positions, national values, and the instruments of law and society, and beliefs that shape the way problems are constructed and resolved. The problem and the solutions, the systems of understanding and describing problems and solutions, and the ways of thinking about the problems and solutions all shift and drift, and invariably create multiple accounts, each being imperfect and only a stage in solving a problem. In a super-complex problem it may not be possible to introduce feedback and influences across time and sectors, only to recognize the multiple systems operating under different conditions in distinct countries and cultures; non-fit and lack of cross-reads are inevitable. Embracing these diverse and often divergent realities becomes the task during the development of progressive policies and practices that are to reach beyond the particular settings and characteristics of specific terrorist incidents or group actions.

Although studies of terrorism have evolved rapidly, sometimes as if entirely separate from other areas of scholarship like criminology or forensic mental health, there are clear interlinkages about the causation of violence in general, and political violence and war more specifically, as well as identifying vulnerabilities. The marginalized are at greater risk of being the victim of violence and a perpetrator, criminality, and social hazards like homelessness, poor housing, and poverty; all argue for a *dynamic matrix* approach, whereby we evolve interlinked bodies of evidence separately, in linkages and then as a complex whole systems, which do not operate in linear, simple, or predictable waya. Thus multiple drives and multiple outcomes can be linked or reinforce one another, dependent on a myriad number of biographical and contextual influences. Cognitive styles and affect and emotional motivations are personal, located within families, social groups, and society. The cognitive and emotional vulnerabilities and sources of resilience can thus be entirely unique, or clustered. Or individuals can come to similar understandings by selecting similar thinkers or influencing through group process, and coercion, dependent on group pressures to confirm and secure an identity and power, if disempowered in other ways.

If a complex set of drivers were to be understood, we will be in a better position to formulate, develop, test, and anticipate effective complex solutions. The current difficulty is that a complex systems approach is difficult to grasp, evaluate, evidence, or even implement across a number of stakeholders holding often very divergent and contrasting—and perhaps even contradictory—perspectives, or so it seems, especially if each body of expertise is wedded inflexibly to their particular aspect of the structures they study. Contradictions arise in concepts, causal explanations, vocabularies, the motivations for generating counterterrorism narratives, and actions. These can range from extreme and immediate responses to more measured conservative longer-term plans. For example, security agencies will prioritize those at risk of imminent threat, groups or individuals, either known to have advocated for violence, used violence, or linked with violent groups. Criminologists will be interested in re-habilitation and deradicalization of offenders, and judging potential risks on release, when the subjects of concern become security threats, while social and cultural commentators may look for group cohesion and the role of persecu-tion, discrimination, deprivation, and poverty in causation and management. Political scientists will consider international foreign policy, human rights and citizenship, and geopolitical drivers of conflict and violence; health specialists will wish to understand motivations and intervention to reduce the chances of impulsivity or vicarious accidental co-option of the developmentally vulnerable due to youth and inexperience, psychological fragility, social isolation; govern-ments will identify particular features for emphasis and challenge ideologies such as those attributed to religion, which are argued to sanction, at least if not advocate, violence; and these assertions are then refuted by theologians and re-ligious experts. It is difficult to resolve such tensions and perhaps they cannot be eliminated completely.

Even the method of inquiry, statistical analyses, and qualitative research (ethnographic, thematic, realist) each bring with them specific strengths and weaknesses, with varying sensitivities to pick up important influence.

18.3 **Violence and mental health**

The mental health consequences of violence, trauma, and terrorist incidents consistently show higher rates of specific mental illnesses in people exposed to adverse incidents then the unexposed [2, 9, 10]. Yet, research must necessarily focus not on entire populations, but on those who are especially vulnerable to violence in the first place, owing to precarity and disadvantage, placing them at greater risk, as well as those more likely to suffer mental illnesses, owing ei-ther to family histories, previous experiences of mental illness, or the very risk factors that predispose people to precarity. Thus, refugees are especially likely to be exposed to violence, and then to develop mental illnesses such as depres-sion, anxiety, and post-traumatic symptoms as a consequence [11]. People ex-posed to violence in the workplace are likely to develop depression, anxiety, and burnout [12]. Intimate partner violence, coercion, and manipulation lead to greater risks of mental illness, and psychological treatments seem to be helpful. Sexual violence is also more common at times of conflict and war, leading to mental illnesses [13, 14]. Human trafficking and exploitation is also associated with violence and the consequent mental illnesses [15]. War and conflict, in general, also affect soldiers and civilians, with both groups showing higher rates of mental illnesses, especially post-traumatic stress disorder and complex dis-orders, including psychosis and depression, conditioned again by additional risks like a family history of mental illnesses [16, 17]. Thus, it should be no surprise, then, that people exposed to terrorist violence—either as direct victims or by witnessing or indirectly involved—will be at greater risk of mental illnesses, partly mediated by negative attitudes and fears of recurrence [18–20]. Specific country data emphasize subgroups in precarious positions to be especially at risk, for example, refugees, minorities, the poor, and young people at critical stages of development [20–24].

18.4 **Violent extremism and mental health**

A less developed set of hypotheses suggest that different mental states make it more likely for some people to turn to violence [25, 26]. At one level, criminality is part of the definition of antisocial personality disorder, although societal constructions of personality and self vary across cultures, and thus disorder definitions must also vary; for example, personality disorders are less commonly diagnosed among black and minority ethnic groups, and are better recognized if a structured instrument is used rather than clinical opinion, and even U.S. and UK practices differ in this regard [27, 28]. Personality disorder and psychopathy are thought to lead to repeated offending, an inability to learn from experience, and callous unconcern. Yet, other mental illnesses, like psychoses, can include command hallucinations or delusional beliefs, including anger, which may lead to violence. However, it is difficult to conceive people suffering such severe illnesses would be sufficiently well organized or compliant to participate in organized networks [29]. Thus, all data should be considered as related to a particular context or niche, and a particular intermediary pathway and a related mechanism; if we can understand mechanisms and contexts, and these map onto each other in a consistent way, and then on the outcome—be it organizing groups or suicide bombing or threats—our collective efforts are more likely to succeed. Hence, the need for networks of excellence and collaborations across disparate and ostensibly diverse bodies of knowledge. This requires more developmental research, which will frustrate policymakers who need practical options now, and not in the future, following a 10-year research programme. Yet, such research programmes are necessary, awaiting the policy opportunity when a new approach is possible. Thus, the policy and criminal justice priorities often immediate solutions to long-standing, difficult, and life-threatening challenging scenarios that are charged to prevent or mitigate.

18.4.1 **A dynamic matrix of causation and prevention**

What might a dynamic matrix of super-complexity look like? By assembling this particular group of remarkable thought leaders, we wish to make just as remarkable a leap to connect previously isolated pieces of research and practice. We seek the help of readers and experts in the sciences and humanities to help identify missing features in this matrix, and to add to the data in an ongoing collaboration.

Listing the areas of concern risks us simplifying and representing them as single interests, so each of the following should be read as being in dynamic linkage with all others at all times, so that the influence of one is conditioned by the influence of another element.

- Cultural psychiatry: explanatory models, health beliefs, cultural and ethnic identity, micro-identities, acculturation, religiosity, conflict, discrimination, migration, and intersectional lens.

- Qualitative research, ethnography and anthropology, sociological and biographical narrative interviews, grounded theory, realistic reviews, rapid policy reviews, epidemiology, systematic reviews, and clinical trials, too.

- Technologies of persuasion and incitement: how psychiatrists, lawyers, and other professionals make judgements about militant and non-militant groups, and attempt to justify violence on cultural and political grounds.

- The role of digital media and communities leverage through digital communications.

- Criminology and emotional resilience as a response to recruitment into terrorism.

- Ensuring criminal justice responses are just and mindful of the structural drivers of terrorism and the way it is perceived, labelled, and addressed. This has implications for policing by citizenship and consent.

- Parallels and contrast across extremist groups: for example, the English Defence League, and the narratives of recruitment, drawing parallels with Islamic groups.

- Equifinality and multifinality: violent radicalization has many paths to it and multiple trajectories to multiple outcomes, and poor mental health, attitudes, and beliefs, and motivations may be one factor.

- Community connections and social capital to counterextremists, including the notion of political engagement and skills to negotiate disagreement.

- Tensions in counterterrorism actions that are effective and use particular narratives of causation and the alienation of communities that need to be part of the solution and intelligence through which we overcome future threats and recruitment to terrorist causes.

- Counterterrorism policy and legislation co-opting public institutions with other functions (health, teaching) creating ethical and professional challenges, exposing skills deficits and capacity issues, and undermining the core role of those institutions.

◆ Youth services: can they work with security agencies constructively or is the tension and inherent contradiction too great? Examples of good practice exist, like cultural consultation and cultural mediation.

◆ Police cultural competence: policy and community response must be aligned and can be complementary for effective counterterrorism and security measures.

◆ Collectivism and individualism lead to different drivers of terrorism but also different responses, some being better suited to reach the potentially radicalized.

◆ Biographies of convicted terrorists offer a rich picture not only of their actions in terrorism but their motivations before, and their plight after—sometimes years after. What can we learn about reconciliation and regret that can be promoted in the public gaze, rather than only focus on the terrorist motivation narrative, subject to binary thinking.

◆ Moral injury: among victims and society, and among perpetrators.

◆ What is the right political process to resolve inter-group and political violence and conflict? How do skills in emotion and communication, group dynamics, and psychological function contribute?

◆ What drivers of conflict related to identity and history might be anticipated and corrected if misused as a 'chosen trauma' or latent identity that is reactivated in specific times of conflict?

◆ What transitional justice arrangements are helpful as a mechanism to reduce the risk of further conflict and violence.

◆ Moral and ethical considerations of the sharing economy and digital media if used for threat and for counterterrorism.

◆ Digitalization of human communications and biographical narrative: implications for identity and group belonging and loyalty in virtual globalized communities.

◆ Sociological and cultural theories that explain the drivers of political extremism, linked to heritage and place identity; and theories that propose particular preventive interventions or deradicalization programmes.

◆ An infinite number of possible and multiple influences with differing levels of resolution, measured in different ways, and changing over time, and visible to some not others, and contested by different parties, having more or less political salience or cultural congruence.

18.4.2 **Preventive contexts and interventions**

Radicalization, a process by which individuals come to support terrorism and extremist ideologies associated with terrorist groups, is also invoked to explain how citizens come to attack their own country and either support terrorist organizations or kill on their behalf. This is a priority for many governments around the world. Prevention of such acts is therefore incredibly important in public policy. The Prevent duty for England and Wales is enshrined in section 29 of the Counter-Terrorism and Security Act 2015 in that certain 'specified authorities' must have due regard in the exercise of their functions to the need to prevent people being drawn into terrorism. The authorities include prison and probation services, the health sector, schools and registered child care providers (excluding higher and further education), and the police. Similar guidance exists for Scotland. Extremism is defined (in Prevent duty 2011) as vocal or active opposition to fundamental British values, including democracy, the rule of law, individual liberty, and mutual respect and tolerance of different faiths and belief, as well as calls for the death of members of the armed forces, whether in the UK or overseas. Terrorism is defined in the UK by the Terrorism Act (2000) as an act that endangers or causes serious violence to a person or people; causes damage to property; or interferes with or disrupts electronic systems. The use of threat must be designed to influence government or to intimidate the public for the purpose of political advancement, or religious or ideological cause. Training, monitoring, leadership and partnerships, inspections, implementation, and enforcement are all applied.

The specific approaches adopted require judgement by clinicians and teachers and other professionals in law enforcement around the risks posed by any one individual or a group, depending on intelligence, depth of knowledge about their biographies, and links with criminality or propensity to violence; known or alleged contact with extremists groups is clearly important.

However, many people not in contact with terrorist groups and with no background of concern are considered suspect if some characteristics are overly emphasized, for example religion, or protest against international foreign policy or disagreement with the legislation; and the lack of understanding and knowledge of their religious positions, acculturative processes and identity, and reasons for lack of social and political engagement and isolation makes it difficult to make precise judgements. Concerns are then expressed through a high index of suspicion followed-up by referral to an appropriate panel and discussion with law enforcement if necessary. This process has the potential to draw disproportionately on public resources from other important core tasks areas of public life (education, health), and for misclassifications, while also creating a culture whereby discussion of beliefs and ideologies is rapidly pathologized and criminalized and then later subject to investigation rather than permitted as a developmental opportunity for young people to consider their position and beliefs and critically examine them in the face of challenge.

In the realms of psychiatric care and in those with mental illnesses, there are disquieting disputes about the role of mental health or illness in terrorist offending and whether teachers and health workers should be co-opted to be counterterrorist agencies [30, 31], although risk assessment and forensic considerations are part and parcel of the work of forensic and general psychiatrists [29, 32], as well as many other health, social care, and educational professionals [33, 34].

18.5 What interventions help reduce radicalization?

Regrettably, given the super-complex nature of terrorism and typologies of extremism, a range of solutions has developed through trial and error, by testing in real-world scenarios with little evaluation by experimental trial designs given the ethical and logistic challenges of undertaking such research. Furthermore, informed practice and expert consensus is all that many practitioners rely on in the absence of an evidence base. Probation agencies and law enforcement, including the police, are experts in offender management in general and are well placed, although better knowledge of cultural and religious antecedents and motivations is needed. A systematic review by the Youth Justice Board in 2012 found little compelling evidence of what works to prevent radicalization [31], other than outreach and engagement projects, including youth community programmes that challenge ideologies, and empower young people; other potentially valuable approaches included deradicalization programmes in Islamic countries and tackling right-wing extremism, although these required better evidence. A related concurrent evaluation of 48 programmes in the UK [35] examined processes of what works and for whom, and proposed the following for the projects they reviewed:

◆ Deliver Preventing Violent Extremism (PVE) projects through community-based organizations with a proven track record of delivering PVE interventions.

◆ On the secure estate:

- only use targeted PVE interventions, restricted to young people most at risk of radicalization with multiple PVE-specific risk factors;
- include PVE as a core resettlement activity on release;

- focus on preventing Islamic-inspired violent extremism rather than other forms of 'extremism' (focus of UK situation at the time);
- do not refer for offending risk factors, but for specific PVE-related risk factors (e.g. perception of injustice, hatred towards an out-group, frustration, persecution, and identity confusion).

◆ Develop interventions:

- to challenge extremist ideology through debate and discussion around theology; these should be delivered in an informal setting through community-led debates;
- to promote independent thinking and cognitive skills for critical on extremist narratives, enabling challenge.

◆ PVE projects should be clearly distinguishable from other social policy goals such as community cohesion.

Some of these conclusions supported the Prevent programme and reflect the focus of UK policy at the time, but there was, perhaps, a failure to embrace wider complexity, for example the relevance of community cohesion as critical at times of conflict; the relevance of non-secure state actors, although the youth justice board was perhaps especially interested in the secure estate; and the greater attention paid to Islamic-related radicalization rather than consider extremism more generally to be a greater problem, as the two are linked and we can learn from both.

Other important interventions include using counternarratives to promote inter-faith dialogue, and challenge terrorist propaganda and justifications for violence; and inoculation in general and not challenging terrorist propaganda but presenting a particular perspective to support citizenship responsibilities and the fair and democratic and politically engaged approach to conflict resolution [36]. Moral disengagement, promoting socialization and social roles and life skills are promising deradicalization approaches, and offer a theoretically plausible set of processes for decriminalization that are also useful for other types of serious offending [37]. It is inevitable, as social media dominates global communications and can be used for recruitment [38], and, as such, it can also be used to actively mitigate the encouragement of people to enter terror networks [39].

A recent rapid review investigated the effectiveness of approaches to identify who is vulnerable to violent extremism—and efforts to reduce the risk of recruitment and radicalization [40]. The findings were that the evidence is inconclusive on *actionable insights*. Only 13 studies were found, of which three examined effectiveness. Few were in low-income countries and few offer a gendered perspective. Gender—both the structural and cultural shaping of masculinity and femininity—and culturally shaped roles are exploitered by terrorist organizations is not well researched. There are also gendered impacts [41], with women often being exploited or sexually violated in times of crisis; indeed, terrorist organizations promote men as martyrs, protectors, and enforcers, and women as victims, or women as fulfilling culturally stereotypes roles, or women's roles to support male martyrdom [42]. Recruiters can also reinforce masculinity in recruitment videos [38].

No general causal model or theory can be established, and causal links between risks and outcomes are unclear. The conclusions, as argued by the authors and editors of this volume, is that radicalization is a process within an individual, affected by various contextual factors, interactions, and influences, including group belonging, beliefs, and motivation, which all interact dynamically with the characteristics of the individual. All of these must sit alongside the Countering Violent Extremism and PVE policies in the United States and UK, respectively, that locate extremism in the wider nexus of what drives violence and conflict more generally.

Finally, deradicalization programmes are a priority for convicted offender rehabilitation programmes, and their content, varies from country to country. The Radicalisation Aware Network, that is European Union funded, collated all the interventions available and the evidence narratives (https://ec.europa.eu/home-affairs/what-we-do/networks/radicalisation_awareness_network_en)   as examples of good practice, given that the evidence base remains weak—as demonstrated by many systematic reviews. The weak evidence base reflects the methodological challenge of evaluation of interventions for rare outcomes, for idiosyncratic contexts and individual biographies, and for differing criminal and societal systems, and efforts to solve super-complex problems with inappropriate methods.

We demonstrate in this volume that an approach to better definition and understanding that requires commensurate super-complex and systems-based approaches to interventions. The greatest risk remain in offenders or potential offenders with known links, motives, and the means and mindset to commit violence and terrorist offences, or support such actions.

We hope the thought leaders in this volume have shifted and revised the issues for a new wave of counterterrorism responses, including the prevention of extremism; relevant actions for appropriate country contexts, including good governance, progressive social cohesion policies, and cultural and immigration policy; and considered approaches to prevention that retain the essence of societal involvement in solving societal problems, while at the same time permitting—indeed encouraging—innovative sector-specific solutions. Understanding the variety of mechanisms and conditions for the generation and prevention of violence and terrorism may be a more fruitful area of study across diverse contexts. We thank the authors for helping us evolve a progressive and connected new approach, and implore readers to move towards a progressive and effective response. Irrespective of which sector is of interest to each of us, we propose that ensuring societal engagement and citizenship consenting to act in culturally appropriate and effective ways that do less harm than good is essential to a credible response.

References

1. **Aggarwal NK.** Questioning the current public health approach to countering violent extremism. Global Public Health 2019;**14**:309–17.
2. **Murthy RS, Lakshminarayana R.** Mental health consequences of war: a brief review of research findings. World Psychiatry 2006; **5**:25–30.
3. **Bhui KS, Hicks MH, Lashley M, Jones E.** A public health approach to understanding and preventing violent radicalization. BMC Medicine 2012;**10**:16.
4. **Snyder S.** The simple, the complicated, and the complex: educational reform through the lens of complexity theory. Available from: https://www.oecd.org/education/ceri/WP_The%20Simple,%20Complicated,%20and%20the%20Complex.pdf [accessed 7 August 2020].
5. **Wang Y, Xue H, Esposito L, Joyner MJ, Bar-Yam, Y, Huang TT-K.** Applications of complex systems science in obesity and noncommunicable chronic disease research. Advances in Nutrition 2014;**5**:574–7.
6. **Bar-Yam Y.** Improving the effectiveness of health care and public health: a multiscale complex systems analysis. American Journal of Public Health 2006;**96**:459–66.
7. **Finegood DT, Karanfil O, Matteson CL.** Getting from analysis to action: framing obesity research, policy and practice with a solution-oriented complex systems lens. Healthcare Papers 2008;**9**:36–41.
8. **Riley BL, et al.,** Knowledge to action for solving complex problems: insights from a review of nine international cases. Health Promotion and Chronic Disease Prevention in Canada 2015;**35**:47–53.
9. **Cuartas J, Leventhal T.** Exposure to community violence and children's mental health: a quasi-experimental examination. Social Science & Medicine 2020;**246**:112740.
10. **Lee H, Kim Y, Terry J.** Adverse childhood experiences (ACEs) on mental disorders in young adulthood: latent classes and community violence exposure. Preventive Medicine 2020;**134**:106039.
11. **Scoglio AAJ, Salhi C.** Violence exposure and mental health among resettled refugees: a systematic review. Trauma Violence Abuse 2020. DOI: 10.1177/1524838020915584.
12. **Rudkjoebing LA, Bungum AB, Meulengracht Flachs E, Hurwitz Eller N, Borritz M,** et al. Work-related exposure to violence or threats and risk of mental disorders and symptoms: a systematic review and meta-analysis. Scandinavian Journal of Work, Environment & Health 2020;**46**:339–49.
13. **Santos AGD, de Souza Monteiro CF, Feitose CDA, Veloso C, Nogueira LT, Andrade EMLF.** [Types of non-psychotic mental disorders in adult women who suffered intimate

partner violence: an integrative review]. Revista da Esccola de Enfermagem da USP 2018;**52**:e03328 (in Portuguese).

14. **Ba I, Bhopal RS.** Physical, mental and social consequences in civilians who have experienced war-related sexual violence: a systematic review (1981–2014). Public Health 2017;**142**:121–35.

15. **Ottisova L,** et al. Prevalence and risk of violence and the mental, physical and sexual health problems associated with human trafficking: an updated systematic review. Epidemiology and Psychiatric Sciences, 2016;**25**:317–41.

16. **Greer N, Sayer NA, Spoont M, Taylor BC, Ackland PE, MacDonald R,** et al. Prevalence and severity of psychiatric disorders and suicidal behavior in service members and veterans with and without traumatic brain injury: systematic review. Journal of Head Trauma Rehabilitation 2020;**35**:1–13.

17. **ÓConghaile A, Smedberg DL, Shin AL, DeLisi LE.** Familial risk for psychiatric disorders in military veterans who have post-traumatic stress disorder with psychosis: a retrospective electronic record review. Psychiatric Genetics 2018;**28**:24–30.

18. **Leiner M, Peinado J, Villanos MTM, Lopez I, Uribe R, Pathak I.** Mental and emotional health of children exposed to news media of threats and acts of terrorism: the cumulative and pervasive effects. Frontiers in Pediatrics 2016;**4**:26.

19. **Comer JS, Bry LJ, Poznanski B, Golik, AM.** Children's mental health in the context of terrorist attacks, ongoing threats, and possibilities of future terrorism. Current Psychiatry Reports 2016;**18**:79.

20. **Richman JA, Cloninger L, Rospenda KM.** Macrolevel stressors, terrorism, and mental health outcomes: broadening the stress paradigm. American Journal of Public Health 2008;**98**:323–29.

21. **Tucker P, Pfefferbaum B, Nitíema P, Wendling TL, Brown S.** Intensely exposed oklahoma city terrorism survivors: long-term mental health and health needs and posttraumatic growth. Journal of Nervous and Mental Disease 2016; **204**:203–9.

22. **Gelkopf M, Solomon Z, Berger R, Bleich A.** The mental health impact of terrorism in Israel: a repeat cross-sectional study of Arabs and Jews. Acta Psychiatrica Scandinavica 2008;**117**:369–80.

23. **Bleich A, Gelkopf M, Melamed Y, Solomon Z.** Mental health and resiliency following 44 months of terrorism: a survey of an Israeli national representative sample. BMC Medicine 2006;**4**:21.

24. **Kim D, Albert Kim YI.** Mental health cost of terrorism: study of the Charlie Hebdo attack in Paris. Health Economics 2018;**27**:e1–14.

25. **Misiak B, Samochowiec J, Bhui K, Schouler-Ocak M, Demunter H, Kuey L,** et al. A systematic review on the relationship between mental health, radicalization and mass violence. European Psychiatry 2019;**56**:51–9.

26. **Dom G, Schouler-Ocak M, Bhui K, Demunter H, Kuey L, Raballo A,** et al. Mass violence, radicalization and terrorism: a role for psychiatric profession? European Psychiatry 2018;**49**:78–80.

27. **McGilloway A, Hall RE, Lee T, Bhui KS.** A systematic review of personality disorder, race and ethnicity: prevalence, aetiology and treatment. BMC Psychiatry 2010;**10**:33.

28. **Hossain A. Malkov M, Lee T, Bhui K.** Ethnic variation in personality disorder: evaluation of 6 years of hospital admissions. BJPsych Bulletin 2018;**42**:157–61.

29. **Bhui K, James A, Wessely S.** Mental illness and terrorism. BMJ2016;**354**:i4869.

30. **Hurlow J, Wilson S, James DV.** Protesting loudly about Prevent is popular but is it informed and sensible? BJPsych Bulletin 2016;**40**:162–3.

31. **Reed S.** The Prevent programme: an ethical dilemma for teachers as well as psychiatrists. BJPsych Bulletin 2016;**40**:85–6.

32. **Bhui K.** Flash, the emperor and policies without evidence: counter-terrorism measures destined for failure and societally divisive. BJPsych Bulletin 2016;**40**:82–4.

33. **Wright NM, Hankins FM.** Preventing radicalisation and terrorism: is there a GP response? British Journal of General Practice 2016;**66**:288–9.

34. **Taylor L, Soni A.** Preventing radicalisation: a systematic review of literature considering the lived experiences of the UK's Prevent strategy in educational settings. Pastoral Care in Education 2017;**35**:241–52.

35. **Board YJ.** Process evaluation of preventing violent extremism programmes for young people Available from: https://dera.ioe.ac.uk/16233/1/preventing-violent-extremism-process-evaluation.pdf [accessed 7 August 2020].

36. **Carthy SL, Doody CB, O'Hora D, Sarma KM.**e PROTOCOL: counter-narratives for the prevention of violent radicalisation: a systematic review of targeted interventions. Campbell Systematic Reviews 2018;**14**:1–23.

37. **Ozer S, Bertelsen P.** The moral compass and life skills in navigating radicalization processes: examining the interplay among life skills, moral disengagement, and extremism. Scandinavian Journal of Psychology 2020. DOI: 10.1111/sjop.12636.

38. **Bhui K, Ibrahim Y.** Marketing the "radical": symbolic communication and persuasive technologies in jihadist websites. Transcultural Psychiatry 2013;**50**:216–34.

39. **Ganesh B, Bright J.** Countering extremists on social media: challenges for strategic communication and content moderation. Policy & Internet 2020;**12**:6–19.

40. **Department for International Development.** Identifying groups vulnerable to violent extremism and reducing risks of radicalisation. Available from: https://assets.publishing.service.gov.uk/media/5d7f5b7c40f0b61c7cd6ffe9/VE_REA_Identifying_and_intervening_with_at_risk_groups_Sept_2019_FINAL_with_Annex.pdf [accessed 7 August 2020].

41. **Ghosh PW, McGilloway N, Ali A, Jones E, Bhui K.** Violent radicalisation and recruitment to terrorism: perspectives of wellbeing and social cohesion of citizens of Muslim heritage. Sociology Mind 2013;**3**:290–7.

42. **Brown KD, Rahman F, True J.** Conflicting identities: the nexus between masculinities, femininities and violent extremism in Asia. Available from: https://www.undp.org/content/undp/en/home/librarypage/democratic-governance/the-nexus-between-masculinities-femininities-and-violent-extremism-in-asia.html

Index